Why do some slim—*while others starve themselves and can't lose an ounce?*

How does a woman's metabolism differ from a man's?

What should women eat before *they become pregnant?*

Why do women turn to sugary, high-fat food when they're depressed, angry, or tense?

These are just a few of the many questions answered in *Food and You*—the ideal companion for any woman who wants to know more about food and how it affects her body and mind.

If you want to take control—and take more pleasure in eating good, nutritious food—this is the guide you need. *Food and You* teaches women how to make peace with food . . . and with themselves.

FOOD AND YOU

FOOD AND YOU EDITORIAL STAFF

Managing Editor: Sharon Faelten

Staff Writers: Sarí Harrar, Barbara Loecher

Contributing Writers: Linda Konner, Betsy Bates, Judith Lin Eftekhar, Andrea Warren

Assistant Research Manager: Carol Svec

Project Researcher: Susan E. Burdick

Researchers and Fact-Checkers: Christine Dreisbach, Valerie Edwards-Paulik, Carol J. Gilmore, Deborah Pedron, Sally A. Reith, Sandra Salera-Lloyd, Anita Small, Bernadette Sukley, John Waldron

Cover and Book Designer: Debra Sfetsios

Studio Manager: Joe Golden

Layout Designer: Eugenie S. Delaney

Cover Photographer: William Abranowicz

Photo Editor: Susan Pollack

Illustrator: Barbara Fritz

Senior Copy Editor: Jane Sherman

Production Manager: Helen Clogston

Manufacturing Coordinator: Melinda B. Rizzo

Office Staff: Roberta Mulliner, Julie Kehs, Bernadette Sauerwine, Mary Lou Stephen

RODALE HEALTH AND FITNESS BOOKS

Vice President and Editorial Director: Debora T. Yost

Art Director: Jane Colby Knutila

Research Manager: Ann Gossy Yermish

Copy Manager: Lisa D. Andruscavage

FOOD AND YOU

EVERYTHING A WOMAN NEEDS TO KNOW ABOUT
LOVING FOOD—FOR BETTER HEALTH,
FOR A BEAUTIFUL BODY AND FOR
EMOTIONAL SATISFACTION

By Sarí Harrar, Barbara Loecher, Linda Konner and
the Editors of *Prevention* Magazine Health Books

Edited by Sharon Faelton

BERKLEY BOOKS, NEW YORK

FOOD AND YOU

A Berkley Book / published by arrangement with
Rodale Press, Inc.

PRINTING HISTORY
Rodale Press, Inc., edition published 1996
Berkley edition / July 1998

The Penguin Putnam Inc. World Wide Web site address is
http://www.penguinputnam.com

ISBN: 0-425-16323-7

BERKLEY®
Berkley Books are published by The Berkley Publishing Group,
a member of Penguin Putnam Inc.,
200 Madison Avenue, New York, New York 10016.
BERKLEY and the "B" design
are trademarks belonging to Berkley Publishing Corporation.

PRINTED IN THE UNITED STATES OF AMERICA

10 9 8 7 6 5 4 3 2 1

NOTICE

This book is intended as a reference volume only, not as a medical manual. The information given here is designed to help you make informed decisions about your health. Keep in mind that nutritional needs vary from person to person, depending on age, sex, health status and total diet. The information here is not intended as a substitute for any diet or treatment that may have been prescribed by your doctor. If you suspect that you have a medical problem, we urge you to seek competent medical help.

CONTENTS

PART 2: FOOD AND YOUR HEALTH

x   *Contents*

PART 5: FOOD AND YOUR MEALTIME STRATEGY

FOREWORD

I'm really impressed with *Food and You*. The authors provide
a most thorough and enjoyable review of everything women
need to know about food. Today's health consumer must be
an educated consumer. Managing both her eating habits and
exercise patterns will clearly add up to more healthy, happy
years for any woman.

Food and You offers excellent advice and many useful resources for today's woman, who all too often finds herself
sandwiched between conflicting demands and juggling multiple tasks. Smart food choices and exercise can help manage
stress-induced feeding frenzies—to say nothing of away-
from-home meals dictated by business travel.

I think this will be an important book for many women.

Jean L. Fourcroy, M.D., Ph.D.
President, 1995–1996, American Medical Women's Association

INTRODUCTION

"Pass the cookies—
my diet starts tomorrow"

Eavesdrop on any conversation between a woman and her friends, and more than likely the talk will turn to food. Do these comments sound familiar?

"I was bad today—I had a *huge* lunch!"

"Oh, I was good. No junk food."

"I've *had it* with diets. Real women can't look like fashion models! We've got to eat."

"I skipped breakfast and had two doughnuts and coffee at work—boy, was I jittery!"

"It was the most *romantic* dinner—lobster and champagne, cappuccino and chocolate torte."

"What can I believe about weight gain and health? Some studies say a few pounds are okay, but I just heard we shouldn't gain an ounce after high school. Who's right?"

"I don't know. But please pass the cookies—my diet starts tomorrow!"

A RELATIONSHIP LIKE NO OTHER

No doubt about it. Women have a unique physical and emotional relationship with food. It's fuel for our busy days and nights, nutrition for our minds and bodies and raw material for "building" babies and nourishing our young.

But that's just the beginning.

For this book, we asked hundreds of women what food really means in their lives. Our informal survey became an intimate conversation about the pleasure of delicious meals, the struggle to maintain a healthy weight and the powerful psychological grip that food can exert on our lives. These real-life stories bear out what hundreds of doctors, psychologists, weight-loss experts and nutritionists from across the country told us about women's relationships with food.

- More of us than ever are overweight. According to the Centers for Disease Control and Prevention in Atlanta, one out of three adult women is overweight today. Thirty years ago, it was one in four.
- Most of us are dieting—again. Look at the women around you, at work, church or the supermarket. According to a survey done for the American Dietetic Association (ADA), one in three is currently on a weight-loss program, and two out of three have tried at one time or another to shed extra pounds. But the diets don't seem to work. Three-quarters of current dieters in the ADA poll admitted they'd tried to lose weight in the past.
- We know *more* about healthy eating but are doing *less*. Among women ages 35 to 54, nearly 70 percent say it's important to select healthy foods, but just over 40 percent put their dietary smarts into practice. We're missing out on vital nutrients. Adult women need 1,000 to 1,500 milligrams of calcium a day, for example, yet less than half of us get enough to protect our bones from osteoporosis.
- We may overeat for emotional reasons. If you stuff down anger with ice cream, grab a doughnut to soothe yourself after a stressful day or sneak a muffin when no one's watching, you're not alone. The experts told us that emotional issues are often the reason we overindulge—and choose sugary, high-fat foods. The consequences? Weight gain, stifled feelings and a feeling of never being satisfied.
- We don't like our bodies. An astonishing 62 percent of the women surveyed in one Gallup poll said they want to be thinner—yet many admitted they're *not* overweight. The

shapes and sizes of our bodies can be a constant preoccupation. Nineteen percent of the women in the poll said their weight depressed them; another 13 percent worried about it all the time.

REAL WOMEN NEED FOOD, NOT GUILT

Food: We love it, we hate it, we need it. It's a dilemma shared by thousands of women every day, in kitchens and office lunchrooms, restaurants and grocery stores, dining rooms and fast-food drive-throughs.

If anything, the dilemma is more perplexing than ever. Why? First, we're around food all the time. Our traditional, nurturing roles as the household grocery-shoppers and meal-preparers haven't changed much—even if we hold down full-time jobs outside the home. Second, we're constantly bombarded by messages to be thin. The fashion industry's image of ideal female beauty has only gotten skinnier through the years. You see this idealized yet unrealistic visage everywhere—on magazine covers, TV shows and in the movies—except in your own mirror.

"If you look at any of the women's magazines in the checkout line in the grocery store, they really present some interesting dilemmas for women," notes Sandra Campbell, Psy.D., clinical director of the Eating Disorders Program at the Brattleboro Retreat in Vermont. "They tell you to bake a triple chocolate cake for your family, and on the next page they tell you how to lose 20 pounds. It's a pretty confusing message."

You *can* sort it out and make food your ally for good health, glowing good looks and emotional well-being. In this book you'll discover effective ways to form that alliance. You'll learn how to meet your unique nutritional needs—and put cravings to work *for* you, not against you.

And you'll also be inspired by the success stories of women just like you.

Women like Jane P., a *Food and You* survey respondent, who conquered emotional eating and lost 215 pounds. "If I don't take care of me first, I won't have a life," she says. "No matter what, I won't let myself cope with a difficult situation now by eating."

Or Karen M., who knows how to nurture herself. "Whenever I leave the house with my two daughters," she says, "our bag is packed with healthy snacks like fruit, raisins and whole-grain snack bars."

And Fran K., a firm believer in the power of small pleasures. "You can't deny yourself," says Fran, who's maintained a 15-pound weight loss for the past three years. "Treat yourself to small amounts of 'forbidden' food, or you'll feel deprived and give up. For me, it's half-and-half in my coffee and a few small pieces of chocolate every day!"

FOODS YOU CAN LOVE

Red, juicy strawberries for dessert. Crunchy broccoli on your lunchtime salad. Whole-grain breads and low-fat cheese for a snack. A tall, cool glass of milk at bedtime. And now and then, a little bit of chocolate.

What makes foods like these the focus of "for women only" eating plans recommended by experts in the growing field of women's health? Quite simply, the power to help us heal or relieve many health problems, protect our bodies from the threat of major illness and make us look and feel our best.

Specifically, they're rich in nutrients like folate, to lower the risk of cervical cancer, colon cancer and cardiovascular disease. Calcium, for strong bones and better blood pressure control. Iron for energy. And vitamin C, beta-carotene and other antioxidants for cancer protection. High in fiber and low in fat, they will also help protect you from colon or breast cancer, as well as heart disease, the number one cause of death among women. And if health problems such as fatigue, constipation, water retention or yeast infections concern you, you'll find lots of food-based healing techniques here as well.

You'll see why snacking (yes, snacking!) may help ease the painful symptoms of premenstrual syndrome. How eating breakfast is an important weight-control strategy. Why choosing colorful fruits and vegetables can be more important than taking vitamin supplements. How cutting back on caffeine could raise your energy levels. Why a Mediterranean diet could help you control diabetes. And when red meat is a smart nutritional choice.

You'll even discover why a little chocolate now and then is a good idea. Thanks to monthly shifts of our reproductive hormones, women often crave it. Have a bite or two—it can satisfy your hankering without causing weight gain.

But we don't eat simply to satisfy hunger pangs. You'll discover ways to recognize and overcome emotional eating habits, as well as some powerful self-help tools for fulfilling your inner needs—for intimacy, achievement, respect or simply fun. There are tips for making the most of holiday celebrations without gaining an ounce and for traveling without hauling extra pounds home with your souvenirs.

The results? You'll be free to truly nourish yourself—and savor each meal enjoyed with family or friends or all by yourself—without guilt, fear or embarrassment.

"We, as women who have taken care of others for so many years, need to feed ourselves as if we were someone we were taking care of," says Nan Kathryn Fuchs, Ph.D., a nutritionist in Sebastopol, California, and author of *Overcoming the Legacy of Overeating*. "We need to love ourselves as much as we love our partners, our children and our best friends."

This is the book that shows you how.

FOOD
AND YOU

PART 1
FOOD AND YOUR EMOTIONS

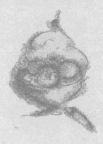

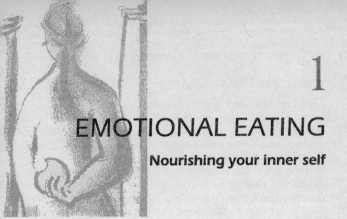

1

EMOTIONAL EATING

Nourishing your inner self

Jane P.'s six children are tucked in bed. The last fiery argument with her husband is extinguished. As she has on many previous nights, she huddles at the kitchen table, "eating all night long," she told us in our *Food and You* survey. Chocolate. Homemade bread. Leftover spaghetti.

"I ate whatever there was," recalls Jane, now 56. "I could never get enough."

Sue K.'s self-esteem was as fragile as a porcelain teacup. Sharp words and imagined slights sent her racing to the freezer for ice cream (lots of it). "I was eating to push down anger and depression," Sue, 50, a photographer's assistant, told us. "I thought I needed a goody, a treat. Years later I realized eating was really a punishment—I was making myself fatter."

Barbara M., 47, a busy manager at a utility company, roars up to a convenience store after work. She's just finished a big project, and once again, it's treat time. She picks a hefty slice of cheesecake.

"It feels good at the time," Barbara told us. "But the next day when your skirt won't button anymore, you say 'Oh my God, why did I do that?' "

EMOTIONAL ANESTHESIA

Like Jane, Sue and Barbara, most of us turn to food once in a while to satisfy emotional needs—to fulfill a hunger of the heart or quell what Sandra Campbell, Psy.D., clinical director of the Eating Disorders Program at the Brattleboro Retreat in Vermont, calls a hunger of the soul.

It's not that our stomachs are growling. We may be angry, depressed, anxious or sad or feel our self-esteem has been punctured. We may be avoiding intimacy. We may eat during lulls in our hectic schedules—like when we walk through the door after work. And sometimes munching goes along with procrastinating, so we eat to avoid paying the bills or making a decision. Or we may even be pleased with ourselves and, like Barbara, celebrate the occasion with a treat.

Crunchy potato chips when we're angry. Sweet, soft fudge, muffins or ice cream when we're upset. Sometimes even our choices reflect our feelings.

"Emotional eating is a way to manage overwhelming feelings," says Dr. Campbell. "Some women literally fill themselves up with food, and it becomes an emotional anesthetic."

Who's most vulnerable? Studies show that so-called restrained eaters—women who diet or strictly control food intake to maintain a low weight—seem especially susceptible, responding to strong feelings by reaching for something to eat. Yet no one is immune.

"Women say to me, 'Look at me: I'm smart. I'm managing my business. Look at me: I'm an architect. Look at me: I'm a marriage counselor, I save marriages. I can move mountains. But I can't keep my mouth shut to food,' " says Connie Roberts, R.D., manager of nutrition consultation services and wellness programs at Brigham and Women's Hospital in Boston. "Eating is an arena over which they feel they have no control."

A SUBSTITUTE SEDATIVE

If you're feeling particularly blue on occasion, there's no real harm in taking solace in a pint of soft double-chocolate-chip ice cream—*if* it happens once in a blue moon. Eating in response to emotional cues can release tension.

The key is to not overeat, which in itself can cause guilt. "By overeating and then feeling guilty about it, you create another tension. This is how a vicious cycle develops," says Roberts. Routinely using food to distract yourself from, disguise or detour around inner feelings has definite physical and psychological downsides, says Mary Anne Cohen, director of the New York Center for Eating Disorders and author of *French Toast for Breakfast: Declaring Peace with Emotional Eating*.

The downsides? Guilt and shame about enjoying food and an empty, never-satisfied feeling because needs for love, passion, independence, self-confidence, achievement, freedom or a sense of belonging are not being truly satisfied.

"Emotional eating is like a red flag going up, telling you that there's something deeper you need to attend to," says Dallas physician Frank Minirth, M.D., co-author of *Love Hunger: Recovery for Food Codependency*.

The upside? Breaking patterns of emotional eating will leave you free to experience your true feelings, to more easily reach and maintain a healthy weight and to savor food to the fullest—even the occasional goody—without guilt or fear.

"The range of foods a person likes tends to increase as they stop compulsive overeating and become healthier with food," says Hoyt Morris, Ph.D., director of the Oklahoma City Center for Eating Disorders. "The sense of taste often tends to become more pronounced. Foods taste better."

WHAT TRIGGERS EMOTIONAL EATING?

When Ronette Kolotkin, Ph.D., a clinical psychologist and director of behavioral programs at the Duke University Diet and Fitness Center in Durham, North Carolina, asks women in her weight-control classes to describe how food satisfies them, the answers are rarely about nutrition. Food, they say, is: A best friend. Unconditional love. Comfort. Escape. A pick-me-up. Sexual fulfillment. A tranquilizer.

When Dr. Kolotkin asks which emotions would make them stray from a well-balanced diet and regular exercise program, two are at the top of almost every list: anger and stress. "Yet few women are aware of the connection between what we eat and how we're feeling, unless they really look for it," says Dr. Kolotkin. So let's take a look.

Keep a food/mood diary. Angry and stuffed? Write it down. Uncovering those connections is the first step toward curbing problem eating and satisfying buried emotional needs, says Edward Abramson, Ph.D., professor of psychology at California State University in Chico and author of *Emotional Eating: A Practical Guide to Taking Control.*

"Carry a small notebook or 3-by-5 card in your pocket or wallet," he says. "Then, if you find yourself eating unnecessarily and it seems related to an emotional experience, write down what you ate and what you were feeling or thinking and note your location and who was around you."

After you've monitored emotional eating for a week or so, patterns may begin to emerge. Perhaps you eat when you're depressed or anxious or angry or bored or lonely. In some cases, food can even be a substitute for sex and intimacy.

"Sex is more than the physical climax—it's about warmth and comfort and nurturing," says Dr. Abramson. "Similarly, food is about more than having a full tummy—it's satisfying emotionally, too. So there is a parallel."

The next step is to uncover the "automatic thoughts" that make you worried or self-critical—thoughts that may prompt you to reach for food because you need comfort or a quick escape.

Ask yourself why you reach for food when you do. "Maybe you're anxious because you're getting ready to host a big party on Saturday night. You worry that there won't be enough food and everyone will dislike you; that no one will come and you'll be a social failure; that no one will talk to each other and you'll feel awkward," says Dr. Abramson. "These thoughts can contribute to a stressed or anxious feeling. If you can teach yourself to be a little more realistic, the feelings don't have to be quite so intense and negative."

Identify the triggers that make you eat. Using your food/mood diary—or mentally reviewing your personal emotional eating patterns—pick out recurring interactions with people or situations that send you running to the candy machine, suggests Dr. Minirth.

Eat regularly, not impulsively. Dr. Kolotkin says you can also uncover triggers by eating on a regular schedule. "An unaware emotional eater is probably popping something in her mouth often,'' she says. ''But if you eat on schedule, then find yourself wanting food an hour after lunch, you can say 'Wait. This isn't necessary. What's going on here?' ''

A LOVE/HATE RELATIONSHIP

But how do mashed potatoes and double-fudge brownies become what Jane P. called ''my friend, my god, my lover''? Experts say the answers may come from our growing-up years, our brain chemistry and even our adult habits.

''It starts at birth,'' notes Sheryl S. Russell, R.N., Ph.D., a psychotherapist in Knoxville, Tennessee, who studies women's eating issues. ''If a baby is crying, she gets food. So food becomes linked to alleviating discomfort. We carry that into childhood—say, if you get a cookie when you scrape your knee.''

For children and young women living in a sometimes harsh and confusing world, their relationship with food may be the only one in which they don't fear abandonment or criticism, notes psychotherapist Mary Anne Cohen. For many people, trusting food seems to be safer than trusting people, she explains. Food is never demanding or abusive—and it never rejects us.

An overeater who craves carbohydrate-rich foods when depressed or anxious may be attempting to increase brain levels of serotonin, a naturally occurring substance that regulates mood, notes Judith Wurtman, Ph.D., nutrition research scientist at the Massachusetts Institute of Technology in Cambridge and author of *Managing Your Mind and Mood through Food*. Through a series of natural chemical reactions in the body, carbohydrates allow more of the amino acid tryptophan to enter the brain, causing more serotonin to be released and thus relieving negative moods.

But the ''blue mood, more food'' syndrome can be an endless cycle. In a study of eight overweight emotional eaters between the ages of 28 and 54, Dr. Russell found that when the women felt rejected, it ''precipitated feelings of anger, betrayal, depression and isolation, and those feelings started the cycle of eating all over again.''

THE FOOD/MOOD QUIZ

Getting a handle on emotional eating is the very first step toward successful weight control and true eating enjoyment—not to mention real emotional satisfaction, says clinical psychologist Ronette Kolotkin, Ph.D., director of behavioral programs at the Duke University Diet and Fitness Center in Durham, North Carolina. But how can you tell if you are an emotional eater? See if the following statements, suggested by experts, are generally true for you.

1. I often eat for reasons other than hunger. ☐ Yes ☐ No
2. When I am overwhelmed, I very often eat to find relief. ☐ Yes ☐ No
3. I usually eat to calm myself down. ☐ Yes ☐ No
4. When I am angry with someone, I turn to food. ☐ Yes ☐ No
5. Whenever things feel out of control, I eat more. ☐ Yes ☐ No
6. If someone dislikes me or puts me down, I often turn to food to feel better. ☐ Yes ☐ No
7. When I'm happy, eating makes me feel even happier. ☐ Yes ☐ No
8. When I want to reward myself, I usually choose food, as my reward. ☐ Yes ☐ No
9. Food is more than nutritional fuel. It's my best friend, my comforter, my escape, a source of unconditional love. ☐ Yes ☐ No
10. If I'm lonely or bored, I'll overeat and feel better. ☐ Yes ☐ No

If you answered yes to five or six of these questions, food is moderately important in your emotional life, says Dr. Kolotkin. If you have seven or more yes answers, food has a central role in your emotional life. You may eat to avoid unpleasant feelings or as a substitute for love, intimacy, achievement or even fun, she says. Keeping a food/mood diary and using other tactics suggested in this chapter to prevent emotional eating episodes may help you meet those needs—and avert feeding frenzies and weight gain.

Dr. Russell says the eating cycle often starts in a surprising place: with feelings of boredom, loneliness and emptiness. Behind it often lurks low self-esteem, she notes. When a woman is feeling like that, a "triggering" event may cause strong negative emotions—and lead her to turn those emotions, especially anger, against herself.

"The feelings that come with anger are scary," Dr. Russell says. "A woman is brought up to be a people-pleaser, not to confront." So she eats. And for a moment, things are better. But the cycle's not over. Soon she may feel guilty and angry with herself for eating. Self-esteem drops. If she's overweight, she may also be ridiculed or rejected by others. She may isolate herself and begin feeling lonely, bored and empty again.

"If we could bolster self-esteem so a woman wouldn't feel so vulnerable, it would help," Dr. Russell says. "Or if a woman can start recognizing that vulnerable state of loneliness, boredom and emptiness and find support to help her get through it in a positive way, it would help, too."

Jane, who conquered her emotional eating habits and lost 215 pounds, says, "If I don't take care of me first, I won't have a life. No matter what, I won't let myself cope with a difficult situation now by eating."

HOW TO HALT A FEEDING FRENZY

Overcoming emotional eating can be especially challenging for women who are faced with conflicting messages about food, weight and body image. "How do we make sense of a culture that promotes slenderness, yet advertises seeking comfort through food?" asks Dr. Campbell.

Still, you can sort it out—even when the desire seems overwhelming, say experts. If you feel drawn to the candy machine or the refrigerator when you know you are not hungry, experts suggest the following quick rescue techniques.

Talk to yourself. "Tell yourself 'This feeling will pass whether I eat or not,' " says Cohen. One reason some women cannot tolerate discomfort is that they are sure the discomfort will last forever. You need to realize that feelings have a beginning, a middle and an end, explains Cohen. You must understand that your depression *will* end.

Solve the problem. What's prompting you to reach for food at the moment? A tight work deadline? A conflict with a spouse? A crying child? Try to focus on solving the problem, rather than avoiding it with food, suggests Dr. Minirth.

Take a time-out. For ten minutes, resist the urge to nosh and ask yourself what's going on. Take the opportunity to figure out what's behind that craving, says Dr. Campbell. And make it a habit to tune in to your inner feelings at these times.

Reach out and call someone. A brief phone call to a friend or relative may distract you and provide the emotional connection you really crave, says nutritionist Connie Roberts. "You don't have to tell them you were about to eat four chocolate cupcakes," she says. "Just chat. It helps."

Delay. In advance, come up with a list of alternative activities to do when the eating mood strikes, suggests Dr. Abramson. At work, tack the list to your calendar. Distractions that usually work include reading your mail or flipping through the newspaper. At home, sew a button on that skirt that's been out of commission for months. Polish your navy blue shoes. Repot your favorite fern. Do one small thing—but make it an activity that can compete with eating. (Cleaning the oven probably won't cut it.)

Enjoy new treats. Celebrating a personal achievement? Had a good day at the office? Lost five pounds? Indulge in a manicure, pedicure or facial; take a bath in your favorite bath salts; relax with a new book; sign up for a low-fat cooking course.

"I suggest women try things they used to like as kids, or just try new things," says Dr. Kolotkin. "One woman started horseback riding again. Another joined a soccer league for enjoyment."

Practice safe snacking. We all need an emotional pick-me-up once in a while. Try satisfying your need with tasty foods that don't load on the calories. This approach also keeps you from fearing the foods you desire.

"I have patients practice buying one chocolate truffle and enjoying it to the utmost," says Roberts. "Sometimes denying yourself the one thing you want can lead to eating more calories somewhere else."

Plan. If you must eat, tell yourself in advance what snacks you'll turn to when emotion-driven episodes occur, says Roberts. Possible examples, she says, include a muffin with jelly or air-popped popcorn. Picking and choosing what you do instead of eating anything in sight reminds you that you are still in control.

FEED YOUR HEART, NOURISH YOUR SOUL

After keeping a food/mood diary for a couple of weeks, says Dr. Abramson, you'll probably be able to identify specific feelings that make you eat. Here's how to deal with them.

Don't beat yourself up. Pay close attention to your inner voice—and give yourself positive messages, not self-criticism.

"We think 450 to 1,200 words a minute. If you turn your thoughts against yourself, it's like a laser beam on the heart that will literally destroy you," says Dr. Minirth. "Be realistic. If you make a mistake, ask yourself what you can learn from it. If you're having a difficult time, don't say 'I'm done for.' Instead, tell yourself 'This is tough on me right now, but things will work out.' "

Confide in others who are supportive. Talk with friends and family or join a support group, such as Overeaters Anonymous. "Many emotional eaters feel ashamed of their feelings and thoughts," says Dr. Kolotkin. "They may live in environments where they feel controlled and judged and criticized. It's so helpful to have supportive friendships, people who can say 'Oh, I know what that feels like, too. You aren't alone.' "

Listen to your anger. We may have grown up hearing that anger is not polite or fearing an angry parent. As a result, "our own anger can be terrifying," says Dr. Campbell. "Women have a challenging time learning about all the shades of gray of anger."

Learn them by using time-outs before eating to see if, in fact, you are angry. Then what should you do? Dr. Russell suggests talking it out with a friend—a neutral third party—before confronting the object of your anger. Why? It may keep you from blowing up.

Make time for self-reflection. If you're always busy meeting the needs of your spouse, your children and your boss, when do you meet your own? Make time to ponder, to keep a journal, to clarify your goals and priorities—to respond to your inner self.

"If you don't stop and reflect, you're going to ignore a lot of emotions," notes Dr. Kolotkin. "And if you ignore emotions when they're mild, they'll only get stronger and hit you over the head. But if you monitor your emotions regularly, they won't loom so large."

Learn—and look ahead. One emotional eating episode is not the end of the world, says Dr. Russell. Learn from it.

Ask yourself a few questions, says Dr. Minirth. "Were you angry about something? Should you have been more direct? Did something trigger old wounds?" Self-reflection will help you steer clear of the emotional eating cycle.

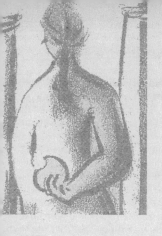

2
STRESS
Calm nervous nibbling

Judy D., an executive assistant at a busy East Coast airport, has a secret weapon for coping with 12-hour workdays, an impatient boss and high-anxiety deadlines.

"Gummi Bears!" laughingly says this 55-year-old, who responded to our *Food and You* survey.

"When things get really hectic in our office, we all gravitate toward junk food," says Judy. "One day we went through a five-pound bag of Gummi Bears. No kidding! And Gummi Bears get us through a lot of bad days."

So do doughnuts brought by co-workers and coffee from the cafeteria. "Under stress, we stuff our faces," says Judy, referring to the women she knows. "It's very consoling."

WOMEN, STRESS AND HIGH-PRESSURE MUNCHING

Stress? We all know it well. It can hit at any time. In the morning, the car won't start, the babysitter's sick, you're out of milk, and you *have* to be at work on time. At night, you argue with your husband. The next day, you're cooking a holiday dinner for 12 and—simultaneously—cleaning the house.

"Stress is very individual," explains Paul J. Rosch, M.D.,

clinical professor of medicine and psychiatry at New York Medical College and president of the American Institute of Stress, both in New York City. "The same experience could make one woman feel anxious and have no impact on another. That's because stress comes from feeling a lack of control, and different people feel they lack control in different situations."

Yet experts see some common ground when it comes to women and their experiences with stress.

First, women experience unique stress due to role conflicts. "We're trying to do it all," says Sylvia Gearing, Ph.D., a clinical psychologist in Dallas and author of *Female Executive Stress Syndrome*. "The bottom line is, women feel they are in a particularly challenging time of our history. We don't have clear rules. Do we stay at home? Work? How will we raise the children?" Men are less apt to face conflicting demands.

Fifty-four percent of women polled in a National Health Interview survey said they routinely experience moderate or severe stress. Mental and emotional stress can raise a woman's blood pressure, deposit more fat around her tummy, lower her immunity and, if she's past menopause, increase her risk of heart disease.

Second, while both women and men may respond to tense times by overeating, there's evidence that women turn to food more often in stressful moments and more often choose sugary foods, washed down with copious amounts of coffee to keep them going.

You may sip extra coffee, tea or caffeinated soft drinks to perk up after an anxious night's sleep, says Scottsdale, Arizona, dietitian Tammy Baker, R.D., a spokesperson for the American Dietetic Association. You might reach for a candy bar or other snack food because it's convenient, because you get a quick (but short-lived) energy boost from the sugar or because you were too busy for breakfast—and now you feel famished.

This nervous eating is a "double-edged sword," says Nicholas Hall, Ph.D., director of the psychoneuroimmunology division at the University of South Florida Psychiatry Center in Tampa. "It's natural to seek food under stress—your body is gearing up for a fight-or-flight response, the increase in adrenaline production and other physiological changes triggered by stress. Your body needs energy. It's a biochemical urge." Yet what we eat can render us less able to function at our peak when the going gets tough—at the moment and in the future.

FIGHT, FLIGHT OR FIG NEWTONS?

Red alert! Your body's age-old fight-or-flight response is swinging into high gear. Instantly, stress hormones pour into the bloodstream, sharpening your senses, raising your blood pressure and quickening your heart rate. Muscles tense. Breathing grows shallow.

You're prepared to fend off a saber-toothed tiger or run from marauding cheetahs. But the trouble is, twentieth-century stresses—from traffic jams to coordinating the Little League car pool to caring for kids and aging parents—elicit the same response. And this takes a toll on your body.

"Back in the Stone Age, if you were trying to outrun that saber-toothed tiger, you'd be expending a large amount of energy. An important mechanism in your body would kick in and you'd find food to fuel the intense physical exercise. Your body's needs balanced out, and intake would equal what you were expending," says Dr. Hall. "Today everything's different. We usually don't have a physical release from stress. But we may still want to eat. In contrast to previous eras, you don't even have to expend energy in order to acquire food. You can have a pizza at your door in 15 minutes just by punching seven numbers into the telephone."

Stress-induced feeding frenzies can wreck the most well-intentioned eating plans. Overweight women report that stress is one of the top two reasons they overeat, says Ronette Kolotkin, Ph.D., clinical psychologist and director of behavioral programs at the Duke University Diet and Fitness Center in Durham, North Carolina.

Sugary snacks, too much caffeine, overeating and skipping meals can leave you tired, irritable, jittery and mentally unfocused—just when you most need to feel alert and energetic.

"If a woman is under stress constantly, she must take the time to take care of her body," says Georgia Hodgkin, R.D., Ed.D., associate professor in the Department of Nutrition and Dietetics at Loma Linda University in California. "The key is to set aside time and energy for good meals and good snacks,

REACH FOR AN ORANGE—AND A TOWELETTE

It's Hell Week at work. And what's piling up in your trash can, orange peels or candy wrappers?

Chances are, it's candy wrappers.

"Under stress, people grab whatever they can get their hands on; often that's junk food," says Carla Wolper, R.D., a nutritionist at the Obesity Research Center at St. Luke's Hospital and the Center for Women's Health at Columbia-Presbyterian Hospital, both in New York City. "No one stops and says, 'Gee, I could really use a couple of oranges right now.' "

But oranges might be just what you need, says Nicholas Hall, Ph.D., director of the psychoneuroimmunology division at the University of South Florida Psychiatry Center in Tampa. When stress comes knocking, oranges (and other foods rich in vitamin C) have an especially important place in a woman's diet, say researchers.

Scientists have long known that physical stress depletes stores of vitamin C, says Paul J. Rosch, M.D., clinical professor of medicine and psychiatry at New York Medical College and president of the American Institute of Stress, both in New York City. The impact of emotional stress is less clear, "but there's little doubt emotional stress increases production of substances known as free radicals, by-products of cellular oxidation that can damage the immune system and accelerate aging," Dr. Rosch says. "Vitamin C is an important antioxidant—that is, it blocks the action of free radicals and protects against their damage."

Besides oranges, other top sources of C include berries, kiwifruit, broccoli, tomatoes, brussels sprouts, potatoes, cantaloupe and grapefruit. If you decide to snack on an orange or other fresh fruit, though, be prepared. "Fresh foods *are* trickier," notes Georgia Hodgkin, R.D., Ed.D., associate professor in the Department of Nutrition and Dietetics at Loma Linda University in California. "Just keep moistened towelettes (like baby wipes) around so you don't get your computer all sticky."

plus get plenty of sleep, exercise and relaxation. The payoff is, you'll feel at your best.''

Eating properly can be important, says Dr. Rosch. ''The more you perceive that you're in control, the less you feel threatened under stressful situations,'' Dr. Rosch says. ''Knowing that your diet is good and your nutritional needs are being met can help strengthen your sense of control.''

EATING TACTICS FOR TOUGH DAYS

To feel good—and good about yourself—on stressful days, doctors and nutritionists suggest the following steps for taking charge of nervous eating.

Start with breakfast. You wouldn't start a cross-country road trip with an empty fuel tank, says Dr. Hodgkin, so why begin a stressful day on an empty stomach? For a breakfast that supplies steady energy and enough calories to hold you until lunch, she suggests a low-sugar, high-fiber cereal with skim milk, fruit or fruit juice and a slice of toast, a bagel or an English muffin spread with a tablespoon of peanut butter or fat-free cream cheese.

Think twice about caffeine. Some studies show that a little caffeine can increase alertness. But drinking coffee, tea or other caffeinated beverages is apt to leave you feeling jittery and irritable in the long run, says Dr. Hodgkin. In fact, researchers at Duke University have found that caffeine can actually stimulate the body's fight-or-flight response to stress. So if you're feeling pressured, drinking caffeine may aggravate matters, say experts.

''You have to be aware of how you react to caffeine,'' says Dr. Rosch. ''Some people need a good strong cup of coffee to get them going in the morning, and they're fine. Others get so jittery after consuming caffeine, it's counterproductive.''

Eat mini-meals. ''By eating several small meals, you will have more consistent blood sugar levels, and you won't get the sluggish feeling that comes with digesting a big meal,'' says Baker. She suggests eating breakfast, followed by fruit and low-fat yogurt at midmorning, a sandwich made with low-fat lunch meat and a salad for lunch, fruit, veggies or low-fat microwave popcorn in the afternoon, and a moderate dinner.

Keep your hand out of the sugar bowl. High-sugar foods make blood sugar levels rise, prompting an infusion of insulin that ushers the sugar into your cells—dropping blood sugar levels, says Dr. Hodgkin. "If you eat candy or sugary baked goods alone, without protein or fiber-rich foods, there won't be anything left in reserve to maintain an even blood sugar level," she says. "When blood sugar levels drop, you can feel irritable, tired and unhappy—the last thing you need under stress."

Plan for snack attacks. If you must have a snack, avoid high-fat, high-calorie snack machine fare by bringing your own treats, suggests Dr. Hodgkin. Stock a desk drawer with apples and oranges, low-fat microwave popcorn or single-serving boxes of crunchy, low-sugar cereal. Tote a small bag of prewashed and peeled baby carrots.

Drink water first. "As we get older, we lose our sense of thirst," says Dr. Hodgkin. "Sometimes when we think we're hungry for a snack, we really need a drink of water." Before you snack, walk to the water fountain for a long sip, suggests Dr. Hodgkin. We need at least eight glasses of fluid a day. Without it, even mild dehydration can leave you feeling fatigued and even headachy.

Delay. Crave a packet of chocolate-covered raisins when a deadline looms? Wait ten minutes and the urge may pass, says Carla Wolper, R.D., a nutritionist at the Obesity Research Center at St. Luke's Hospital and the Center for Women's Health at Columbia-Presbyterian Hospital, both in New York City. "Or have a nice cup of caffeine-free tea. Or take a short break. Distracting yourself for ten minutes could be all you need," she says.

Avoid high-fat lunches and dinners. A high-fat lunch can leave you fighting off sluggishness for the rest of the afternoon, says Baker. And because your body digests fat slowly, a high-fat dinner could actually interfere with a good night's sleep, she says. So try to keep the fat content at both meals to less than 30 percent of total calories. (For more specific guidelines, see chapter 46.)

Unwind wisely. Pouring yourself a couple of beers, a glass or two of wine or a couple of cocktails after a hard day could become a habit, especially if the bad days outnumber the good. So can using alcohol as a sedative to lull you to sleep. Experts warn that relying on alcohol to deal with tension could lead to alcohol abuse.

There's another reason to be wary of the bottle. Researchers at the University of Pittsburgh have found that women may actually feel the effects of a cocktail less when they're under stress, and it may take an extra drink or two in order for them to relax. And with alcohol, more is definitely not better, especially since women are usually more sensitive to the effects of alcohol.

If you're in the habit of using alcohol to unwind, sit down with a cool nonalcoholic drink instead—an alcohol-free mock cocktail (like cranberry juice and club soda) or a tropical juice spritzer, made with a half-and-half mixture of tropical juice blend and seltzer, suggests Baker.

Breaking a drinking habit isn't easy—you may need the help of a supportive friend or relative or a 12-step group like Alcoholics Anonymous.

COPING WITH TENSION—WITHOUT FOOD

Stress is an unavoidable consequence of life, says Dr. Rosch. "There are some stressors you can do something about and others you can't hope to control or avoid. The trick is in learning to distinguish between the two, so you can use your time and talents effectively, rather than being constantly frustrated."

Experts suggest these ideas for fixing the stress you can control and accepting unavoidable stress.

Figure out what's bugging you. "Over and over, people say stress and anger make them overeat," Dr. Kolotkin says. "We try to help them see the stress patterns behind the eating and to control the eating by easing the real cause of the stress."

Decide what you can deal with, and forget the rest. List the most stressful situations in your life, suggests Dr. Rosch. Then list the ones you can change (like leaving too late for work in the morning) and the ones you can't (like getting caught in the daily traffic jam at the toll-booth).

"Prioritize the stressful events that you can control and outline destressing action plans," says Dr. Rosch. "And remember that a lot of stress is due to faulty perceptions. Ask yourself if your worst fears would really come true in a situation you find stressful.''

Defuse. Even when pressed for time, you can take three minutes to defuse a stressful situation—and derail the need to eat, says Dr. Kolotkin. How? Wash your face in the rest room and tell yourself you won't let stress drive you to the candy machine. Step outside for some fresh air. Close your office door and stamp your feet, punch a pillow, turn on a relaxation tape for a few minutes or call your home answering machine and vent about what's happening.

Balance thinking and feeling. Under stress, we may consciously recognize that we're not at fault or not in trouble, but our emotional selves may not, says Dr. Gearing. "There may be some feelings stirring about in there that you can calm," she says. "Remind yourself that this will pass, it will be over soon. Continuing to obsess will not help—it only takes energy away from doing what you have to do."

Get your daily requirement of play. Unwind, suggests Connie Roberts, R.D., manager of Nutrition Consultation Services and Wellness Programs at Brigham and Women's Hospital in Boston. Set aside playtime—and don't use it to run errands or buy groceries. "Go to an art museum, see a movie, take a walk with a friend," she says. "This helps two ways—you've taken some control by organizing an activity for yourself, and then you get to enjoy it."

Exercise. A physical workout can energize and relax you. Strenuous exercise, says Wolper, may also counter stress by releasing endorphins—body chemicals that contribute to a feeling of well-being.

Know your trigger points. The ultimate stress-control strategy is to know yourself, says Dr. Kolotkin.

"Look for patterns," she says. "If you start crying every Sunday night and find you're eating all night long, it could very well be that you're having some feelings about your job and things aren't right," she says. "Sometimes we have to either accept that this is a stressful job and find less stressful work, or take steps to make the job more tolerable. The same is true of relationships. Ultimately, you have two choices—change the situation, or accept it."

3

RECREATIONAL EATING

For a good time, dial f-o-o-d

Click goes the remote control unit. Crunch go the Fritos. For Jane P., who responded to our *Food and You* survey, watching television unleashed a wild desire to munch.

"As soon as the TV came on, I'd drag out the chips and the popcorn," Jane says. "It was fun. But I'd be so intent on watching *Roseanne* or *Monday Night Football* that I wasn't aware that I was eating."

Food *is* fun. Yet when recreational eating becomes a habit, the good times can add extra pounds—and subtract enjoyment from your life. If devouring a bag of chocolate chip cookies serves as a form of play and self-expression, you may be missing out on more satisfying experiences.

"Food is no substitute for real, honest-to-goodness fun," says Ronette Kolotkin, Ph.D., a clinical psychologist and director of behavioral programs at the Duke University Diet and Fitness Center in Durham, North Carolina. "Chances are, if you watch children at play and call them in to eat lunch, the typical response is 'Do we have to? We're having too much fun!'

"In contrast, adults often think they're not supposed to play anymore. So instead, I hear women say to their friends all the time, 'Let's have lunch,' " Dr. Kolotkin says.

PLAY DATES, LUNCH DATES

Whether you indulge in "viewing and chewing" like Jane, eat when you're bored or unwind with food after a hectic day, recreational eating can easily become a habit, says Edward Abramson, Ph.D., professor of psychology at California State University in Chico and author of *Emotional Eating: A Practical Guide to Taking Control.*

"If you do something often enough, you don't think about it," Dr. Abramson says. Then a cue like switching on the television or arriving home after work may trigger the desire to eat. Certain messages program us to think of food as recreation, says Dr. Kolotkin. "Fun-size" chocolate bars seduce you in the convenience store checkout line. Chewing gum promises to "double your pleasure, double your fun." Neon signs with flamingos and palm trees lure you into taco stands with the promise of a late-night tryst with a taco. "We get a lot of messages about using food for fun," says Dr. Kolotkin.

Replacing recreational eating with fun activities can open up new worlds of enjoyment, notes Dr. Kolotkin. It can also free you to savor food as a true pleasure, says Connie Roberts, R.D., manager of nutrition consultation services and wellness programs at Brigham and Women's Hospital in Boston.

"Food can be a wonderful experience," says Roberts. "Some women think their food troubles stem from enjoying food too much. The key is to have fun with food, without guilt."

LOOKING FOR FUN IN ALL THE RIGHT PLACES

Experts suggest these ways to balance food and fun in your life.

Redefine fun. Recreational eating may be a substitute for something you'd really like to do, says Dr. Kolotkin. Ask yourself what activities intrigue you or what you enjoyed in the past. Then go for it! One woman counseled by Dr. Kolotkin joined a community soccer league. Another started horseback riding.

Make social "play dates." Rather than going out for pizza, tacos or dinner with your friends, do something active—bowl, see a movie, go dancing or roller-skating. "I encourage people

---

BORED? STAY OUT OF THE KITCHEN

"Help yourself to some crackers!"

Left alone with brimming bowls of wheat crackers and a researcher's casual invitation to snack, 60 women students from California State University in Chico proved something you may have long suspected: When we're bored, we eat more.

In the study, half the women did a boring task—copying the letters *CD* over and over again. The others wrote stories. Women in the "boredom" group ate up to seven times more crackers.

Researcher Edward E. Abramson, Ph.D., professor of psychology at the university, says the link between a dull moment and the desire for, say, doughnuts, may be a natural one. But you don't have to fall for it.

One logical solution, says Dr. Abramson, is to relieve the boredom with an interesting task. But if you can't escape a tedious chore, don't do it where the food is.

"I tell students they should try to do their boring homework in the library—where there's no food," he says. "One woman I know used to iron in the kitchen. She'd get very bored and end up eating. I suggested she do her ironing away from the kitchen. Now she irons in the garage."

---

to deliberately think of things to do rather than get together and eat," Dr. Kolotkin says. "They laugh at first, but it really is fun."

Truly satisfy yourself. To break routine "bored eating," Dr. Abramson suggests having another activity ready for boring afternoons or evenings or other dull times. A woman he counseled realized she was bored and ate for fun after work. Now she gardens instead.

Uncover your "view and chew" style. Does watching TV bring out the snacker in you? Dr. Abramson suggests paying attention to when and how this happens: After 45 minutes? During the commercials? Use the information to sever the view-and-chew connection. After your program is over, take up another activity, like reading or a hobby. Or if you get up during commercials or between programs, avoid the kitchen.

Plan light snacks for boring moments. The most common times of a day for recreational eating are from 3:00 to 4:00 and 8:00 to 9:00 P.M., says Roberts. Plan a low-calorie, fun-to-eat snack for those moments, she suggests. (In chapter 54, you'll find 50 snacks with 100 calories or less.)

Savor the food you eat. Small amounts of the most decadent foods—a sliver of cheesecake, a chocolate-covered cherry, a small dish of premium ice cream—can be fun without packing on the pounds, says Roberts. The secret is to have your fun in small doses.

Toss out temptation. Keep your home and work environment "safe," advises Roberts. If you are prone to recreational eating and you keep snack food around, you *will* eat it. The temptation will be there—you will hear those chocolate-covered peanuts calling to you. "You need to be an environmental engineer," says Roberts. "Don't keep those tempting foods around."

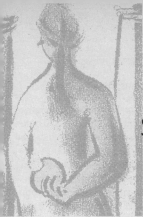

4

SNEAK EATING

Freedom from guilt

Deft as a cat burglar, Cathy B. remembers snitching a plate piled high with her favorite Christmas cookies and diving under the dining room table. Hidden by her mother's fanciest tablecloth, she devoured all the cookies.

"I ate till I was sick, and the whole time I was afraid someone would find me," recalls Cathy, now 35, a new mother and administrative assistant who responded to our *Food and You* survey. "I was in my twenties and had just lost a lot of weight. I didn't want to be seen eating sweets because I had always been the fat one in the family."

Nearly every woman hides out to eat sometimes—and savors the experience. But if, like Cathy B., you go to great lengths to keep your snack attacks hidden from view, you often eat in private, and you feel guilty or ashamed afterward, then you may be trying to quell unmet emotional needs through "closet eating," says Ronette Kolotkin, Ph.D., clinical psychologist and director of behavioral programs at the Duke University Diet and Fitness Center in Durham, North Carolina.

SAVORING FOOD IN SOLITUDE

A woman who eats on the sly can devour hundreds or thousands of calories in a short period of time, says Connie Roberts, R.D., manager of nutrition consultation services and wellness programs at Brigham and Women's Hospital in Boston. "She may feel like she's in a stupor afterward and think she can somehow lull herself to sleep with food," she says.

With sneak eating, quantity isn't the real issue. Even consuming small amounts of food on the sly may indicate that you have a problem.

"Sneak eating is about feeling judged and criticized, probably way beyond the issues of food and weight," says Dr. Kolotkin. "Often it means we feel we're being judged and criticized about ourselves and our life choices by close family like mothers, fathers, brothers or sisters." Sneak eating may spring from direct or indirect comments about our relationships, appearance, job, hairstyle or other personal qualities, she explains.

The impulse to crunch covertly may also spring from shame, says Mary Anne Cohen, director of the New York Center for Eating Disorders and author of *French Toast for Breakfast: Declaring Peace with Emotional Eating*. "Any time what you do with food would humiliate you if someone else knew, you're dealing with a shame-based eating problem." You can feel shame because you're angry or sad or jealous, or even because you feel sexual, she says.

When families shame children about their emotions or their needs, it becomes very easy to turn to food as a diversion or to fulfill an emotional need. Eating on the sly may easily become a lifelong habit, Cohen says. After all, "our relationship with food is like no other—food never laughs at us, never abandons us, never pokes fun at us, never abuses us, never leaves us," she says.

Then there's the flip side. Eating cookies under the dining room table can also have what Dr. Kolotkin calls "a delightfully sinful aspect" that makes the habit hard to break. "You know it's naughty," she says, "but you're doing it anyway. You think you're getting away with something or getting back at someone. But it really can't solve the underlying problems."

COME OUT OF THE CLOSET

Sneak eating is as much a potential problem for your self-esteem as it is for your waistline, say experts. "There is delight while you eat, but afterward there is shame and guilt—about the eating and about who you are as a person," Dr. Kolotkin says. "That's why the pattern must be stopped."

To help break the pattern of sneak eating, experts offer the following tips.

Keep track. Jot down, day by day, what you ate in private. Simply monitoring—not judging or criticizing—makes you more aware of what you're doing, says Roberts.

"Write it on a piece of paper, or just keep the candy and snack-food wrappers in a bag," she suggests. "The idea is, this is objective information that shows you in black and white what you're really doing. Simply being aware of how you eat in private can help you cut down on the frequency and the calories."

Go public. Instead of huddling in the kitchen with a half-gallon of ice cream, order two scoops at the local ice-cream parlor. Instead of ordering a late-night pizza, go out on the town with your family and enjoy one together, suggests Dr. Kolotkin.

The experience may be a lifetime first for a woman who has never consumed a "forbidden food" while the world watches. "For some, openly eating their coveted food triggers anxiety," says Dr. Kolotkin. "Others experience an immediate feeling of freedom—that they really can do this, it's really okay."

Slowly cut back. If your hidden treats are giant-size, scale down gradually. "If you have no trouble polishing off half a package of Oreos, eating just two may be very difficult. You may feel deprived and keep on eating," says Roberts. "Move slowly. If you tend to eat eight cookies, go to six for a while."

The ultimate goal? Finding the right small "dose" of a favorite food that's just enough to comfort you if you need it.

"I tell patients to think about aspirin. Do they take the right dose? Of course. Do they take more to feel even better? No—because they know there could be side effects," says Roberts. "Well, it's the same with food. Find out what the right dose

THE SNEAK-EATING QUIZ

Perhaps you indulged in a chocolate-crunch bar on the way home from work yesterday, then felt embarrassed when your husband discovered the crumpled wrapper in your car. Or maybe you sneaked an extra slice of cake while viewing a late-night movie—after everyone else went to bed.

Are these harmless treats, or have you slipped into the sneak-eating trap? To find out, take the following quiz, suggested by clinical psychologist Ronette Kolotkin, Ph.D., director of behavioral programs at the Duke University Diet and Fitness Center in Durham, North Carolina, and Hoyt Morris, Ph.D., director of the Oklahoma City Center for Eating Disorders. (If a question is generally or always true, check yes. Otherwise, check no. Be honest.)

1. Do you hide your eating from others? □ Yes □ No
2. Do you keep eating problems, like overeating, a secret? □ Yes □ No
3. Do you lie about how much you eat? □ Yes □ No
4. Do you hide food? □ Yes □ No
5. Do you find it difficult to eat high-calorie or high-fat foods in the presence of others? □ Yes □ No
6. Do you feel ashamed, guilty or depressed after an episode of sneak eating? □ Yes □ No
7. Do you isolate yourself from others if and when you feel fat? □ Yes □ No
8. Do you feel judged or criticized about your weight, body size or eating habits by parents, siblings, your spouse or close friend? □ Yes □ No

If you answered yes to four or five of these questions, says Dr. Kolotkin, sneak eating may be of moderate concern. If you have six or more yes answers, it's a serious concern. To break sneak-eating habits, says Dr. Kolotkin, follow the tips recommended in this chapter.

is—the amount that makes you feel comforted without side effects like weight gain.''

Look deeper—and accept yourself. On a deeper level, sneak eating may be an expression of anger and rebellion felt toward people who criticize and judge us for who we are, says Dr. Kolotkin. Ask yourself who, now or in the past, has harshly judged you—for your appearance, your lifestyle, your friends, your job.

''It's most important to work within yourself, accepting the parts of yourself that feel unacceptable,'' says Dr. Kolotkin. ''Tell yourself 'I accept that I have big thighs and I'm always going to. I can eat in public. I have the right to eat ice cream like everybody else. I have the right to be imperfect, weak or vulnerable or to do things that don't conform to my family's expectations.' ''

Open up. Let friends and family know who you really are—don't hide by isolating yourself or feeling that you must be perfect. But start with small steps, suggests Cohen. Disclose a small revelation to a friend or family member, then watch his or her reaction. It's important to reveal yourself to people who will accept you as you are.

Reach out. Women who sneak eat tend to think that they are all alone. ''Eating problems are considered diseases of isolation, because many people have come to learn that trust in food is safer than trust in people,'' says Cohen. ''The road to recovery is about connecting with people we can feel safe with.''

If you are finding it hard to open up and trust others, consider some group support, says Dr. Kolotkin. ''Seeing others who have struggled the way you have can help,'' she says. One group recommended by Dr. Kolotkin is Overeaters Anonymous. To find out if there is a group in your area, look under Self-Help/Support Groups or a similar heading in the Guide to Human Services in your telephone book. ''Overeaters Anonymous is a good support group for any eating problem, including sneak eating,'' says Dr. Kolotkin.

5

DREAMS

What food images and themes reveal

One woman repeatedly dreamed that a giant poached egg was pursuing her. Another found herself eating cardboard in her dreams. Then there was the woman who, more than once, dreamed of mouth-watering strawberries surrounded by a high-voltage electric fence.

"The woman who dreamed she was chased by the egg was truly terrified by this dream scenario," says Patricia Garfield, Ph.D., California psychologist, dream expert and author of *Women's Bodies, Women's Dreams* and *Creative Dreaming*, among other books on dream analysis. "The egg was all wobbly and gooey and was going to catch and engulf the woman."

In more than two decades of research and experience in dream interpretation, countless women have revealed their dreams to Dr. Garfield. And food images have figured prominently in those dreams.

THE LOGIC BEHIND THE BIZARRE

Illogical as dream images may seem—runny eggs, cardboard dinners and such—dreams can tell us things about ourselves that our conscious minds don't or won't reveal, say Dr. Garfield and other dream experts.

Dreams about food can unveil buried feelings of neglect or simply remind us that we went to bed hungry. They can unmask problems we've been ignoring, such as overeating, and can even help us find solutions, says Dr. Garfield.

What might you learn from an image of a giant poached egg, you wonder?

"As the woman talked about her dream, it came out that as a child, she had been force-fed," says Dr. Garfield. "She had to eat every scrap on her plate no matter how little it appealed to her. The poached egg was a symbol of an engulfing, messy situation with her parents that was still pursuing her."

Both past events—like childhood traumas—and present circumstances influence our dreams, says Dr. Garfield. If we're hungry, thirsty or cold or have to use the bathroom, these feelings affect the content of our dreams.

As you might expect, when we're hungry or feeling deprived of favorite treats, we often dream of food, Dr. Garfield says. A study of women with anorexia and bulimia, for example, found they had frequent dreams in which they needed to eat but couldn't for some reason. Other research showed that conscientious objectors who'd put themselves on semi-starvation diets to protest the draft had recurring dreams of food.

"When I first became a vegetarian, I tended to have dreams about eating meat," says Allan Siegel, Ph.D., a California psychologist and author of *Dreams That Can Change Your Life*.

What about the woman who saw herself eating cardboard? Further reflection revealed that the cardboard diet symbolized the strict diet she'd adopted. "What she was eating was so plain and unappealing, subconsciously, that she felt she might as well be eating cardboard," Dr. Garfield explains. The woman's dreams were telling her the strict diet wasn't going to satisfy her over the long haul.

Women who have love/hate relationships with food (love to eat it but hate the thought of what it might do to their figures) are particularly likely to dream of food in symbolic guise, says Robert Van de Castle, Ph.D., a clinical psychologist, professor emeritus in the psychiatry department at the University of Virginia Medical Center in Charlottesville and author of *Our Dreaming Mind*.

"If a person has developed strong waking feelings about food, these can carry over into her dreams," Dr. Van de Castle says. "For this person, food's become so emotionally loaded a subject that she dreams about it in disguise."

After overeating, one woman Dr. Garfield interviewed dreamed she was trying to change clothes in a tight cubicle—reflecting a fear of growing too large.

WHEN FOOD IMAGES REPRESENT EMOTIONS

Just as nonedibles like cardboard can represent food in dreams, food can represent nonedibles. Often it symbolizes affection, love, romance or sex, Dr. Van de Castle says. We might dream, for instance, that we're eating a birthday cake when we want some tenderness.

Most of us turn to food for comfort every now and then during our waking hours, so it only makes sense that we sometimes turn to food for comfort and affection while dreaming, Dr. Van de Castle explains.

Fruit, it turns out, may be heavily laden with such symbolism. The woman who dreamed of wild strawberries behind an electric fence ultimately concluded that the berries were a symbol of sexual gratification. Since this gratification was lacking in her marriage, the berries in the dream were forbidden, off-limits behind the electric fence, Dr. Garfield says.

As for sex, there are enough similarities between the acts of eating and intercourse to explain the erotic potential of dream-world phallic symbols such as bananas, Dr. Garfield points out. Hot dogs, cucumbers, pickles and corn on the cob are other common dream symbols for the penis. Beverages may represent ejaculate, and a cherry, slang for the hymen, may stand for female genitals, Dr. Garfield notes.

In all dreams, context is key. While dreaming of forbidden fruit may suggest a lack of sexual or emotional fulfillment, dreaming that you're eating a delicious bowl of fruit salad can suggest just the opposite—sexual or emotional satisfaction, she explains.

Dr. Siegel says women's dreams about food may also give clues to changes and challenges in current relationships.

HOW TO REMEMBER YOUR FOOD DREAMS

"Dream recall is a learned skill. Anyone can do it," Dr. Garfield promises. Women tend to be better at remembering dreams than men are, though, so you probably have an edge. These pointers can help you do even better.

Set your internal dream recorder. The power of suggestion is powerful indeed. Telling yourself that you *will* remember your dreams—before you nod off—will increase the odds that you'll recall them upon awakening, Dr. Van de Castle says.

When you first wake up, don't move. "If at all possible, lie still after you awaken, and keep your eyes closed," says Dr. Van de Castle. Don't even move your eyelids. "It seems that, with the act of movement, dreams vanish," he says. So commit the dream to memory immediately.

Recite your dream aloud. "When you wake up, your dreams are still accessible, stored in your short-term memory," Dr. Van de Castle explains. "Putting your dreams in words helps transfer the dream from your short-term memory to your long-term memory."

Describing your dreams aloud or silently to yourself can store them for future recall, says Dr. Garfield.

Keep a dream notebook. Better yet, write down your dreams, says Dr. Garfield. Jotting down whatever fragments of a dream you remember on awakening can also bring back earlier parts of the dream that aren't immediately accessible, she adds.

"If you write down what you remember, that acts like a hook; it will bring back preceding scenes and dreams," she says. Or you may want to recite the dream image into a tape recorder.

Dig below the surface. When food images evoke strong emotions—as they do for so many women—probing behind the obvious can be illuminating.

Say you dream that you go to the store for an ice cream cone, says Dr. Van de Castle. "To begin with, ask yourself whether you feel guilty about eating the cone," he says. "If you find out the cone costs $3.50, ask yourself if you think that's too expensive. Consider whether you ordered a small cone or a triple scooper. All these things give you ideas about how you feel about food—like whether you feel guilty about eating, whether you suspect you're paying too high a price (in terms of health) for what you eat, whether you're eating too much."

Start at the beginning. "The beginning of a dream often tells you what issue you're dealing with," Dr. Van de Castle says. "Focus on key people and objects, the setting and what's taking place at the start."

Look for keys. In a dream that bombards you with fast images of people and objects, how do you decide which ones are key? Look for repetition and for patterns, says Harold Roger Ellis, Ph.D., a psychologist in Hicksville, New York, and author of *Dream Drama*.

Keep in mind that symbols in dreams may have multiple meanings, and you may discover new meanings as you ponder the images in the dream. Say you dream you're drinking a milkshake in your car. You suspect the dream is about affection (symbolized by the shake) rather than wanderlust (the car), but you aren't sure. So try a little test. If affection (the shake) is central, there should be other people and objects in the dream that are also associated with love and caring—like your favorite grandmother or your childhood teddy bear. If the dream is chock-full of highways and maps, though, odds are you may do better turning your attention to the wanderlust/car theme.

Pay attention to context. When interpreting a food image in a dream, advises Dr. Siegel, you need to pay attention to the surroundings and other details.

Consider the nightmare that plagued a woman in one of Dr. Siegel's studies. A few weeks before her wedding—an elaborate affair that required a lot of stressful planning—she dreamed the waiters at the reception were serving her guests canned spaghetti, straight from the cans.

The woman and her fiancé had a solid relationship, so in that context it wouldn't make sense to interpret the canned spaghetti as a symbol of love that was, say, "canned" or "makeshift." What did the nightmare pasta mean, then? After she and her fiancé talked about the dream, he remembered that they'd shared a can of spaghetti on one of their first dates. They'd gone camping, eaten the spaghetti right from the can and had a wonderful time. The dream spaghetti was a reminder that they'd enjoy their wedding more if it were less pretentious, Dr. Siegel says.

Get graphic. Always pay attention to detail—the surroundings, the smells and even the tastes in your dream, says Dr. Garfield. Smells and tastes in dreams are often connected to basic emotions. What people or situations do your dream flavors and scents remind you of?

Consider both the literal and the figurative clues. Sometimes a Cheerio is a Cheerio. Sometimes it's a wedding ring.

If you wake up famished and remember going to bed on an empty stomach, dreaming about food simply means you're hungry for food. But if you're having some relationship trouble, the food is more likely to symbolize something more. "Always consider both the subjective and objective meaning," Dr. Siegel says.

Review your waking week. Your dreams are commentaries on what's happening to you while you're sleeping (whether you're hungry, for example) and what's happened to you in the past, often the recent past.

When interpreting a dream, ask yourself what transpired during the previous day or week. What happened with your relationships, your job, your health? In particular, focus on things that may have upset or moved you.

"Try to figure out what was the unfinished emotional business," Dr. Van de Castle says. "It's the things that upset us that go underground and get moved over toward the subconscious. At night, your mind brings these things up for review in dreams. Dreams are, in a sense, little memos you made to yourself during the day."

Once you identify the people and events that upset or moved you during the week, ask yourself whether they bear any similarity to the people and events in your dream.

Apply the tingle test. When there are many possible interpretations to a food dream, how do you decide which interpretation is right?

"If you get a tingle inside when you think or hear it, you've touched on something potentially meaningful,'' Dr. Siegel says.

Revise the ending. Not only can we learn to interpret our dreams, say Dr. Siegel and his colleagues, we can learn to change the endings of recurring ones. And that can work to our advantage. Studies show that people feel more encouraged and more competent after waking from dreams in which they experience success.

Say you repeatedly dream of overeating, for example. Before going to sleep, review the dream in your head until you get to the ending. Then visualize your own, more satisfactory finale, Dr. Garfield suggests, even if you have to write it out. Odds are, you'll dream a similar thing, with the new ending, says Dr. Garfield.

If you succeed in changing a dream that finds you overeating to one that finds you eating reasonably, you may have a better chance of improving your diet, she suggests.

Of course, if you think changing your dream solves the problem, you're dreaming, warns Dr. Siegel. You still have to make a wide-awake effort to avoid the potato chips and fries— or do whatever else your dreams are telling you to do.

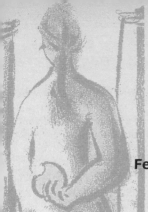

6

SELF-ESTEEM

Feel better about your body

As with so many women, weight was always a big issue in Joni Johnston's family—especially if you were female.

Joni's mother worried about gaining weight. So did her grandmother. So Joni learned early about the "need" to be superthin. In fact, Joni's compulsion about her weight began in elementary school—around the time her parents signed her up for her first beauty pageant. It followed her through high school and college, and all the while she was dieting and exercising compulsively. She constantly compared herself to other women and was obsessed with her weight. Her self-esteem went up and down with the numbers on the scale.

Dieting and obsessing. Obsessing and dieting. It wasn't until Joni finished graduate school that she realized what a psychological toll all this diet and anxiety was taking on her self-esteem. She decided to turn it into a mission to help others with the same problem.

"All this anxiety about our bodies takes a lot of energy out of women," says Johnston, who now has a doctoral degree in psychology and is a clinical psychologist in Dallas, where she specializes in treating eating disorders, body image problems and depression.

Few women, it seems, are happy with their bodies. In one

Gallup Poll, 19 percent of women surveyed said they were depressed because of their weight. Another 13 percent said they worried about it all the time. And a staggering 62 percent, including many who acknowledged they weren't even overweight, said they wanted to be thinner.

Women's dissatisfaction with their bodies is considerably more prevalent now than a generation ago, says Judith Rodin, Ph.D., former chairman of the psychology department at Yale University, currently president of the University of Pennsylvania in Philadelphia and a recognized authority on body image.

Why? Ours is a society that is increasingly preoccupied with appearance and weight, observes Dr. Rodin. Magazine covers, TV shows, music videos and movies tend to feature very, very thin women over those with more realistically filled-out figures.

"The media now expose us to this single 'right' look, and the beauty industry promises that anyone can attain it," writes Dr. Rodin, author of *Body Traps: Breaking the Binds That Keep You from Feeling Good about Your Body*.

Truth be told, though, it's the rare woman who fills the bill naturally. The industry standard is artificially high, set by images of models and celebrities who have the means to hire a personal trainer, spend thousands of dollars on cosmetic surgery and have their photographs airbrushed to perfection. Holding them up as role models only means you're setting yourself up to let yourself down. Dr. Johnston's advice: Let your *own* body be your guide.

UNHEALTHY OBSESSION

A better body—and better body image—is a worthwhile goal if you're truly overweight. If you're susceptible to diabetes or heart disease or some other weight-related disorder, getting in shape is in your best interest. But your pancreas and arteries don't care if you're not perfect.

And some of us aim for a weight so low it's downright unhealthy. We grow ever more miserable trying to shrink to a size 8 when our genes—making their intentions known through our appetites, metabolisms and bone structure—declare we should wear size 10 or 12.

Or we focus so intently on our bodies that the view becomes distorted. We imagine fat where there is bone, says Ann Kearney-Cooke, Ph.D., a psychologist in Cincinnati who specializes in treating eating disorders. Studies show that the longer we focus on our bodies, the more critical we become. And research at Michigan State University in East Lansing has found that most of us consider ourselves heavier than we actually are.

All this can have serious repercussions, says Dr. Johnston, author of *Appearance Obsession*. A negative body image can make you self-conscious, socially anxious and depressed. It can erode your self-esteem and the quality of your life.

"As little girls, women realize they're rewarded more when they look nice," agrees Debbie Then, Ph.D., a researcher at the University of California at Los Angeles and a social psychologist whose specialty is treating body image problems. "How a woman feels about her body really dictates how she feels about herself and how she experiences the world."

In extreme cases, body dissatisfaction can lead to serious eating disorders such as anorexia and bulimia. But it doesn't have to go that far to cause problems.

In pursuit of thinness, many of us commit to impossible diets and unrealistic exercise regimens. "People try diets which are unrealistic and unhealthy to maintain," says April Fallon, Ph.D., assistant professor of psychology at the Medical College of Pennsylvania in Philadelphia.

Eventually we buckle under. We eat the forbidden brownie, skip the 90-minute workout—and end up feeling even worse about ourselves, says Dr. Kearney-Cooke.

Compounding the problem, she says, is the fact that restrictive diets and exercise regimens can leave little room for other things that can make us feel good about ourselves—like the companionship and support of other people.

"The achievement of looking good can get so demanding that you miss out on connections with others," Dr. Kearney-Cooke says. She cites, for example, women who turn down dates because they feel they should stay home and exercise.

Especially vulnerable, says Dr. Kearney-Cook, are women who are perfectionists. A weight problem makes them feel ineffective or isolated. This in turn can lead to feelings of depression, says Dr. Johnston. A study at Cambridge University in England, for example, found that most of us are more likely to feel bad about our bodies when we feel depressed. Low self-esteem is the inevitable result.

ESCAPE THE BODY TRAP

The low self-esteem/bad body image syndrome is what Dr. Rodin calls the body trap. Fortunately, there are ways to wiggle out of it.

Pay attention. What's contributing to your dissatisfaction with your body? Ads that promise slimness and success for everyone (all for the low price of a three-month supply of the latest diet drink)? Scrutinize these influences with a critical eye, Dr. Kearney-Cooke suggests.

"It's useful for women to trace the history of their body image and get a sense of why they're so concerned with their bodies," she says. Once you understood *why* you're preoccupied with your body, Dr. Johnston says, you may be able to get some perspective and control.

Get in shape—but get real. You're not made of Silly Putty—moldable into any shape you desire. It's useful to understand the extent to which your body can, and can't, be made over, says Dr. Rodin.

At the same time, say experts, it's important to treat your body well.

"When you give your body what it really needs, including moderate exercise, healthful foods, sensual pleasures and relaxation, your body will respond by treating you better," Dr. Rodin writes. "I've seen person after person look healthier, and walk with a lighter, more confident step, when they break their body traps."

Pamper yourself now. Don't wait until you've lost weight to buy yourself that new suit or get that new haircut, says Dr. Then. You'll feel better about yourself if you do it now. And that will help you view your body less critically and encourage you to make other positive changes in your eating and exercise regimen.

Just say "Thank you." Accepting compliments is not only

polite, it's good for you, says Kathy Bowen-Woodward, Ph.D., a clinical psychologist in Virginia Beach who specializes in women's issues. Whatever you do, she says, don't contradict the compliment-giver. What you say about yourself affects how you feel about yourself.

Put physical beauty in perspective. Yes, we're often judged on appearance, says Thomas Cash, Ph.D., professor of psychology at Old Dominion University in Norfolk, Virginia. But while beauty may open some doors, attributes like self-confidence and geniality are what make the biggest difference in our lives. Keep that in mind and make a point of paying at least as much attention to your pleasing attributes as to ones you don't like, he says. Other people notice all these aspects of you, not just your thighs.

Expand your persona. "You need to look at yourself and think, what is it that is unique and valuable about me?" says Dr. Fallon.

You're a fabulous soprano? A talented writer? A great friend? Give yourself credit. And diversify, to use all your talents. Join the church choir. Write short stories. You get the idea.

"If I feel good about myself because I'm a good writer or singer or have developed friendships with people who value me, I'm less preoccupied with my body," Dr. Bowen-Woodward says.

Be your own best friend. Examine your critical assumptions about your body, Dr. Cash adds. "Ask yourself 'When people see me, do they really think, My God, she's got big hips!' And if they do, does that mean they won't like you? Do your friends pity you for having big hips? Not likely." Thinking through your assumptions about your appearance, says Dr. Cash, will help you see how off-base many of them really are.

Ignore the beautiful people. If you compare yourself to fashion models, stop. The same goes for singers and actresses.

Expecting to look like a cover girl without benefit of an airbrushing is setting yourself up for a self-esteem problem, says Dr. Then. In fact, she conducted a scientific study measuring the impact of fashion magazines on the women who read them. By the time the women in the study had paged

SHEILA'S STORY
What We Can Learn

Of all the women who responded to our *Food and You* survey, no one exemplifies the principles of rebuilding weight-related esteem more than Sheila M., a 35-year-old mother of two who was overweight all her life and gained added weight during pregnancy. Here, experts in dieting and self-image comment on Sheila's story.

WEIGHT ISN'T EVERYTHING

"When I was growing up, carrying extra weight was always a negative thing, even though all the women in my family were a little overweight," Sheila told us. "After my second pregnancy, I was heavier than before. I still am," says Sheila.

"Initially, I felt a little uncomfortable," she says. "But I didn't obsess about it. I felt I had a lot of other good things in my life. I think you can sort of devalue all the other good things because you happen to be a little heavier at one time."

Why it works: Focusing on body weight and dieting can leave little room for other things that can make us feel good about ourselves, says Ann Kearney-Cooke, Ph.D., a psychologist in Cincinnati who specializes in treating eating disorders.

SLOWER IS BETTER

"I have about 30 pounds to lose from the pregnancy, but I'm going to do it slowly rather than starve myself for a month and gain it all back," says Sheila.

Why it works: "Losing weight only to regain it takes a real toll on your self-image," says C. Wayne Callaway, M.D., an obesity specialist at George Washington University in Washington, D.C. To lose slowly, you have to make sustained changes in behaviors. "No gimmick will do it," warns Dr. Callaway. By losing slowly, you don't set yourself up for the inevitable regain. So Sheila's approach is smarter in the long run.

WALK MORE, EAT LESS

"For exercise, I'm walking," Sheila told us. "And I'm trying to eat a healthier diet. If I go to dinner, I get salad for an appetizer, whatever I want for a main course but no butter, and for dessert, I have coffee.

"You can't go out to dinner and say 'I'm not going to eat a thing,'" she says. "That sort of thing becomes a downer. And you become a downer to everyone else."

Why it works: Exercise burns calories, controls appetite, promotes weight loss and boosts self-esteem, according to Debbie Then, Ph.D., a researcher at the University of California at Los Angeles and a social psychologist whose speciality is treating body image problems.

TAKE PRIDE IN YOUR PROGRESS

"I'm not waiting until I lose weight to buy new clothes or other nice things," says Sheila. "I have to live my life as it is now. It makes no sense to wait until I'm perfect, because I'm never going to be perfect."

Why it works: "Keep in mind that women look good in bigger sizes, too," says April Fallon, Ph.D., assistant professor of psychology at the Medical College of Pennsylvania in Philadelphia. And treating yourself well enables you to feel better about yourself, says Dr. Then.

through to the back cover, two-thirds of them felt worse about themselves.

"If you want to see what women really look like, stop looking at the TV and go to a mall or look around at work," Dr. Kearney-Cooke advises.

Lighten up. Dr. Cash also suggests relaxation techniques—like deep, rhythmic breathing—to soothe yourself when you're in situations that make you anxious about your appearance. If looking in the mirror makes you anxious, for instance, use deep breathing to relax when you do.

Don't crash diet. Trying to lose? Think "slow" and "permanent."

"If you do undertake weight reduction, give yourself a chance to keep it off," says C. Wayne Callaway, M.D., an obesity specialist at George Washington University in Washington, D.C. Translation: Don't try to lose by cutting way back on calories. Studies show that exercise plus eating sensibly are your best bets for permanent loss.

Give yourself the gift of exercise. Set aside time for an exercise regimen you really enjoy, whether it is walking, dancing or aerobics class. It burns calories *and* it boosts your self-esteem.

"When you carve out time to do something for yourself, you're saying 'I'm important,' " Dr. Then says. "That makes you feel better."

Research shows regular exercise can lift depression about the way you see yourself, says Dr. Then. And exercise will help you control your appetite and lose weight—if you need to, she says. But don't commit to a regimen that's so demanding you can't enjoy it. Dr. Callaway says three 30-minute sessions each week are enough to make a difference.

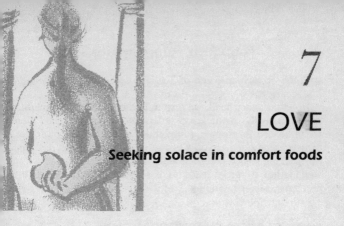

7

LOVE

Seeking solace in comfort foods

"In the end, I always want potatoes," the heroine of Nora Ephron's *Heartburn* confides when, seven months into her second pregnancy, her husband announces he has fallen for another woman.

Heartbroken but still hungry, she turns to mashed potatoes for solace. "Nothing like mashed potatoes when you're feeling blue," she muses. "Nothing like getting into bed with a bowl of hot mashed potatoes already loaded with butter and methodically adding a thin cold slice of butter to every forkful."

We've all been there—in bed with a bowl of mashed potatoes or a pint of double-fudge ice cream or a big bag of Doritos, spooning up comfort or munching to our heart's content.

Turning to food when we want some comfort, some affection, some love is only human. Even men do it—although they may not feel as guilty about it as most women do, says Joel Yager, M.D., professor of psychiatry at the University of California at Los Angeles. "For women, who are very conscious of what they're eating and how it will affect their appearance, it's a bigger issue," he says.

But it shouldn't be, says Dr. Yager. There's no reason to feel guilty. There's nothing wrong with comforting ourselves with the occasional batch of Toll House cookies—as long as it's occasional.

If, on the other hand, we turn to pistachio fudge and marble pound cake to soothe every everyday disappointment, then we're headed for trouble, says Linda Smolak, Ph.D., professor of psychology at Kenyon College in Gambier, Ohio. Habitually seeking solace with Ben and Jerry can easily lead to overweight, but it rarely leads to a solution to the underlying problems, says Dr. Smolak.

FOOD IS LOVE: A CHILDHOOD LEGACY

We learn to equate food with love in infancy. When our mothers held us to feed us, with breast or with bottle, we were nurtured both nutritionally and emotionally.

"For babies, food and love are synonymous," says Nan Kathryn Fuchs, Ph.D., a nutritionist in Sebastopol, California, and author of *Overcoming the Legacy of Overeating*.

"It's a common child-rearing practice to use food to silence a fussy baby," says David G. Schlundt, Ph.D., assistant professor of psychology and medicine at Vanderbilt University in Nashville. "You pick the baby up, hold it, talk baby-talk to it, placate the child with food. That's a very powerful experience—children learn to associate eating with comfort."

For many of us, our parents (and extended family of grandparents, aunts and uncles) reinforced the association as we got older, comforting us with chocolate bars when we skinned our knees or flubbed our lines in school plays, says Dr. Schlundt.

The "food is love" association can be particularly ingrained if family members find it difficult to express their feelings in other ways—by saying "I love you," for instance. If chocolate cake is served as a means of expressing love in your household, you may be more likely to cut yourself a slice when you feel low or to offer one to the people you love when they need reassurance and comfort, says Dr. Smolak.

Our culture as a whole sanctifies the food/love bond, adds Dr. Smolak. At first communions, bas mitzvahs, graduations, weddings, christenings—all the events we associate with closeness—we celebrate with food.

"We have cultural rituals, things like Thanksgiving, where

we sit around with our family and friends and overeat," Dr. Smolak says. "Strong bonds form over food."

Says a young woman who works as an artist, "Rice pudding reminds me of my Nana. When I'd go visit my Nana, she'd always make rice pudding for me."

DATELESS DINNERS

In courtship, too, we mingle love and food. We cook fancy dinners for the men we love. We enjoy fancy dinners they cook for us. A fancy dinner out is the epitome of a perfect date. Virtually every culture endows certain foods, such as oysters and red wine, with the power to inflame the heart. According to legend, the amorous Madame de Pompadour fed her paramours chocolate, truffles and celery soup to make them simmer.

All these links draw us to food when we want love. And food never runs away when we approach, says Gail Post, Ph.D., a clinical psychologist in Jenkintown, Pennsylvania. "And eating doesn't involve having to ask anyone for anything—something women often have trouble doing."

Food never turns us down after consulting its appointment book. It never breaks a date. Food is ever accessible, ever agreeable, even when husbands and lovers and friends are not.

And it seems so safe when other approaches to love and closeness may seem scary, says Lillie Weiss, Ph.D., adjunct associate professor of psychology at Arizona State University in Tempe and co-author of *Women's Conflicts about Eating and Sexuality*. After all, ice cream can't give you herpes.

"I have a lot of single women friends who've given up on men and turned to food," says Robin K., one of the women who responded to our *Food and You* survey. Dr. Post is not surprised. "It's simpler, more convenient and may feel emotionally safer," she says.

Food also absorbs your attention and distracts you from feelings of loss and loneliness, says Dr. Schlundt.

WOMEN'S TOP TEN COMFORT FOODS

What do the following foods have in common?

- Grilled cheese sandwich with tomato soup
- Oreos and milk
- Hot cocoa
- Macaroni and cheese
- Apple pie
- Mashed potatoes
- Waffles
- Oatmeal
- Rice pudding
- Ice cream

Those foods were most often named as "comfort foods" by women who responded to our *Food and You* survey. Other, less predictable entries included such diverse favorites as lettuce with hot bacon dressing, salmon, artichoke hearts, nectarines and water chestnuts.

"Specific foods bring back specific memories of good times," says Joel Yager, M.D., professor of psychiatry at the University of California at Los Angeles. "They remind us of our mothers, our grandmothers or other favorite people who served us food and comforted us. By association, the foods comfort us."

Given that legacy, it's no wonder we turn to food when we need solace.

A NATURAL MOOD ELEVATOR

Aside from the emotional connotations food carries, there are strictly biological reasons for its soothing effect. An empty stomach is uncomfortable, a full one can be calming, says Jennifer Kennedy, M.D., director of the Eating Disorders Program at the Menninger Clinic in Topeka, Kansas. And eating itself is engrossing. According to Dr. Yager, foods like cake and cookies, which are rich in carbohydrates, may also stimulate brain chemicals that soothe and relax us.

When German researchers fed chocolate milk to baby rats, levels of feel-good endorphins in the animals' bodies shot way up. "Endorphins are natural painkillers," explains Adam Drewnowski, Ph.D., professor and director of the Human Nutrition Program at the University of Michigan in Ann Arbor.

WHEN FOOD ISN'T THE ANSWER

While it's okay to turn to a bowl of mashed potatoes for comfort now and then, that can't be our only recourse in tough times, says Dr. Weiss.

It would be nice if you could simply pick up a good cheesecake after your lover runs off with his old girlfriend or your husband or best friend has grown distant, and feel fulfilled. But a cheesecake can't hold up its end of a conversation, make you laugh, drop forgotten lunches at your office and share intimate secrets. For true love and affection, says Dr. Weiss, food can't compete with human companionship.

"If what you really want is a hug, and instead you're gorging and feeling bad afterward, that's destructive," says Dr. Weiss.

Turning to food for nurturing can become a way of avoiding relationship problems that we should solve, says Dr. Post. If we're always choosing unfulfilling relationships, for example, we need to ask ourselves why and figure out how to steer clear of them. Maybe we need to stop dating men who are fearful of commitment. If our husbands and friends seem distant, maybe we need to speak up and tell them so. We need to explain what we want from them, ask for affection or find out why they pull back.

"It's often easier to reach for food so we don't have to risk speaking up and saying what we want," Dr. Post says.

By the same token, if we rely on serving food to demonstrate our affection, we may need to learn different ways of showing others that we care.

"I loved to cook, so I cooked. And then the cooking became a way of saying 'I love you,' " Ephron's heartstruck heroine realizes after the shock of her husband's defection has begun to fade. "And then the cooking became the easy way of saying 'I love you.' And then the cooking became the only way of saying 'I love you.' I was so busy perfecting the peach pie that I wasn't paying attention."

WHEN FOOD BECOMES THE PROBLEM

Clearly, habitually turning to food won't solve our problems. What's more, it can create some new ones, like overweight and low self-esteem, says Dr. Smolak. And it can also set the stage for an eating disorder.

"It's not always a problem to eat when you want comfort but aren't hungry, just as it's not always a problem to sleep when you're feeling lazy but not tired," Dr. Smolak says. "But when it starts to damage your health because you've gained so much weight or you start to feel it's out of control or you worry that people will find out what you eat or how much or you start to think about purging—taking laxatives or forcing yourself to throw up, or both, which is potentially very dangerous—then you have a problem."

So you solve it. The first step, of course, is realizing that you've got the problem. If you do, rest assured that you can deal with it. Here are some pointers.

Don't deprive yourself. You're more likely to turn to food for comfort if your diet leaves you feeling deprived, Dr. Smolak suggests. You can't go very long with a menu that allows you a cup of cottage cheese, a lone lamb chop and a slice of dry toast daily. Before long, you're feeling deprived, upset and primed for a binge. If you want to slim down, don't crash-diet—cut back on fat and sugar. (For more information on how to diet sensibly, see chapter 49.)

Keep a diary. Do you curl up with a jumbo bag of sour cream and onion potato chips every time you have a fight with your husband or mother or friends? Check it out. Keep a diary, jotting down what you ate and what prompted you to eat it.

"We call this monitoring," says Katherine Halmi, M.D., professor of psychiatry at Cornell University Medical College in New York City and director of the Eating Disorder Program at the New York Hospital, Westchester Division, in White Plains. "It's very effective. You note whether you're feeling depressed, angry or excited when you eat. Note your stress level. Consider how you handled the situation. Analyze the positive and negative consequences of your behavior. And write it all down and look for a pattern."

Find solutions that don't involve food. Once you've identified a situation that makes you turn to food for comfort, you need to come up with a different response. If your boss chews you out and makes you feel unappreciated, think about other ways to deal with it, strategies that don't involve eating. Weigh the pros and cons of each alternative.

"If you have a run-in with your boss, instead of eating a candy bar to soothe yourself, draft a memo that calmly presents your point of view, call the boss back to resolve the issue or (even better) discuss the situation with a co-worker and come up with a plan for addressing this," Dr. Schlundt says.

Share your feelings. If you want your husband or friends or children to give you a hug now and then, let them know, says Dr. Post. Conversely, show the people you love how you feel about them. Don't rely on giving them a batch of cookies to express how you feel. Tell your children, your partner and your close friends the positive feelings you have for them.

Seek out support. Sometimes the problem is that there's no one around to talk to. If loneliness drives you to eat, a support group like Overeaters Anonymous can be helpful, Dr. Smolak says. In fact, a support group can be a great resource even if there is someone to talk to at home. It's often easier to discuss difficult circumstances with people who share them.

Treat yourself well. Instead of reaching for food, do something nice for yourself—take time out for a walk, soak in a warm tub, play your favorite CD or call a friend, Dr. Smolak suggests.

"There are all kinds of ways you can restore emotional balance without using food, drugs or alcohol," adds Dr. Schlundt.

Use self-talk. Words are powerful things. By repeating an affirmation that focuses on the solutions you can use instead of overeating when you feel unloved, you actually make it less likely that you'll turn to the pantry for nurturing, Dr. Fuchs says. Try repeating the following for five or ten minutes every day: "I handle my problems well. I eat food to nourish myself." Or come up with your own affirmation. Just remember to put it in the present tense, even if this is not what you are now doing. In time, you will.

Have a backup plan in the pantry. Sometimes you do everything you can to make yourself feel better, but you still feel bad, says Dr. Schlundt. Perhaps someone you loved died, and you're feeling the loss keenly. If you know you're going to turn to food, and you've got a weight problem or there's some other reason a bag of chips could jeopardize your health, be prepared.

"Realistically recognize that sometimes you're going to get something to eat when you feel bad," Dr. Schlundt says. "But don't assume 'All hope is lost; I may as well eat a half-gallon of ice cream.' If you're going to give yourself permission to eat to feel better, eat things that don't have a bad impact, like low-fat foods. I had one woman I worked with get low-calorie frozen ice pops and keep them in the freezer. They had 15 calories each. I told her she could eat the whole box anytime she wanted. That was her safety net."

8

MOTHERS

The true source of your food attitude

Folklore leaves a rich legacy of images that equate mothering with food. In rural Java, farmers call rice "Rice Mother" and believe the shoots they plant are pregnant with grain the way a mother is pregnant with a child.

Indonesian folk traditions also speak of "the Mother of Rice," the largest ear of rice in the field, which is harvested first and stored in a special rice shed. This Mother of Rice will keep the shed well-filled with rice until next year's harvest.

In North America, Native American stories relate the life and death of "Corn Mother," a woman who becomes food to save her children from starvation. And Greek mythology tells of a "Mother Earth."

In many cultures, mothers and food are inextricably linked, says Nan Kathryn Fuchs, Ph.D., a nutritionist in Sebastopol, California, and author of *Overcoming the Legacy of Overeating*. And with good reason. As infants, says Dr. Fuchs, we're breast-fed directly by Mom or often bottle-fed by her. Mothers introduce us to food. They teach us what and how to eat. When we grow older they prepare our meals. So from birth onward, our mothers shape our eating habits and attitudes.

"The person who prepares the food, feeds us and makes

and breaks the rules about food is most influential," says Dr. Fuchs. "In most households that's still the mother."

As we grow up, other families, peers, teachers and spouses all influence our eating habits and attitudes, says Dr. Fuchs, but not in quite the same way our mothers do.

MODELING MAMA

As daughters, we tend to pattern our behavior after our mothers'. Their eating habits, their attitudes toward food and their feelings about their bodies influence our own habits, attitudes and feelings, says Jennifer Kennedy, M.D., director of the Eating Disorders Program at the Menninger Clinic in Topeka, Kansas.

"Most of us identify more strongly with the parent of the same gender," says Dr. Kennedy. "So mothers are very important in shaping how we nourish ourselves."

If our mothers were constantly complaining about the size of their thighs, dieting or bingeing on "fattening" foods they usually considered forbidden, we may be inclined to do the same, says Linda Smolak, Ph.D., professor of psychology at Kenyon College in Gambier, Ohio. If they ate whenever they were angry or needed comfort or wanted to reward themselves, we may follow their lead in that respect, too.

But there's a wild card in the interplay between mother and child: We may mimic Mom's eating habits and food attitudes, or we may do the opposite, says David G. Schlundt, Ph.D., assistant professor of psychology and medicine at Vanderbilt University in Nashville. If our mothers overate and were overweight, says Dr. Schlundt, we may diet compulsively so we don't end up overweight, too. If they dieted incessantly, we may eat with abandon, regardless of how much we weigh.

Given the high value our society places on thinness, though, abandoning control is a less common response, says Dr. Smolak.

"A mom's dieting probably contributes to her daughter's early dieting," she says. "And some data suggest that dieting early in life contributes to a lifetime of chronic dieting."

In a similar vein, research at Yale University has found that teenage girls with eating disorders are more likely to have mothers who are preoccupied with their weight and dieting.

PRESSURE ADDS POUNDS

Of course, what our mothers *say* about our eating habits and weight affects us too, says Dr. Smolak.

Even "gentle" kidding and well-intentioned remarks such as "You'd look so pretty if you just lost a few pounds" can cause problems, Dr. Smolak says.

"Research suggests that this kind of teasing and criticism leads to body dissatisfaction, dieting and eating problems," she says.

When Japanese researchers compared teenage girls who had eating disorders with those who didn't, they found the first group far more likely to have moms who were critical of their weight or encouraged them to diet. Nearly half said their mothers had urged them to lose weight. Girls who merely suspected that their mothers thought they were fat or ate too much were also more likely to have eating problems.

"This kind of influence can create a chronic dieter or someone who gets into a pattern of dieting and bingeing," Dr. Schlundt says. "Or sometimes it makes the kids all the more determined to eat whatever they want and not give in to the parental pressure to diet. There's no way to know why a child reacts in one way or another."

TOO MANY RULES

In general, the fewer restrictions our mothers (and others) put on eating, the better, says Dr. Smolak.

"American families tend to have a fair number of rules around eating," she says. " 'You can only eat at designated mealtimes,' for example, or 'You have to clean your plate.' "

Research suggests that too many rules aren't such a good idea. Scientists at the University of Illinois, for instance, found that preschoolers whose mothers let them decide how much to eat were less likely to overdo it than those whose moms dictated how much food they could have.

Offered nutritious foods and left to their own devices, children seem to have an innate ability to read their bodies' hunger signals and eat appropriately, according to the researchers.

If your mom or dad always made you clean your plate, you may have lost this ability, Dr. Schlundt says. The same may apply if they insisted you eat by the clock—at, say, 8:00 A.M., noon and 6:00 P.M. sharp—and not according to your body's hunger signals, which go off every four hours or so. Ditto if your parents rewarded you with goodies all the time or said "I love you" with milk and cookies.

"To an extent, trying to get children to eat when they're not hungry can encourage an eating problem, like compulsive eating or emotional eating," Dr. Smolak says.

THE EMOTIONAL CHARGE

The evidence is sketchier, but the emotional climate in your family may also contribute to your relationship with food as you grow up.

"Women whose parents can't provide support and affection or are abusive may become compulsive eaters or binge eaters," Dr. Smolak says. They may turn to food as an alternative source of comfort.

On the other hand, growing up amid a great deal of family conflict can raise the odds that we'll become chronic dieters, Dr. Kennedy says. In a household where everything seems out of control, strictly monitoring what goes into our bodies can become a way of exerting some degree of control over our lives, she explains.

LEAVING EATING PROBLEMS BEHIND

Many of the eating habits we practiced as children stay with us as adults. So subconsciously, our mothers (and influential others) continue to influence the way we eat long after we've struck out on our own, says Dr. Fuchs.

But they don't have to. If you don't want to spend your life dieting the way your mother did, you *can* stop, says Dr. Fuchs. If you want to stop bingeing on cookies (which she denied herself or you), you *can*. You *can* change the bad eating habits that are seeded in your childhood. Here's how.

Forgive your mom. Rather than blame her for putting you on a diet when you were a kid or for constantly criticizing your weight, forgive your mother and move on, Dr. Fuchs advises.

It may help to talk things over with your mom and get to the bottom of the matter, she says. Odds are your mom learned what to eat and what to feed her kids, from her mother, who learned from her mother, and so on, Dr. Fuchs says. And there may have been extenuating circumstances.

"Sometimes you can find out why she did what she did," says Dr. Fuchs. "I asked my own mother, 'Why, when you knew I was trying to lose weight, did you make all those creamed foods like turkey á la king and tuna á la king?' She said, 'I was trying to stretch the food to feed all of us.' I said, 'Forgiven.'"

Don't worry, though, if you can't (or don't want to) hash things out with your mother, says Dr. Fuchs. "It's not always necessary. Sometimes we don't want to relive the past," she says. "People can spend so much time reliving that they can't get on with a solution."

Acknowledge that you make mistakes, too. This may help you empathize with and forgive your mom, says Dr. Fuchs. "We all make mistakes," she says. "Think of what it's like to not be forgiven for a mistake you've made."

Unload the emotional baggage. The anger and resentment that accompany blame can really weigh you down, says Dr. Fuchs. Forgiveness can lift the weight. "So, for your own sake, forgive your mom," she adds.

Remind yourself that you're not your mother. At least once a day, tell yourself: "I am not my mother; I eat to nourish my body," Dr. Fuchs suggests, or try some similar affirmation.

Affirmations are statements that we make to ourselves, about ourselves, to change our outlook and behavior, she explains. These statements may not be true just yet. But the idea is that, by repeating them, you change your attitude and then your actions so they become true.

Value yourself. Your identity goes beyond the numbers on a scale or measuring tape.

"Don't define yourself solely in terms of how thin you are or how few calories you've eaten," says Dr. Smolak. "Your contributions—at work or to your family or community—are all valuable.''

Take an inventory of your contributions and attributes. "List all the things you do at home—like take care of your children, your garden, your animals—and at work," Dr. Smolak says. "Then look at the list. When you think about it, all the different things you accomplish have nothing to do with your weight or shape."

Accept compliments willingly. Most of us don't really hear compliments we're given, let alone accept them graciously, Dr. Smolak adds. "Comments like, 'You did a really good job' or 'Where'd you learn to paint so beautifully?' seem to go right by a lot of women," she says. "Pay attention to compliments. Whatever you do, don't answer by saying, 'It was nothing' or 'Oh, it's really a mess.' Just say 'Thank you.' Accept compliments as further reminders of your many good qualities."

Make time for yourself. Treat yourself like the valuable person you are by setting aside time for yourself, says Dr. Smolak. "Even if it's just half an hour a week, this time should be yours to do with as you please," she says. "Spend it relaxing in the tub, reading your favorite author, daydreaming or, even better, reviewing your accomplishments."

Break the cycle. Don't leave your kids a legacy of bad eating habits and attitudes, Dr. Smolak says. Set a good example. Eat nutritious foods—when you're hungry. Kids do what we do, not necessarily what we say, adds Dr. Smolak.

Keep "smart food" around the house. "Kids tend to eat what's available," Dr. Smolak says. "So if you don't have chocolate cake in the house, but you have carrots, they're more likely to eat carrots."

Show your kids you love them. Remember to show affection, says Dr. Schlundt. Hold your kids. Help them with their homework. Listen to them. "They don't need chocolate cake," he says. "They need you."

9

EATING DISORDERS

Help for the diet- and weight-obsessed

You might call it food phobia: While most women grapple with a bona fide need to cut calories and lose excess weight to improve their health, women with anorexia, bulimia or binge-eating disorder go to the extreme, obsessing over diet and weight until they put themselves in serious danger.

Consider the story of Sheri G., one of the women who shared her experiences with us in the *Food and You* survey. Sheri never thought she was thin, even after she'd lost so much weight that she was too frail to stand up. She still worried about getting fat, even after she'd become so emaciated that she was blacking out regularly. She was afraid to gain a pound, even after her weight dropped to 45 pounds.

For nearly six years, doctors and therapists told Sheri she had an eating disorder. But she wasn't convinced. Only teenagers had eating disorders, she told herself, and she was 41.

NOT LIMITED TO TEENS

Though most women with eating disorders develop symptoms by their twentieth birthday, you're never too old for anorexia, bulimia or binge-eating disorder, says Andrea Bloomgarden,

Ph.D., director of out-patient services at the Renfrew Center, a women's mental health facility and research center specializing in eating disorders, based in Philadelphia.

"I don't think there are any good studies telling us how common eating disorders are among women over 30," says David Herzog, M.D., associate professor of psychiatry at Harvard Medical School and director of the Harvard Eating Disorder Center. "But they're not uncommon. At least a third of the people we see at our clinic are 30 and older."

Those with anorexia suffer from self-induced starvation. Theirs is a *non*eating disorder, really. It's not uncommon for anorexic women to prepare gourmet feasts for others but not eat a bite themselves.

Women with bulimia binge uncontrollably, then purge, either by vomiting, swallowing fistfuls of laxatives or diuretics or exercising past the point of exhaustion.

Other women experience episodes of uncontrolled eating, or bingeing, without purging, which are known as binge-eating disorder.

These destructive behaviors constitute some of the most perplexing syndromes in women's health. Women with eating disorders find themselves lost in a looking-glass world of distorted body image, food obsession and self-starvation. Yet oddly enough, say experts, they deny to themselves that they have an eating disorder. Many women may realize they have a problem, but they avoid acknowledging the fact that their eating (or noneating) behavior leaves them dangerously unhealthy.

Many of the 30- and 40-something women Dr. Herzog and his colleagues treat developed eating disorders in their teens, long before bulimia and anorexia were household words. Others first developed the problem in their thirties or forties, often after a major life change—pregnancy, divorce, a grown child leaving home or the death of a parent, for instance.

Still others, says Dr. Herzog, relapse in their thirties and forties—often following those same life changes and crises—after overcoming eating disorders that first appeared in adolescence.

JUST THIN, OR ANOREXIC?

Eating disorders are most successfully treated before they become ingrained, say experts. So it's best to recognize disordered eating early on. A variety of symptoms may point to anorexia, bulimia or binge-eating disorder.

"Take a hard look," says Andrea Bloomgarden, Ph.D., director of outpatient services at the Renfrew Center, a women's mental health facility and research center specializing in eating disorders, based in Philadelphia. "Most women with eating disorders are secretive, to avoid detection."

The following profiles can help determine if your eating behavior may be putting you at risk.

Anorexia. Not to be confused with women who are naturally slender, women with anorexia experience dramatic, often rapid weight loss. "Women with anorexia become emaciated—they look like skin and bones to the rest of the world, but feel fat," says Dr. Bloomgarden. They diet yet deny they're hungry. They tend to be finicky eaters, eating certain foods only at certain times or serving themselves tiny portions, often spending a lot of time cutting up and rearranging the food on their plates. Some alternate between periods of self-starvation and bouts of bingeing and purging.

Binge-eating disorder (BED). Women with this disorder typically binge a couple of times a week or more, eating a lot of food at once (most of a cake, for instance, not just a couple of pieces).

"They may eat normally in front of others," says Marjorie Crago, Ph.D., a research specialist in eating disorders at the University of Arizona College of Medicine in Tucson. "But after meals, they eat the leftovers and clean other people's plates. They can't stop."

Bulimia. Women with bulimia purge by vomiting, taking laxatives or diuretics and sometimes giving themselves enemas. Some vomit even after a normal meal, heading for the bathroom after the last bite. Occasionally the vomiting becomes involuntary, and they can't keep themselves from

purging after eating. They may exercise compulsively to
burn off what they've eaten.

They'll binge by themselves, often hoarding food in out-
of-the-way places like closets or even cars.

Many women with bulimia are often of normal weight.
But their weight can fluctuate noticeably, says Dr. Crago.

If friends have encouraged you to get help for your eating behavior and you've ignored them, consider that their
concern may be well-founded.

GREAT EXPECTATIONS

Men develop eating disorders, too. But nearly 90 percent of
those with anorexia and bulimia—both potentially life-
threatening—are women. The numbers aren't that surprising,
Dr. Bloomgarden says. Women are still bombarded with far
more messages that it's imperative to be thin than men are.
(In recent years, however, an increasing emphasis on a thin,
fit male physique has coincided with an upswing in the incidence of eating disorders among men.)

For the last 25 years, American popular culture has em-
braced an extremely thin ideal for women, notes Vivian Meehan, R.N., D.Sc., president and founder of the National
Association of Anorexia Nervosa and Associated Disorders
and director of the Center for Eating Disorders at Highland
Park Hospital in Illinois. According to one study, women's
magazines include ten times as many ads and articles promoting weight loss as men's magazines do.

Another factor in the feminization of disordered eating is
the difference in what little girls and boys learn as they're
socialized, says Dr. Meehan. "Men aren't taught that the way
their bodies look is important to the same degree that women
are," she says.

Among adult women, the culture's fascination with youth
(and the age bias that goes with it) may also figure into eating
disorders, says Pat Donahoe, Ed.D., director of counseling and
psychological services at Montana State University in Boze-
man. Like it or not, thinness is equated with youth, and women
who try to lose weight by purging or starving or going on the

restrictive diets that can precipitate binges may do so out of fear of aging, Dr. Donahoe says.

NOT JUST ABOUT WEIGHT

To suggest that eating disorders are caused solely by a desire to be thin would be misleading, says Dr. Bloomgarden.

A woman may diet because she wants to be thinner. But she doesn't endanger her health by bingeing and purging or starving herself unless there's some other underlying problem, Dr. Bloomgarden says. Some possible causes, she says, include poor self-image, inadequate stress-management skills, a sense that everything is out of control, a fear of conflict with family or underlying depression.

An eating disorder can begin innocently enough, she says. A woman loses a few pounds through dieting and gets the usual kudos from friends and family. Then she gets hooked: Longing for more reinforcement, she may continue to diet—to the point of starvation. Or she may start to binge and purge. The regimen of strict dieting or a pattern of bingeing and purging may afford some sense of control, an anchor that keeps her from feeling adrift amid chaos. So she sticks with it. Or she may cling to the regimen because it keeps her mind off other problems that seem unsolvable. She may feel overwhelmed by the thought of confronting problems such as a bad marriage or difficulties encountered at work, says Dr. Bloomgarden.

Some women feel helpless, stuck in a situation they cannot change. And some, explains Dr. Bloomgarden, would rather sacrifice themselves than confront the people or situations that make them unhappy. These women feel they do not have the power to influence unsatisfactory situations. Food offers a form of comfort or a false sense of control.

With binge eating, women may overeat habitually to comfort themselves, says Dr. Meehan, or to bury "unacceptable" feelings like anger, explains Marjorie Crago, Ph.D., a research specialist in eating disorders at the University of Arizona College of Medicine in Tucson.

In some cases, the weight gain that accompanies chronic

bingeing serves a purpose. The extra weight makes a woman feel less vulnerable to sexual advances or may provide a general feeling of security, says Dr. Bloomgarden.

The anorexic's androgynous look can offer a similar sense of protection, explains Sandra Campbell, Psy.D., director of the Eating Disorders Program at the Brattleboro Retreat in Vermont.

Major life changes and crises often trigger eating disorders because they exacerbate feelings of helplessness, insecurity, anger, fear and incompetence, says Dr. Bloomgarden. Unfortunately, many women don't recognize this. They don't *consciously* try to bury their angry feelings with food or boost their self-esteem by losing weight or gain a sense of control by adhering to a regimented diet. They simply feel comforted while overeating or feel a sense of reward when they're losing weight or sticking to their diet plan. So they keep it up, even when they find themselves on the brink of starvation or bingeing and purging so often that there's little time for anything else. Since they don't consciously shift their attention to weight and eating, they can't understand their preoccupation with either—or break free of it.

"A good number don't have a clear sense of why this is going on," says Jennifer Kennedy, M.D., director of the Eating Disorders Program at the Menninger Clinic in Topeka, Kansas. "Their struggle is quite painful."

A SERIOUS OBSESSION

If untreated, eating disorders can cause serious complications, says C. Wayne Callaway, M.D., an obesity specialist in Washington, D.C.

Anorexia and bulimia can lead to osteoporosis, heart damage and even death. A diet deficient in calcium will cause bone loss. And both self-starvation and purging can play havoc with the levels of electrolytes (sodium and potassium) in a woman's body. Since these minerals regulate vital functions like heartbeat, these changes can lead to heart rhythm abnormalities. Rhythm abnormalities are one of the most common causes of death among people with eating disorders, says Dr. Callaway.

Binge-eating disorder often goes hand in hand with obesity,

A SELF-TEST FOR EATING DISORDERS

This quiz, developed by researchers at The Toronto Hospital, can help you identify signs of disordered eating. For each statement, select the answer that most accurately describes you.

1. I am terrified about being overweight.
   ☐ Always ☐ Usually ☐ Often ☐ Sometimes ☐ Rarely ☐ Never

2. I avoid eating when I am hungry.
   ☐ Always ☐ Usually ☐ Often ☐ Sometimes ☐ Rarely ☐ Never

3. I find myself preoccupied with food.
   ☐ Always ☐ Usually ☐ Often ☐ Sometimes ☐ Rarely ☐ Never

4. I have gone on eating binges where I feel that I may not be able to stop.
   ☐ Always ☐ Usually ☐ Often ☐ Sometimes ☐ Rarely ☐ Never

5. I cut my food into small pieces.
   ☐ Always ☐ Usually ☐ Often ☐ Sometimes ☐ Rarely ☐ Never

6. I am aware of the calorie content of foods that I eat.
   ☐ Always ☐ Usually ☐ Often ☐ Sometimes ☐ Rarely ☐ Never

7. I particularly avoid foods with a high carbohydrate content (such as bread, rice and potatoes).
   ☐ Always ☐ Usually ☐ Often ☐ Sometimes ☐ Rarely ☐ Never

8. I feel that others would prefer if I ate more.
   ☐ Always ☐ Usually ☐ Often ☐ Sometimes ☐ Rarely ☐ Never

9. I vomit after I have eaten.
   ☐ Always ☐ Usually ☐ Often ☐ Sometimes ☐ Rarely ☐ Never

10. I feel extremely guilty after eating.
    ☐ Always ☐ Usually ☐ Often ☐ Sometimes ☐ Rarely ☐ Never

11. I am preoccupied with a desire to be thinner.
    ☐ Always ☐ Usually ☐ Often ☐ Sometimes ☐ Rarely ☐ Never

12. I think about burning up calories when I exercise.
    ☐ Always ☐ Usually ☐ Often ☐ Sometimes ☐ Rarely ☐ Never

13. I am told that other people think that I am too thin.
    ☐ Always ☐ Usually ☐ Often ☐ Sometimes ☐ Rarely ☐ Never

14. I am preoccupied with the thought of having fat on my body.
    ☐ Always ☐ Usually ☐ Often ☐ Sometimes ☐ Rarely ☐ Never

15. I take longer than others to eat my meals.
    ☐ Always ☐ Usually ☐ Often ☐ Sometimes ☐ Rarely ☐ Never

16. I avoid foods with sugar in them.
    ☐ Always ☐ Usually ☐ Often ☐ Sometimes ☐ Rarely ☐ Never

17. I eat diet foods.
    ☐ Always ☐ Usually ☐ Often ☐ Sometimes ☐ Rarely ☐ Never

18. I feel that food controls my life.
    ☐ Always ☐ Usually ☐ Often ☐ Sometimes ☐ Rarely ☐ Never

19. I display self-control around food.
    ☐ Always ☐ Usually ☐ Often ☐ Sometimes ☐ Rarely ☐ Never

20. I feel that others pressure me to eat.
    ☐ Always ☐ Usually ☐ Often ☐ Sometimes ☐ Rarely ☐ Never

21. I give too much time and thought to food.
    ☐ Always ☐ Usually ☐ Often ☐ Sometimes ☐ Rarely ☐ Never

22. I feel uncomfortable after eating sweets.
    ☐ Always ☐ Usually ☐ Often ☐ Sometimes ☐ Rarely ☐ Never

23. I engage in dieting behavior.
    ☐ Always ☐ Usually ☐ Often ☐ Sometimes ☐ Rarely ☐ Never

24. I like my stomach to be empty.
    ☐ Always ☐ Usually ☐ Often ☐ Sometimes ☐ Rarely ☐ Never

25. I enjoy trying new rich foods.
    ☐ Always ☐ Usually ☐ Often ☐ Sometimes ☐ Rarely ☐ Never

26. I have the impulse to vomit after meals.
    ☐ Always ☐ Usually ☐ Often ☐ Sometimes ☐ Rarely ☐ Never

To determine your score: For question 25, give yourself a 0 for answering "always," "usually" or "often," 1 point for "sometimes," 2 points for "rarely" and 3 points for "never." For all other questions, give yourself 3 points for "always," 2 points for "usually," 1 point for "often" and 0 for "sometimes," "rarely" or "never." To interpret your score: A total of 20 or more is cause for concern and a reason to discuss your attitudes toward food with your physician or a counselor.

which is life-threatening in itself: As many as 30 percent of obese women in weight-loss programs report bingeing. Obesity boosts a woman's risk of heart disease, diabetes, high blood pressure and some types of cancer.

A woman with anorexia, bulimia or binge-eating disorder often doesn't recognize that she has an eating disorder. If she does, she doesn't know how to escape it, because she doesn't know why she developed it in the first place. Severe weight loss or purging only complicates the problem because it affects the brain's ability to think rationally. The only cure is to seek professional help, says Dr. Bloomgarden.

Most experts recommend a combined strategy of individual, group and family psychotherapy and nutritional counseling. Sometimes hospitalization is necessary to stabilize a woman's weight and eating habits. The sooner treatment begins, the better the odds of recovery.

The odds of a full recovery were against Sheri, the woman mentioned earlier. She'd starved herself for six years. But she succeeded nevertheless. After checking into a treatment center, she gained 30 pounds in the first two months. And, for the first time in years, she was able to think rationally. Most important, she learned that her real problem was a feeling of low self-worth that had dogged her since childhood.

"I no longer need to strive to be this perfect individual," says Sheri. "I can cope with the ups and downs."

PREVENTION PRIMER

Understanding the symptoms of anorexia, bulimia and binge-eating disorder and what leads to the disorders is half the battle, says Dr. Bloomgarden. The other half is seeking help and ultimately addressing the underlying problems driving the disorder. Experts offer these tips for preventing eating disorders (or dealing with worrisome signs of an existing problem).

Shun low-calorie diets. About 80 percent of women with bulimia say they first binged and purged while on a restricted diet, according to researchers. If you need to lose weight for health reasons, says Dr. Donahoe, consult a nutritionist, who can design the right, healthy plan for you.

Set realistic goals. Ask your doctor or check height and weight tables to find out what weight is healthy for you, Dr. Crago says. Never shoot for a weight lower than that. (To find your ideal weight, see chapter 44.)

When you reach your goal, stop. "If you get to your goal weight after dieting and then decide to set your goal ten pounds lower, that's a warning sign," Dr. Bloomgarden says.

Watch for the red flags. "If you start wanting to use laxatives or to throw up to lose weight, or you feel horribly guilty when you eat, those are warning signs, too," says Dr. Bloomgarden.

Talk, talk, talk. If something is bothering you, confide in a friend, a support group for women with eating disorders, your clergy or a psychotherapist, says Dr. Donahoe. But don't just talk about your diet, your body and what you eat.

"Talk about underlying issues—your self-esteem, need for (or lack of) control or perfectionism," says Dr. Donahoe. "That's what really needs to be addressed."

Forget Superwoman. No one is the perfect wife, mom, career woman and size 8. Don't expect yourself to be perfect, says Dr. Donahoe. It helps if you know other women who feel the same pressure to achieve the impossible; you can support each other.

"No one can be all things to all people," says Dr. Donahoe. "It's a setup for feeling out of control."

Rethink your body image. When you look in the mirror, focus on parts of your body that you like, not just ones you'd rather trade in, says Dr. Donahoe. The rest of the world looks at the whole package. You're probably a lot more critical of yourself than others are. The best alternative is not to measure your worth by what you see in the mirror. Some studies, notes Dr. Donahoe, have shown that some women overestimate their body size by up to 25 percent.

Burnish your self-esteem. "Find things other than your appearance that make you feel like a valuable, competent person," Dr. Crago says. Give yourself credit for your wit, your panache, your musical talent, your skill at a sport you enjoy, caring feelings toward others, accomplishments at work and so on.

Consider therapy. If you, a friend or a family member has an eating disorder, get professional help. "The problem with all of these disorders is that it is difficult to get over them on your own,'' Dr. Crago says.

All sorts of agencies can help you get help. Call a local hospital or medical school and ask if they run eating disorder clinics. Check with a local university's psychology department. Dial your HMO or doctor and ask for a referral to a specialist nearby. Or get in touch with the local mental health clinic, Overeaters Anonymous or an organization like the American Anorexia/Bulimia Association for referrals to therapists in your area.

Treatment may not be as expensive as you might think. Many insurance plans provide at least some reimbursement for treating eating disorders. Some therapists charge on a sliding scale and offer free services when necessary. There's a good chance your therapist will be able to work out a plan that best fits your needs and budget.

PART 2

FOOD AND YOUR HEALTH

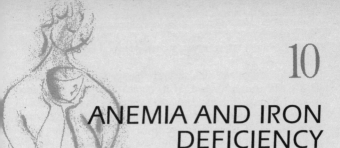

10

ANEMIA AND IRON DEFICIENCY

Pump iron into your diet

The news was unexpected. Blood tests of 300 women working at the University of Texas Medical Branch Hospital in Galveston revealed that one in four—including the doctor who did the study—had iron-poor blood.

"I had no idea I was iron-deficient," says Suzanne McClure, M.D., Ph.D., associate professor of medicine in the Division of Hematology/Oncology at the university. "The signs creep up on you—low tolerance to cold, a tired feeling. Once my iron levels got back to normal, I had significantly more endurance for my daily three-mile run."

While iron-rich foods like lean red meat, kidney beans and dried apricots replenish this energizing mineral, women who are pregnant or have had a baby in the preceding year and those who exercise, diet frequently or eat "on the run" may be missing out.

RUN-DOWN?

Anemia occurs when your blood lacks sufficient red blood cells and hemoglobin (a protein inside the red cells) to deliver oxygen to your body's cells. Anything that limits the number or size of red blood cells severely hampers oxygen delivery. That's where iron (or lack of it) comes into play. Embedded in every hemoglobin molecule are iron particles that bind with oxygen in the lungs and transport it to the heart, muscles and body tissues. If iron stores are low, your body makes fewer and smaller red blood cells, with less hemoglobin.

Women with heavy menstrual flow lose a lot of hemoglobin along with blood. A woman's iron reserves are also subject to depletion by the demands of a growing fetus during pregnancy and by childbirth. It's no surprise then that women with anemia—the final stage of iron deficiency—outnumber men by ten to one. Doctors and nutritionists suspect an estimated 5 to 65 percent of women in their childbearing years may have low iron stores. Less often, anemia may result from a deficiency of vitamin B_{12} or folic acid, infection or inflammation or diseases such as rheumatoid arthritis, lupus erythematosus (an autoimmune disorder) or kidney disease.

HARD TO DETECT, EASY TO CURE

"The three key symptoms of iron-deficiency anemia are lethargy, a feeling of always being cold and difficulty in mental processes," says Henry C. Lukaski, Ph.D., supervisory research physiologist at the U.S. Department of Agriculture (USDA) Human Nutrition Research Center in Grand Forks, North Dakota.

Women with symptoms suggesting anemia or iron deficiency should see a doctor to have their iron status checked. If necessary, the physician may prescribe supplements of iron, B_{12} or folic acid, especially for women who are planning to have children: A pregnant woman who becomes anemic may experience complications such as heart trouble or high blood pressure unless preventive measures are taken. Proper nutrition also helps ensure the birth of a healthy infant.

One problem with anemia is that it doesn't show up on commonly used tests until you're in pretty bad shape, energy-wise.

"If you feel tired a lot, ask your doctor for a serum ferritin test—the only test that looks at how much iron is stored in your body," says nutritionist Elizabeth Somer, R.D., author of

Nutrition for Women. "If the results are low, ask about a supplement."

If you're anemic (or suspect you are), don't reach for supplements without medical clearance. You need to find out the cause of your anemia, advises Janet R. Hunt, R.D., Ph.D., research nutritionist with the USDA research center in Grand Forks. By taking iron supplements, you could mask the true reason for your iron deficiency, thereby prolonging the problem. You may not be anemic at all and build up your iron stores to an extreme.

SECRETS OF AN IRON-RICH DIET

"Women explain away their tiredness with 'Oh, I'm juggling a job and a family' or 'Oh, I'm getting older,' when in fact it could be an iron deficiency," says Somer. "Then they reach for coffee to give them energy when they should be reaching for an iron-rich food."

The Daily Value for iron is 18 milligrams. Some experts believe, however, that women of childbearing age and those with heavy menstrual periods may need slightly more. Postmenopausal women need 10 milligrams a day. Even pregnant women, who usually take doctor-prescribed supplements that provide 60 milligrams of iron, benefit from the additional nutrients in an iron-rich diet, says Somer.

Some nutritionists, like Somer, think it's hard for women who consume less than 2,000 calories a day to get sufficient iron from their diets. You have to eat enough of a wide variety of foods to get the amount of iron you need. However, Somer also has good news: You can maximize the absorption of iron from the foods you eat by choosing them carefully and combining them skillfully.

RED MEAT: THE IRON STATUS SYMBOL

The problem with iron is that your body doesn't absorb all it takes in. Meat and seafood are the top—in fact, the only—sources of heme iron, the kind that's best absorbed by the body. About half the iron in meat is heme iron, of which your body normally absorbs 20 to 34 percent.

PERFECT MATES

Nutritionist Elizabeth Somer, R.D., author of *Nutrition for Women*, suggests two ways to boost iron absorption: Combine meat and plant sources of this vital mineral and eat foods rich in iron and vitamin C at the same meal. Here are some ideas.

MEAT-AND-BEAN COMBOS

- Split-pea soup with a little ham
- Black-bean burritos with ground chicken
- Lentil soup garnished with lean ground turkey
- Broiled chicken leg accompanied by three-bean salad
- Baked beans with low-fat ham
- Tofu stir-fried with chicken

VITAMIN C ENHANCEMENT

- Tofu and broccoli
- Bell peppers stuffed with rice and red beans

THE BEST OF BOTH

- Shish kebabs with very lean beef and green peppers
- Fajitas with chicken and red peppers

"Because they're cutting fat and calories, women tend to stay away from the best source of iron—meat," says Somer. "But there are ways to get iron without adding much fat. It only takes three ounces of extra-lean red meat to improve your iron status. It doesn't (and shouldn't) have to be a huge steak." Here are some other ways to build up your iron stores.

Buy lean meats. Or get cheaper cuts and trim the fat, says Fergus Clydesdale, Ph.D., professor of food science and head of the Department of Food Science at the University of Massachusetts in Amherst. Both strategies offer a healthy, reduced-fat option while allowing the consumption of a good iron source.

Consider fish and fowl. Other important sources of heme iron include a half-cup of raw oysters (five milligrams total

iron), three ounces of skinless chicken (one milligram total),
and three ounces of skinless roast turkey (one milligram total).

You can also get more heme iron into your diet by adding
water-packed tuna to a green salad or some shredded chicken
to soup, or by grilling shish kebabs of very lean beef and
peppers.

Stock your pantry with pintos and kidneys. Rich in folic
acid, pinto and kidney beans are also two of Nature's top plant
sources of iron—and they're a great substitute for meat. A
half-cup of pinto beans has three milligrams of iron, and the
same amount of canned refried beans has a respectable 2.3
milligrams of iron. So pop open a can of your favorite beans,
rinse them and toss them into a green salad. Mash some for a
quick dip. Roll 'em in a flour tortilla for a quick breakfast
burrito.

MAXIMUM IRON WITHOUT MAXIMUM CALORIES

Beans and other plant foods contain nonheme iron, a form that
is absorbed by the body at the rate of 3 to 5 percent. This is
low compared to 20 percent for heme iron, but luckily, researchers have discovered a way to boost absorption of nonheme iron.

Make chili con carne. Any time you add heme iron to a
nonheme food, you help make it possible for your body to
absorb more of the nonheme iron. "Many studies have shown
that adding a small amount of heme iron to any food containing nonheme iron, such as iron-fortified breads and vegetables,
increases the absorption," says Dr. Lukaski. "We think the
fatty acids in the meat may be responsible."

Think orange-ish juice. According to Dr. Clydesdale, vitamin C also helps the body absorb more nonheme iron. It's
another good reason to try those shish kebabs—just enough
meat teamed up with a vegetable packed with vitamin C.

"At a single, real meal of typical food, adding a vitamin C
source increased absorption about 1.7 times," says Dr. Hunt.

Reports on the rate of iron absorption vary because iron
absorption varies with a woman's individual needs. "In general, the more you need," says Dr. Clydesdale, "the more your
body takes in."

Don't overlook cereal. Another fantastic but easily overlooked iron source is ready-to-eat cereal, notes Dr. Clydesdale. These cereals are usually iron-fortified and contain vitamin C. That's just the combination that's needed to increase iron absorption, he explains.

Cook acidic soups and sauces—such as tomato sauce—in a cast-iron pot. This simple act of nutritional alchemy adds additional nonheme iron direct from the pot, says Somer. And the longer the soup or sauce simmers, the more iron it absorbs.

STOP THE IRON ZAPPERS

It would be a shame to pay extra attention to maximizing your iron intake and absorption while inadvertently ignoring factors that could block absorption. Heed these hints.

Go easy on the tannins. Coffee and tea contain substances called tannins that interfere with iron absorption, says Dr. Clydesdale. One cup of java probably won't hinder iron absorption from foods by much. Just don't wash down your iron-supplying food with black tea or coffee.

Don't take an iron supplement with milk or other calcium-rich foods. The two minerals may interact to block iron absorption. Instead, Dr. Clydesdale recommends taking calcium and iron supplements about three hours apart.

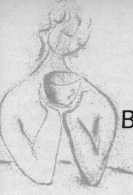

11

BREAST CANCER

Foods that rein in the risk

Pamela. D. breakfasts on nonfat yogurt, opens a can of low-fat soup for lunch and serves up broiled chicken—sans skin—with vegetables at suppertime.

It's a healthy meal plan. But for Pamela, 38, a registered nurse and mother of two, it's also a breast cancer prevention plan.

"I'm considered high-risk," says Pamela. "My mother lost a sister to breast cancer. My father lost two sisters to it, and a third sister survived it. When a mammogram showed some changes in my breast, it was time to do something," she says.

At the High Risk Clinic of the Hollings Cancer Center at the Medical University of South Carolina in Charleston, Pamela learned that her new high-fiber, low-fat diet would help her shed pounds while reducing estrogen levels in her body—a factor tied to breast cancer.

"This is my diet from here on in," she says. "I have to help myself. It can't wait."

CLUES TO AN ANTI-CANCER DIET

Pamela's not alone. Whether due to rising incidence or earlier detection (or both), the odds that the average 45-year-old woman will face breast cancer are about 1 in 96, according to statistics from the National Cancer Institute in Bethesda, Maryland. Luckily, the survival rates look promising. Still, given the choice between surviving breast cancer and preventing it in the first place, women are paying a lot of attention to dietary prevention.

While researchers have not identified all the ingredients of a strategy against breast cancer, many agree on basic dietary building blocks that seem to offer protection along with overall health benefits. This much is known:

- Evidence strongly suggests that cutting alcohol consumption, getting sufficient vitamin A and eating whole grains, fruits and vegetables (particularly broccoli, brussels sprouts and cabbage) help guard against breast cancer.
- Breast cancer rates are lower in Japan, China and low-income regions of the world, where fat intake is also low. Although scientifically controlled studies have yet to confirm that link, most nutrition experts advise women to reduce total fat—particularly animal fat—to less than 30 percent of total daily calories.

"We know that cutting fat, adding fiber and eating fruits and vegetables do something to the body's estrogens that is protective," says Daniel W. Nixon, M.D., associate director for cancer prevention at the Hollings Cancer Center and author of *The Cancer Recovery Eating Plan*. "We're just not sure how it works yet."

A CLOSE LOOK AT THE FAT/ESTROGEN LINK

Estrogen. It sounds crazy, but the same reproductive hormone that regulates our menstrual cycles and fertility—our very ability to have children—also prompts normal breast cells to multiply, mutate and become cancerous under certain circumstances. The longer estrogen circulates in your body, the higher your breast cancer risk, say experts. Studies show that women who menstruate early in life, bear children late or not at all and experience late menopause are at greater risk for breast cancer, due to the estrogen factor.

"Each time estrogen comes into a breast cell, it causes the cell to divide more," explains Brian E. Henderson, M.D., professor of preventive medicine at the University of Southern California School of Medicine in Los Angeles. "Cell division is not a perfect process, particularly for breast cells. They can make a lot of mistakes. Those mistakes can lead to cancer."

But researchers disagree about whether a link exists between dietary fat, estrogen and breast cancer. In the Harvard University Nurses' Health Study (an ongoing study of 115,000 women considered a landmark source of evidence regarding women's health), a comparison of fat intake and breast cancer rates in 89,494 women found no connection, says lead researcher Walter C. Willett, M.D., Dr.P.H., professor of epidemiology and nutrition at Harvard's School of Public Health. In fact, the women who ate the least fat—less than 29 percent of total calories—had slightly higher breast cancer rates than those whose diets contained 49 percent fat.

Other cancer experts, however, do see a link. They point to the results of population studies and of dietary fat/estrogen research for proof.

"If you look at population studies from Japan, breast cancer rates were very low when most people ate 15 percent of their calories from fat," notes David P. Rose, M.D., Ph.D., D.Sc., chief of the Division of Nutrition and Endocrinology at the Naylor Dana Institute of the American Health Foundation in Valhalla, New York. "Now that the Japanese are eating more fat, the breast cancer rates are rising. We think there's a connection, and a good reason for American women to cut their fat intake to 20 or 25 percent of total calories."

And at Tufts University in Boston, researchers monitored estrogen levels of women whose diets contained either 21 or 40 percent of calories from fat. Premenopausal women in the low-fat group had estrogen levels 30 to 75 percent lower than those in the high-fat group. Among postmenopausal women who ate low-fat foods, estrogen levels were 300 percent lower.

A STRONG CASE FOR PHASING OUT FAT

What's a woman to do? Carve the fat out of your diet anyway, say those in the know. The American Cancer Society recommends reducing fat intake from the current average of about 40 percent to 30 percent or less of total calories. Closer to 20 percent may be even better, some researchers say.

"Lowering fat and raising fiber is healthy for other reasons, like preventing cardiovascular disease. Research doesn't show that it necessarily helps with breast cancer, but it can't hurt," says Dr. Henderson.

Part V of this book devotes chapters to ways to switch to a low-fat lifestyle. Here nutritionist Elizabeth Somer, R.D., author of *Nutrition for Women*, offers a few simple strategies you can start to use right now.

- Simmer foods in defatted chicken stock instead of butter.
- Air-pop your popcorn.
- Choose nonfat dairy products instead of whole milk, half-and-half or cream.
- Use nonfat mayonnaise in coleslaw, chicken salad, tuna salad and salad dressings.
- Eat small (two- to three-ounce) portions of meat, preferably mixed with whole-grain rice, noodles or vegetables.

A CRISPER FULL OF CRUCIFERS

Crunching on cabbage, broccoli, brussels sprouts and cauliflower may have special benefits—all contain compounds believed to help the body break down estrogen. "There are over 1,000 possibly preventive chemical compounds in fruits and vegetables," notes Dr. Nixon.

Researchers at Johns Hopkins University in Baltimore have also shown that sulforaphane, a chemical in broccoli, protects animals against the development of breast cancer. Sulforaphane boosted production of anti-cancer enzymes. "The body uses these to detoxify foreign substances, including cancer-causing agents," says molecular pharmacologist Paul Talalay, M.D., director of the Brassica Chemo Prevention Laboratory at Johns Hopkins.

BUT WAIT—THERE'S MORE

Packed with fiber and antioxidant vitamins A, C and E, other fruits and vegetables should star in any cancer-conscious woman's diet, says Jean H. Hankin, R.D., Dr.P.H., nutrition researcher and professor of public health with the Epidemiology Program of the Cancer Research Center of Hawaii at the University of Hawaii in Honolulu.

In a University of Toronto study that followed 56,837 Canadian women, those who consumed the most fiber had a 30 percent reduction in breast cancer risk. Those who ate the most fruits and veggies rich in vitamins A and C had similarly lower risk. Whole-grain cereals also seemed to have a protective effect.

In the Nurses' Health Study, women who ate more veggies—especially vitamin A*f* rich varieties like butternut squash—seemed to have reduced risk. Other rich sources of vitamin A include sweet potatoes, carrots, spinach, fresh tuna and cantaloupe. "Whole foods seemed to have more of an impact than taking a vitamin supplement," says Dr. Willett.

"It wouldn't hurt to have six or seven servings of vegetables and fruits a day," says Dr. Hankin.

OTHER BUILDING BLOCKS OF PROTECTION

Experts also suggest the following food strategies to reduce breast cancer risk.

Say soybeans. You can add soybeans to chili, stir-fry protein-packed tofu in place of meat in a variety of dishes, or even drink soy milk, which can be found in some grocery stores or at health food stores. "Soybeans contain phytoestrogens, which can help block the effects of the estrogen circulating in your body," says Dr. Hankin.

Cairo University researchers saw a 50 percent reduction in breast tumors among lab animals whose diets contained soybeans. Though they weren't sure why it worked, they speculated that insoluble fibers in the soybeans might absorb carcinogens.

Reach for the olive oil. Need a little dressing on the salad greens, a little something to sauté the onions in? Skip the creamy ranch and butter. Think Mediterranean.

"Monounsaturated fats seem to have some protective effect," says Dr. Willett. "In a study we conducted in Spain, women who consumed more olive oil did have lower rates of breast cancer. It's intriguing. We don't know why. But there are many antioxidants in the oil."

Olive oil's potentially protective role was underscored in a study of 2,368 Greek women. Those who consumed olive oil more than once a day had a 25 percent lower risk of breast cancer, according to researchers from the Harvard School of Public Health and the Athens School of Public Health.

Serve up some fish. Put Atlantic herring, canned pink salmon or broiled bluefin tuna—all high in omega-3 fatty acids—on the dinner table. Laboratory evidence suggests that omega-3's inhibit the growth of breast cancer tissue.

Season with garlic? Researchers aren't yet sure what the implications are for the human diet, but they've found cancer-battling compounds hidden within pungent cloves of garlic. John Milner, Ph.D., head of the nutrition department at Pennsylvania State University in University Park, has shown that a sulfur compound in processed garlic inhibits the binding of carcinogens to breast cells, while other compounds inhibit and even kill tumor cells.

"It appears that garlic and related foods play an important dietary role in the cancer process," Dr. Milner says.

Drink less—or not at all. If you're already a teetotaler, no problem. If not, consider restricting beer, wine and mixed drinks to special occasions only, says Dr. Nixon. Many studies suggest that even very moderate alcohol consumption—such as a few glasses of wine a week—may increase breast cancer risk in women. Two drinks a day could increase the risk by up to 70 percent. The type of alcohol does not seem to matter.

"Alcohol increases circulating estrogen levels," says Dr. Willett. "The evidence is pretty clear that cutting down on alcohol probably will reduce a woman's risk somewhat."

Be a calorie miser. There's mounting laboratory evidence that a high-calorie diet may actually stimulate breast cancer cells. Restricting food intake to what you need to maintain a normal weight—or exercising to burn extra calories—could stall the development and growth of breast cancer, says researcher Clifford Welsch, Ph.D., professor of pharmacology and toxicology at Michigan State University in East Lansing.

"It's so consistent and so profound in animal studies that we speculate this would also act in the same manner in humans," Dr. Welsch says. "I truly believe that cutting calories by reducing the amount of food we eat by 20 to 30 percent, combined with cutting fat intake, will reduce the risk."

12

BREAST PAIN

Tactics for periodic tenderness

It's *that* time of the month again.

Your breasts ache—a not-so-gentle reminder that your menstrual period is on its way. Even your flimsiest summer nightgown feels like sandpaper. A hug is agony. And sleeping on your stomach? Forget it.

"No one knows exactly what causes breast pain," says Renee M. BeLieu, M.D., assistant professor in the Department of Obstetrics and Gynecology at the University of Missouri-Kansas City School of Medicine and an obstetrician and gynecologist at the Truman Medical Center in Kansas City. "Hormones may play a role, because most breast pain is cyclical, and hormones can cause other cyclic changes in a woman's body."

Your breasts may swell and feel more lumpy each month as the milk-secreting glands they house multiply and fill with fluid. The swelling can cause mild tenderness to severe pain. After menstruation begins, the fluid is usually reabsorbed and the pain disappears.

Monthly breast pain is often most pronounced in your thirties and forties—and it's fairly common. In one study, two out of three women surveyed reported experiencing monthly breast pain. And while cyclic breast pain usually ends with menopause, breast pain may be a side effect of hormone replacement therapy. The replacement of female hormones with medication, taken either cyclically or continuously, after menopause has been found to be associated with increased breast pain in some women.

Women may also experience other kinds of breast pain, due to pregnancy, a milk-duct infection called mastitis that can occur in breastfeeding mothers or an injury to the breast tissue (such as getting hit in the chest with a flying volleyball). Once in a while, cancer may be the cause. While any kind of pain should be checked out, keep in mind that there are many kinds of tumors that can occur in breast tissue, and not all are cancerous.

"One of the biggest fears of women with breast pain is breast cancer," says Kathleen Mayzel, M.D., director of the Faulkner Breast Center and assistant clinical professor of surgery at Tufts University School of Medicine, both in Boston. "Most of the time, what we find is the pain is simply normal fluid retention." Nevertheless, if you have breast pain, you should talk to your doctor about it, says Dr. Mayzel.

SOOTHING SOLUTIONS

What helps? Soaking in a hot tub up to your chin may ease discomfort, says Rosalind Benedet, R.N., a breast health nurse specialist at the Breast Health Center of the California Pacific Medical Center in San Francisco. When breasts are tender, she says, wear a bra that's one cup size larger than usual—a C instead of a B cup, for example. Or, suggests Dr. BeLieu, you can be professionally fitted for a support bra in the correct cup and body size—one that's neither too loose nor too tight, fits properly and doesn't dig into your shoulders or ride up in back.

If a good soak and a less restrictive bra don't ease your breast discomfort, experts suggest trying one or more of these dietary pain-soothers.

Go low-fat. Restrict your fat intake to no more than 20 percent of total calories, suggests David Rose, M.D., Ph.D., D.Sc., chief of the Division of Nutrition and Endocrinology at the Naylor Dana Institute of the American Health Foundation in Valhalla, New York. In one study, Dr. Rose and his team found that pain eased in women who cut dietary fat.

"Cutting fat may work by reducing levels of hormones, including estrogen or prolactin," he says. "It may be that these hormones influence fluid levels inside the breast. When fluid levels rise, it stretches structures inside the breast."

Be a caffeine watchdog. Many women report that drinking less caffeinated coffee, tea and soda—or eliminating caffeine entirely—brings some relief, says Dr. BeLieu.

In a study conducted at Duke University in Durham, North Carolina, 113 women with painful breasts reduced their caffeine intake to two cups a day or less for six months. Sixty-one percent felt better. "We believe that the chemical trimethylxanthine in caffeine stimulates breast tissue and causes the pain," says researcher Linda Russell, R.N., a certified oncology specialist who works with cancer patients at Duke University Medical Center.

But Dr. Mayzel adds that "some women who come to our clinic say it doesn't work."

Soothe with evening primrose oil. In England, physicians report that among women who've tried evening primrose oil for breast pain, roughly half experience relief. Theoretically, say its proponents, evening primrose oil may relieve breast tenderness by balancing fatty acid levels in the blood. Dr. BeLieu recommends two 500-milligram gel-caps three times a day.

Try E. Vitamin E may also spell relief. While the Recommended Dietary Allowance (the adequate level for healthy adults) for vitamin E is 8 milligrams a day for women, the Daily Value is 20 milligrams or 30 international units (depending on the unit of measure used for the supplement you choose). The safe upper limit is 400 international units (although some experts recommend higher amounts). Check with your doctor about exploring this option—the exact amount may take some trial and error.

Give dietary changes a chance. To distinguish between normal variations in breast pain from month to month and the effects of dietary measures, keep a calendar of your pain cycle for at least three months. Each day, keep a record of pain severity, activity, diet and medications, as well as your menstrual cycle, says Dr. BeLieu. ''Breast pain often comes and goes, and it may be better some months on its own,'' she explains. ''Over a long period of time, you may be able to tell if it is worth the effort or not in reducing your breast pain.''

13

CERVICAL CHANGES

A trio of protective nutrients

There's good news about cervical cancer these days. In the United States, fewer women get it today than 40 years ago. Researchers believe they've found a very common link to this disease: a sexually transmitted infection caused by the human papillomavirus. And apparently the risk is increased in women who have had several children or multiple sexual partners or had their first experience with sexual intercourse before age 18.

Still, cervical cancer is the third leading cause of cancer deaths among American women, behind only lung and breast cancer. So doctors advise women to visit their doctors faithfully (how often depends on your age) to determine if trouble's brewing. What they look for is cervical dysplasia, an abnormal arrangement of cells on the surface of the cervix that can (but doesn't always) lead to cervical cancer.

PROTECTIVE POWER OF FRUITS AND VEGETABLES

In researching the basis of cervical changes, scientists discovered an intriguing dietary link: In several studies, women who consumed more vitamin C, beta-carotene and folate had less cervical dysplasia or cancer.

"It's fairly consistent," says Nancy Potischman, Ph.D., senior staff fellow at the National Cancer Institute's environmental epidemiology branch in Bethesda, Maryland. "It was even true for smokers who ate lots of vitamin C-rich foods. A slightly protective effect existed among the smokers and they had less of a problem, even though smoking puts you at increased risk."

When researchers at the University of Alabama at Birmingham compared the diets of 257 women with cervical dysplasia to those of 133 women without the condition, they found a link between disease and the dining room table: Women who consumed less vitamins A and C and folate had more cervical dysplasia.

Among women who took in the least vitamin C, the risk of cervical dysplasia was 60 percent higher than for women who took in the most, among those who got the least folate, the risk was 40 percent higher, and those who took in the least vitamin A had double the risk.

The researchers speculated that a lack of folate may play a role when cancer cells are forming and that deficiencies of vitamins C and A may promote cancer growth.

When Juliet VanEenwyk, Ph.D., an epidemiologist with the Washington State Department of Health in Olympia, conducted a similar study in Chicago, the results were similar.

"The odds of cervical dysplasia went up as intake of certain nutrients went down," Dr. VanEenwyk says. "The women with the lowest dietary levels of folate and vitamin C were 2.5 and 5 times more likely to have cervical dysplasia, respectively, compared to the women who ate the most."

MENU ITEMS THAT GIVE YOU AN EDGE

How can you diminish the risk of cervical dysplasia and cancer? Experts offer these suggestions.

Heap your plate with beans and greens. Beans—from lentils to pintos—as well as wheat germ and green vegetables like spinach, asparagus and turnip greens are the richest low-fat sources of folate.

Paying attention to folate intake is especially important for women who have taken oral contraceptives, says Dr. Potischman. "Their folate levels begin diminishing."

Reach for C-rich foods. To give yourself the edge afforded by vitamin C, turn to black currants, orange juice, red bell peppers, papaya, strawberries, cantaloupe and broccoli. Getting plenty of vitamin C may be of particular concern for smokers, whose vitamin C levels tend to run low, says Dr. Potischman.

Think "yellow" and "green" side dishes. For vitamin A or beta-carotene, look to carrots, sweet potatoes, pumpkin, spinach, dandelion greens, mangos and cantaloupe. "The evidence is pretty consistent for fruits and vegetables rich in carotenoids," says Dr. Potischman. "They seem to be working as antioxidants here, by enhancing immune reactions."

Strive for a mix of nutrients. "I never think one single nutrient is the key," says Dr. Potischman. Nutrients interact biologically, she notes. A big dose of one—either as a supplement or in food—could throw off an important interaction.

Don't rely on processed foods. "Folate gets lost when food is processed," notes Dr. VanEenwyk. "It's important to rely on fresh foods or freshly frozen fruits and vegetables. There are a lot of nutrients we don't know that much about yet. And like folate, they may be lost in the processing of foods."

14

CHOLESTEROL

Foods that cut the risk

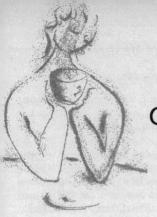

Terry W. was silly about steak, crazy for cheese, indiscreet with ice cream.

For breakfast, Terry told us in our *Food and You* survey, she liked to cozy up to a plate of bacon and eggs with hash browns fried in butter. For lunch, she enjoyed a Burger King Whopper with cheese and extra mayo. For dinner, she relished a thick, well-marbled steak, a baked potato with sour cream, vegetables doused in butter and a bowl of premium ice cream for dessert.

Terry also told us that when a routine blood test showed her cholesterol levels were uncomfortably high, she dropped those eating habits like a philandering boyfriend.

Smart move, say doctors. High blood cholesterol is one of the leading causes of both heart disease and stroke, two of the top three killers of American women. And a diet rich in fatty foods, like cheese and steak and ice cream, is one of the leading causes of high cholesterol, says Debra R. Judelson, M.D., a cardiologist in Beverly Hills and chair of the Cardiovascular Disease in Women Committee of the American Medical Women's Association.

"After I got my results, I made some big changes in my diet," says Terry.

WHAT'S THE FUSS?

Everybody needs a little cholesterol. Your body uses cholesterol, a waxy, fatlike substance transported via the bloodstream, to manufacture cell membranes, certain hormones and
other important body substances.

Too much cholesterol, however, can lead to trouble. In your
bloodstream, excess cholesterol can build up inside artery
walls. In the arteries leading to your heart or brain, cholesterol
buildup can choke off vital blood supplies, causing a heart
attack or a stroke, explains Penny Kris-Etherton, R.D., Ph.D.,
professor of nutrition at Pennsylvania State University in University Park.

GOOD VERSUS BAD CHOLESTEROL

Some of the cholesterol in your bloodstream comes from the
cholesterol-containing foods you eat. Your body manufactures
the rest from the fatty acids in fat, says Donald M. Small,
M.D., chairman of the Department of Biophysics at Boston
University School of Medicine.

Actually, your body produces two types of cholesterol. Before sending cholesterol out into your blood, it encases the
fatty stuff in tiny protein capsules—some thick and heavy,
others thin and light, explains Dr. Small. The light protein
shells contain a lot of cholesterol and are known as low-density
lipoprotein, or LDL. The heavy shells get very little cholesterol
and are known as high-density lipoprotein, or HDL.

Circulating through your bloodstream, it's the cholesterol-
laden LDL that clogs your arteries. The cholesterol-lean HDL,
on the other hand, actually cleans your arteries. In a process
called reverse cholesterol transport, the HDL pulls errant cholesterol from your artery walls and ferries it back to your liver,
where it's broken down into bile and excreted by your intestines, explains Dr. Kris-Etherton.

Your diet, your genetic heritage and whether you smoke,
exercise or are overweight all determine how much of each
type of cholesterol your body produces, adds Dr. Kris-
Etherton.

RUNNING THE NUMBERS

A simple blood test will tell you how much cholesterol (the total of HDL and LDL) and triglycerides, another type of fat, are floating around in your blood. The American Heart Association (AHA) suggests you get an initial cholesterol test at age 20 and have follow-up tests at least once every five years after that. Experts recommend tests that look at your total cholesterol level and your HDL, LDL and triglyceride levels. Your test results will show your cholesterol levels in milligrams of cholesterol per deciliter of blood (mg/dl).

Since HDL helps clean up the LDL mess, a low HDL reading is a tip-off that your body is not repairing the damage caused by LDL deposits and that you need to take action. Data from the ongoing Framingham Heart Study suggest that for every ten mg/dl drop in HDL, women experience a 40 to 50 percent increase in coronary risk.

According to many experts, a desirable total cholesterol level is below 200 mg/dl, a good HDL level is above 35 mg/dl, and a desirable LDL level is less than 130 mg/dl for people without coronary heart disease and under 100 mg/dl for those with heart disease. According to the AHA, triglycerides should fall below 200 mg/dl. Dr. Judelson points out that since the average HDL for women is 50 to 60 mg/dl, a better "desirable" HDL for women is more than 50 mg/dl, and it is prudent for women to aim for this higher target.

A total cholesterol reading over 200 mg/dl or an HDL below 35 mg/dl—or both—warrants remedial changes in your eating and exercise habits, say experts. A total cholesterol reading over 240 mg/dl may warrant changes in both your eating and exercise habits, plus cholesterol-lowering drugs—based on your level of heart disease risk—especially if the high reading is due to very high LDL levels, says Dr. Judelson.

Just make sure your doctor looks at your HDL level in addition to your total cholesterol reading before prescribing a cholesterol-lowering drug, says Bernadine Healy, M.D., a cardiologist at the Cleveland Clinic Foundation in Ohio who, as director of the National Institutes of Health, launched the landmark Women's Health Initiative. Though a total cholesterol reading over 200 may seem troubling at first blush, it may simply reflect a high HDL reading—a desirable marker.

Rather than relying on total cholesterol readings alone, most doctors now calculate the ratio of total cholesterol to HDL. You can calculate your own by dividing your total cholesterol reading by your HDL reading. If the ratio is 3.5-to-1 or lower, you're doing fine.

PAST MENOPAUSE? TAKE HEED

Before menopause, women have average HDL levels higher than men's—55 mg/dl for women versus 45 mg/dl for men—which may be one of the reasons that premenopausal women are less likely to have heart disease.

After menopause, though, women's HDL levels drop closer to a man's level, their LDL levels rise, and their triglyceride levels may rise higher than those of a man the same age. Women aren't immune to heart disease. They just develop problems a decade later than men do, says Dr. Judelson.

Estrogen production seems to afford women added protection against heart disease by simultaneously shoring up HDL levels and keeping a lid on LDL, Dr. Judelson explains. Estrogen also normalizes blood vessel tone, which reduces the likelihood of spasms or irritation to any existing plaque, she adds. When estrogen levels drop off after menopause, women have more problems, unless they are on hormone replacement therapy.

Compounding the problem, other hormonal changes accompanying menopause often cause weight gain, which in turn can also raise LDL and lower HDL, says Margo Denke, M.D., associate professor of internal medicine at the Center for Human Nutrition at the University of Texas Southwestern Medical Center in Dallas and a member of the AHA's Nutrition Committee.

That's why it's particularly important for women to keep tabs on their weight and their cholesterol levels after menopause, says Dr. Denke.

THE RIGHT FOODS

By changing their diet, women like Terry are able to lower their cholesterol levels significantly. Studies show that a healthy diet reduces your cholesterol levels and should slow the progression of heart disease. What's more, eating right may also reverse the buildup of cholesterol associated with coronary artery disease, according to research.

Heart specialists and other authorities advise women who want to lower their cholesterol count to take the following steps.

Watch cholesterol in food. Eating too many foods high in cholesterol will boost your bad LDL levels, says Dr. Kris-Etherton. So limit animal products, particularly egg yolks, liver, kidneys and other organ meats—they're very high in cholesterol.

The AHA suggests you limit daily cholesterol consumption to 300 milligrams. (One egg yolk has 213 milligrams.) If you have heart disease or high blood cholesterol levels that aren't responding to dietary changes, then shoot for no more than 200 milligrams daily, says Dr. Denke.

One study showed that postmenopausal women who reduced their intake of fat and dietary cholesterol to the AHA's recommended levels for three months lowered their blood cholesterol levels by an average of 11 mg/dl.

Eat less fat (and a lot less saturated fat). Both the AHA and the National Cholesterol Education Program of the National Heart, Lung and Blood Institute recommend a diet that limits total fat to less than 30 percent of total calories and saturated fat to less than 10 percent of calories. After menopause, women may do well to lower total fat to less than 25 percent and saturated fat to about 7 percent, says Dr. Judelson.

Why? Fat, particularly the saturated kind found in meat, poultry skin, tropical oils (such as coconut oil), whole milk, butter and other high-fat dairy products raises the levels of bad LDL cholesterol in your blood, explains Mary Felando, R.D., a cardiovascular nutrition specialist in Los Angeles. In fact, say researchers, lowering saturated fat may be even more important to lowering blood cholesterol than cutting dietary cholesterol. Since animal foods are a primary source of both saturated fat and cholesterol, reducing your intake of meat and

DON'T IGNORE TRIGLYCERIDES

If you've had your blood cholesterol tested, the lab report will show your total cholesterol, HDL and LDL levels. It may also tell you the status of your triglycerides, fats that circulate in your bloodstream and, like cholesterol, appear to raise your risk of heart disease.

Like cholesterol, triglycerides are found in dietary fats and oils. So a diet rich in fat can boost your blood levels of both triglycerides and cholesterol, explains Debra R. Judelson, M.D., a cardiologist in private practice in Beverly Hills, California and chair of the Cardiovascular Disease in Women Committee of the American Medical Women's Association. Your body can also manufacture triglycerides from sugars, including the kind found in alcohol. So even if you have a low total cholesterol reading, you may have high triglycerides; you need to have them checked.

High triglyceride levels are bad news because they slow the rate at which your liver clears LDL cholesterol from your blood. That means you have considerably more bad cholesterol traveling in your bloodstream and depositing itself on the inside walls of your arteries, setting the scene for stroke and heart attack. In other words, high triglyceride levels and high LDL cholesterol levels are a dangerous combination.

Ideally, your triglycerides should be 200 mg/dl or lower, says Peter H. Jones, M.D., associate professor of medicine in the Atherosclerosis and Lipid Disorders Section at Baylor College of Medicine in Houston. Readings over 200 mg/dl are cause for concern if your LDL cholesterol levels are also high (over 160 mg/dl). And regardless of your LDL levels, triglyceride readings over 500 mg/dl can be very dangerous, putting you at risk for both heart disease and pancreatitis, a potentially fatal inflammation of the pancreas.

The best way to lower your triglyceride levels—which is also the best way to lower your LDL cholesterol levels—is to cut back on fat.

"The major source of cholesterol and triglycerides in the blood comes from the diet," says Donald M. Small, M.D., chairman of the Department of Biophysics at Boston University School of Medicine.

Here's the rundown on what you can do.

Scrutinize food labels. "Learn what's in the food you eat," says Dr. Small. "If you eat Fritos, you may think you're eating corn, but you're really eating fat. Between 50 and 60 percent of the calories in corn chips and potato chips are from fat. Over 90 percent of the calories in salad dressing are from fat. In fact, the main source of fat in the American woman's diet is now salad dressing. Ice cream is over 50 percent fat. Bacon is more than 75 percent fat. Almost any piece of beef is more than 50 percent fat calories. And most bakery products are loaded with hidden fat. Reading labels can help you find out what you're eating," says Dr. Small.

Give high-fat foods the boot. Once you spot the high-fat troublemakers in your diet, ditch 'em. Remember: Fat is 99 percent pure triglyceride, says Dr. Small, and lots of it will raise your blood triglyceride and cholesterol levels.

"Unless you have a genetic problem, eating a relatively low-fat diet will most likely lower your blood levels of triglycerides and cholesterol," says Dr. Small. The American Heart Association suggests you get no more than 30 percent of your calories from fat.

Cut the sugar, too. Since your body can manufacture triglycerides from sugar, says Dr. Small, a diet high in simple carbohydrates—like table sugar and corn syrup—can raise triglyceride levels (although the effect isn't as pronounced as with dietary fat). Conversely, cutting sugar intake helps lower blood levels of triglycerides. Dr. Small suggests substituting complex carbohydrates, instead—eat a banana instead of a candy bar, for example, or a whole-wheat roll instead of a doughnut.

Cork the bottle. Like sweets, alcohol can boost triglyceride levels. If your blood test shows elevated triglyceride levels, cut out alcohol in all forms, advises Dr. Jones.

Triglycerides won't budge? See your doctor. If you cut back on fat and sugar and don't drink and your triglyceride and cholesterol levels remain high, you may have a genetic predisposition to high blood fat levels and may benefit from medication, says Dr. Small. See your doctor.

high-fat dairy products accomplishes both objectives.

To cut back on the fat and saturated fat in your diet, follow Terry's example. She traded whole milk for skim milk and ice cream for nonfat frozen yogurt. She started eating her vegetables with fresh ground pepper but no butter and her salads with vinegar instead of creamy dressings. She learned to sauté in broth, not butter, and to trim the fat from meat and poultry before cooking. She made red meat a less frequent guest at dinner and turned instead to fish and poultry and vegetarian dishes. When she ate meat, she ate less—never more than six ounces a day—and she got into the habit of buying only the leanest cuts. She found it fun to try vegetarian dishes, like meatless chili or pasta with vegetables. You can do the same.

Serve soy instead of meat. In an examination of several clinical trials, researchers led by James W. Anderson, M.D., at the University of Kentucky in Lexington, found that substituting roughly 1½ ounces of soy protein for animal protein (meat) reduced total cholesterol by about 9 percent, lowered LDL nearly 13 percent and dropped triglyceride levels around 10 percent. Consuming two to three servings of soy products, such as tofu, daily may be enough to achieve lipid-lowering results, according to the researchers.

When you use fat, make it vegetable oil. In most vegetable oils, very little of the fat is saturated. Olive, peanut and canola oils contain mostly monounsaturated fat, which lowers LDL and, according to some experts, may make LDL less susceptible to oxidation than polyunsaturated oils, says Dr. Kris-Etherton. (Oxidation turns LDL into arterial plaque.) Corn, sunflower and soybean oils contain mostly polyunsaturated fat, which also lowers your LDL levels, she adds. Remember to watch your overall fat intake, though, since fat is calorically dense and, if eaten in excess, can cause weight gain and adverse effects on blood lipids.

A study at Baylor College of Medicine in Houston showed that using vegetable oils in a low-fat diet can reduce total cholesterol by 11 percent and LDL levels by 13 percent. Other studies have shown that similar or even greater reductions in total cholesterol levels are possible.

Use a light hand with margarine. High in saturated fat, butter is a bad deal. But studies indicate that margarine may not be much better.

WHAT'S YOUR CHOLESTEROL?

Like a lot of women who responded to our *Food and You* survey, Celeste P. had her cholesterol tested. When she called her doctor's office for the results, she was told her cholesterol was "a little high." A close look at the lab results, however, showed that her HDL cholesterol (the good kind) was a very respectable 62 mg/dl (milligrams per deciliter)— enough to afford a fair degree of protection against heart disease.

Should you have your cholesterol tested? Probably. The American Heart Association advises all women age 20 and older to have the test. Your test results should include, at least, total cholesterol and HDL cholesterol. If your total cholesterol is above 240 mg/dl or your HDL is less than 35 mg/dl, arrange with your doctor to be retested after fasting in order to learn your LDL cholesterol (the bad kind).

If your total cholesterol is between 200 and 240 mg/dl and your HDL is at a desirable level, don't panic: Like Celeste, you should discuss the results with your doctor. Depending on the number of other coronary risk factors, such as smoking, you may have, retesting may be necessary. But if you have fewer than two risk factors, retesting every year may be all that is needed.

If your total cholesterol is lower than 200 mg/dl and your HDL is at a desirable level, congratulations. Get retested after five years.

Also, if you have coronary heart disease, you should aim for an LDL of 100 mg/dl or lower, says Elena Citkowitz, M.D., Ph.D., clinical instructor of medicine at Yale University School of Medicine and director of the Lipid Clinic at the Hospital of St. Raphael in New Haven, Connecticut.

Total Cholesterol (mg/dl)	HDL (mg/dl)	LDL (mg/dl)	Triglycerides (mg/dl)
Undesirable			
240 and higher	Below 35	160 and higher	400 and higher
Borderline			
200–239		130–159	200–399

Total Cholesterol (mg/dl)	HDL (mg/dl)	LDL (mg/dl)	Triglycerides (mg/dl)
Desirable			
Less than 200	Above 45 (average for men); above 55 (average for women); 60 or higher is protective	130 or lower (100 or lower for people with coronary heart disease)	Under 200

Made from mostly unsaturated vegetable oils, margarine is lower in saturated fats than butter is. But it also contains substances called trans-fatty acids—by-products of the manufacturing process that makes margarine solid at room temperature. Trans-fatty acids tend to raise cholesterol levels, so they may be hard on your heart and arteries, too, say some experts.

A study at the Jean Mayer USDA Human Nutrition Research Center on Aging at Tufts University in Boston is one of several that found that trans-fatty acids can increase LDL levels while lowering HDL levels—both of which are undesirable. And the Harvard University Nurses' Health Study (an ongoing study of 115,000 women considered a landmark source of evidence regarding women's health) has reported that even modest daily consumption of trans-fatty acids (four or more teaspoons of margarine) dramatically increases the risk of heart disease in women.

"Margarine may be a little better than butter, but not that much better," says Felando.

If you use margarine instead of butter, the AHA recommends soft or liquid margarine, since they're lower in trans-fatty acids than stick margarine. In addition, they are low in saturated fat, says Dr. Kris-Etherton. And choose "light" margarines, the ones with the lowest fat content per serving, advises Felando.

Dip, don't spread. A better bet would be to dip your bread into olive oil, the way some Italians do, or to lightly spread it with "natural" peanut butter, Felando adds. A study conducted by researchers at two Finnish universities found that replacing margarine with canola or olive oil resulted in lower cholesterol levels. Canola oil led to a 5.7 percent decrease in blood fats, while olive oil led to a 5.6 percent decrease.

Drop the fat from spreads entirely. Better still, cover your toast and bagels with jelly or nonfat cream cheese, Felando says.

Befriend beans. Pinto, kidney, navy and white beans and lentils contain generous amounts of soluble fiber, which appears to lower blood cholesterol, according to research conducted by Dr. Anderson.

For a 15 to 23 percent reduction in cholesterol, aim for one cup of cooked beans a day—in soups, meatless chili and vegetarian baked beans, says Felando. It's best to add beans to your diet gradually and drink plenty of fluids to avoid gastric distress, she advises.

Start your day with oatmeal. Rolled oats and oat bran are also rich in a type of soluble fiber called beta-glucan. If oatmeal doesn't appeal to you, you can select oat breads, muffins and ready-to-eat cereals with significant amounts of oats or oat bran.

Feast on fruits and vegetables. Oranges, apples, carrots and peppers keep your heart healthy in two ways: They're rich in soluble fiber, and they're good sources of antioxidant vitamins and heart-protective plant chemicals known as phytochemicals. These important substances may help prevent certain chemical changes that allow LDL cholesterol to be taken up by your artery walls, says Dr. Kris-Etherton.

A study conducted in India found that a diet rich in fruits and vegetables—along with moderate exercise—reduced LDL levels by 16.9 percent and raised HDL levels slightly. Exercise appears to be particularly effective in raising HDL.

Go for the garlic. Research at Pennsylvania State University in University Park found that garlic can lower LDL levels. Yu-Yan Yeh, Ph.D., a professor of nutrition who headed the study, eats two cloves a day. ''To maximize the benefits, garlic should be crushed,'' says Dr. Yeh. Garlic can be incorporated into soups or salads or when cooking vegetables, he suggests. If you're worried about your breath, commercially available garlic pills will also do the trick, without odor, says Dr. Yeh.

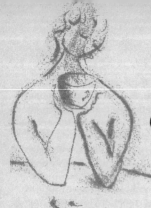

15

CONSTIPATION

Relief is spelled f-i-b-e-r

When poet William Butler Yeats wrote "fine women eat a crazy salad with their meat," it's a cinch he wasn't referring to a smart constipation fighting scheme. But he could have been.

That's because crunchy salads—plus a host of high-fiber fruits, vegetables, beans and whole grains—are the cornerstone of a four-point plan that doctors say relieves that bloated, uncomfortable log-jam in the bowels for nine out of ten women.

The other components? "Exercise, plenty of fluids and getting yourself into a regimen of going to the bathroom regularly," says Barry Jaffin, M.D., a specialist in gastrointestinal motility disorders and clinical instructor in the Department of Gastroenterology at Mount Sinai Medical Center in New York City. "Do all four, and you won't need a laxative."

THE CORE PROBLEM

Doctors estimate that some 12 million Americans are bothered by frequent constipation, which means they have two or fewer bowel movements a week, strain on the toilet or have hard, lumpy stools at least one-quarter of the time, or have a feeling of incomplete evacuation. What can silence the call of nature? A low-fiber diet, taking too many laxatives, the disruptions of travel, pregnancy or hormonal changes during the menstrual cycle, hemorrhoids or the use of iron or calcium supplements, antacids, antidepressants and other medications.

See a doctor if you feel pain, are constipated for longer than seven to ten days or notice blood in your stools. Consulting your doctor is also a good idea if you suspect a prescription medication is the culprit—or if your iron or calcium supplement or an over-the-counter medicine seems to be the cause of your irregularity. "If such is the case, cutting back on the over-the-counter medications (or the iron or calcium) sometimes relieves constipation," notes Dr. Jaffin.

Otherwise, doctors and dietitians say you're probably missing out on fiber—the indigestible plant material that your mother called roughage and one Boston nutritionist nicknamed "the Drano of the digestive system."

"Insoluble fiber, which comes from the skins, husks and stalks of plants and from the covering on bran—like wheat bran—is what really helps out in your digestive system," notes fiber researcher Barbara Harland, Ph.D., a professor in the Department of Nutritional Science in the College of Allied Health Sciences at Howard University in Washington, D.C. "When insoluble fiber absorbs fluids, it expands, making stools softer and larger so the contractions of the intestines have more to push against. Your bowels move better."

While the American Dietetic Association recommends we eat 20 to 35 grams of fiber a day, most American women get less than half that amount. "We eat too many processed foods from which the fiber has been removed," notes Dr. Harland.

A MENU FOR REGULARITY

To relieve constipation, choose whole-grain breads and cereals at breakfast, eat fruit or raw veggies for snacks and spotlight grains, legumes and produce in your lunch and dinner menus, suggests Elizabeth Ward, R.D., a nutrition counselor with the Boston-based Harvard Community Health Plan.

"The easiest way is to include a half-cup of high-fiber cereal at breakfast, which could give you five or more grams of fiber,

THE VEGETARIAN SOLUTION

Doctors notice something enviable about vegetarians: They rarely experience severe constipation. "The extra fiber in a vegetarian diet really helps keep them regular," notes Barry Jaffin, M.D., a specialist in gastrointestinal motility disorders and clinical instructor in the Department of Gastroenterology at Mount Sinai Medical Center in New York City.

With the emphasis on beans, whole grains and nuts for protein, a vegetarian meal plan provides two to three times more bowel-declogging fiber than meat-oriented diets.

Happily, you can enjoy the vegetarian advantage and *still* indulge in your favorite roast turkey or London broil. Just reserve two to three days a week for meatless meals, says Elizabeth Ward, R.D., nutrition counselor with the Harvard Community Health Plan in Boston.

"Try dishes that feature beans, like chili made with kidney or navy beans or black bean stew," suggests Ward. Lentil soup and a salad, red beans and rice, even a peanut butter and banana sandwich on whole-wheat bread are all good vegetarian choices. Or make substitutions: Replace the meat or sausage in your spaghetti sauce or lasagna with spinach or other chopped high-fiber veggies. "You really don't have to be a strict vegetarian to make this work," notes Ward.

topped with a sliced banana for another three grams," Ward says. "Take portable high-fiber snacks—like graham crackers, popcorn or carrot sticks—to work. And if you visit a salad bar for lunch, skip the iceberg lettuce—it has just about no fiber. Instead go for spinach, and include some beans, like chickpeas. Add raw broccoli or cauliflower, too."

If dinner is a hurry-up-and-eat affair, keep frozen vegetables on hand. "Washing and chopping vegetables can really be a chore after a long, hard day," she notes. "This way, you just steam or microwave what you need."

Experts suggest these additional strategies to maximize your fiber quotient.

Choose fiber superstars. Try these fiber-packed foods:

chick-peas (garbanzo beans), with 7 grams per half-cup; kidney beans, with 6.9 grams per half-cup; raspberries, with 6 grams per cup; barley, with 12.3 grams per half-cup; or a fresh pear, with 4.3 grams.

Concoct a fiber-rich topping. Sprinkle a quarter-cup of raisins over cereal or rice for an extra two grams of fiber. Add wheat germ—with four grams of fiber per quarter-cup—to baked goods or hot cereal, says Ward.

Pick a prune, find a fig. Five prunes have three grams of fiber—it's no wonder they're a natural laxative! For a change of pace, Dr. Jaffin suggests eating dried figs; just three give you a whopping five grams of fiber.

Try a fiber powder. "Take one to two tablespoons of a natural fiber supplement like Metamucil, Konsyl or Citrucel mixed with the suggested amount of liquid at about the same time every day," Dr. Jaffin suggests. "This is a good, safe way to make sure you get plenty of fiber." Granulated or flake-type fiber supplements of wheat bran, psyllium seed or soy fiber are available in health food stores. Some doctors have reported rare cases of people whose esophagus became blocked from fiber pills that expanded after being swallowed. Whatever form of fiber you choose, be sure to drink plenty of fluids, especially water.

Fiber up gradually. Whether you're introducing high-fiber foods or supplements, take it slowly, so your system can adjust.

Drink up. Every day, try to down eight, eight-ounce glasses of fluid, says Ward. Water and juice are best. "Without fluid, extra fiber could make you even more constipated," says Dr. Jaffin.

DIABETES

A modern diet for better blood sugar control

At 34, worried by the prospect of diabetes, LaMyra J. began to overhaul her diet. Sugar-free iced tea replaced her favorite apple juice. Low-fat margarine debuted on her toast, and cornflakes landed in her cereal bowl.

"My doctor told me I had a 50-50 chance I'd get diabetes later in life," says LaMyra, a mother of three. "Of course, I don't want to get diabetes. So I changed my eating habits."

Diabetes is a disease that affects the body's ability to produce or respond to insulin, a hormone that allows blood sugar (glucose) to enter the cells of the body and be used for energy. LaMyra was considered at risk for four reasons—she is slightly overweight, has a family history of diabetes, is African American and had gestational diabetes, a temporary condition that can occur during pregnancy. Each factor raised the odds that someday LaMyra would have diabetes permanently.

If that happened, LaMyra's body would be unable to make or properly use insulin, which in turn would cause an increase in cardio-unfriendly blood fats like cholesterol and triglycerides, putting her at greater risk for heart disease, kidney ailments, blindness and circulatory problems. In fact, the risk of heart disease is two to four times higher among women with diabetes than among those without it. So LaMyra was smart to take steps against diabetes early in the game.

MENSTRUATION, FATIGUE AND BLOOD SUGAR CONTROL

Some 8.4 million American women have diabetes. About half know they have it and can control the disease through diet and exercise or with insulin pills or injections. The others can beat diabetes if they pay attention to risk factors and take action early on.

In some ways diabetes affects women differently than men. A few women, like Susan Thom, R.D., a certified diabetes educator in Cleveland, notice that their bodies need more insulin in the week and a half before menstruation begins. Birth control pills can affect blood sugar levels, yet since women with diabetes are at higher risk for infection and intrauterine devices (IUDs) can lead to infections, most cannot use the IUD.

Despite warning signs ranging from excessive thirst and hunger to blurred vision, fatigue and the frequent need to urinate, fully half of the women with diabetes don't even know they have it.

"Too many people walk around with undiagnosed diabetes," says Richard S. Beaser, M.D., assistant section head for internal medicine at the Joslin Diabetes Center and a staff physician at Deaconess Hospital and Harvard Medical School, all in Boston. "Anyone who's at risk should be tested."

What are the risk factors? Overweight; a family history of diabetes; gestational diabetes during a pregnancy; being African American, Hispanic, Native American or Asian; a sedentary lifestyle; high cholesterol or high blood pressure.

HEALTHIER BABIES, HEALTHIER HEARTS

Time was when people thought that eating too many sugary foods caused diabetes, and therefore all you had to do to control diabetes was avoid sugar. Well, dietary control is pivotal, but it's not quite that simple. The goal is to achieve blood sugar levels that are as normal as possible, which is accomplished by looking at the whole diet, not just sweets.

"How you eat is one of the cornerstones for preventing *and* controlling diabetes," says endocrinologist Kathleen Wishner, M.D., Ph.D., associate clinical professor of medicine at the University of Southern California in Los Angeles and president of the American Diabetes Association.

The rewards, says Dr. Wishner, make diabetes management worth the effort. More energy. An end to excessive thirst. More restful sleep, uninterrupted by the frequent need to go to the bathroom.

"Plus," says Dr. Wishner, "there are long-term benefits. Long-standing high blood sugar can lead to very serious health complications (like blindness, kidney disease and circulatory problems). If a woman with diabetes becomes pregnant and her blood sugar is not managed, her child's health is at risk."

Rest assured, a woman with diabetes can get pregnant and give birth to a healthy child—provided her diabetes is under control *before* conception and throughout the pregnancy, says Dr. Wishner. In a study sponsored by the National Institutes of Health that followed 386 women with diabetes through pregnancy, researchers concluded that women with in-control blood sugar were no more likely to miscarry than women without diabetes. And while the risk of birth defects is still two to five times higher, "diabetic women who get nutritional counseling before pregnancy are more likely to have well-controlled diabetes. Excellent blood sugar control before becoming pregnant is essential to having a healthy baby," says Sallie Bartholomew, R.N., diabetes nurse educator at the Endocrine and Diabetes Management Center in Richmond, Virginia. "The real risks of congenital birth defects are in the first six to ten weeks, when the baby is just forming."

In the event you develop diabetes after becoming pregnant (that is, gestational diabetes, a condition that usually resolves after pregnancy), the risks are different, says Dr. Wishner. Your baby could be quite large, and you may require a cesarean section for delivery. Other complications for the baby include low blood sugar, breathing difficulties and jaundice. Mothers with gestational diabetes may develop high blood pressure and more frequent urinary tract infections, says Bartholomew.

WHAT YOU CAN (AND SHOULD) EAT

Whether you're pregnant or not, experts such as Marion Franz, R.D., vice-president of nutrition at the International Diabetes Center in Minneapolis, advocate a three-point plan for diabetes control, to curb the risk of heart disease while tackling blood sugar and holding the line on body weight.

Instead of focusing on sugar, the emphasis is on nutrient-dense, high-fiber carbohydrates and low-fat proteins.

"In 1994, the American Diabetes Association recommended that people with diabetes get 10 to 20 percent of their calories from protein, less than 20 percent from saturated and poly-unsaturated fats and 60 to 70 percent from carbohydrates and monounsaturated fats, because of the latter's beneficial effect on heart health," notes Franz. "Beyond that," she says, "individual diets will vary with a person's weight goals, activity level, and whether they're trying to reduce their cholesterol levels or not." So experts no longer offer one "diabetic diet" for all, says Franz.

Here are some specifics.

Plan your carbohydrates. While everyone needs a certain quantity of carbohydrates for energy, in women with diabetes, too big a dose can send blood sugar soaring, notes Franz.

"Most women with diabetes can eat three to four servings of carbohydrates at a meal, but not more," she says. "A serving is about 15 grams of carbohydrate—the amount found in a glass of milk, a small to medium-size fruit, a half-cup of pasta or three-quarters of a cup of cereal, for example. Keeping the amounts under control helps keep blood sugars even." Which carbs are best? "The least processed," Franz notes. "That means whole grains, fruits or vegetables. If you have the choice of a cookie, a glass of orange juice or an orange for dessert, choose the orange."

Snack early and often. For better blood sugar control, spread breakfast, lunch and dinner over five small meals—or snacks—throughout the day, suggests Franz. "You may not manufacture enough insulin to handle a large meal, but you may make enough for many small ones. The trick is to not overeat."

To eat more frequently without overeating, plan ahead. Franz suggests saving your breakfast fruit for a midmorning

THINK MEDITERRANEAN

Fruity olive oil. Pungent garlic. Crusty whole-grain breads and a riot of brilliantly colored vegetables. Italian, Greek and other Mediterranean foods are a pleasure for the eyes and taste buds.

And now researchers at the Center for Human Nutrition at the University of Texas Southwestern Medical Center in Dallas say Mediterranean food may be the best of all possible meal plans for women with diabetes.

In a study, 42 women and men with diabetes ate one of two diets for six weeks each. One of the diets supplied 55 percent of calories from carbohydrates and 30 percent from fats; the other provided fewer carbs and more fat— 40 percent from carbs and 45 percent from fats. In the second group, the added fat came, in part, from healthy monounsaturated fat like olive oil and avocados—simulating the nutritional makeup of a Mediterranean diet.

The results? Both diets lowered LDL cholesterol, the kind implicated in the development of coronary heart disease. But the regimen that was rich in olive oil had added benefits: blood sugar, triglycerides and levels of VLDL (very low density lipoproteins, which help form LDL) were lowered, while levels of "good" HDL cholesterol (which lowers the risk of heart disease) were maintained. What's more, another study based at the same research center discovered that by consuming a diet rich in olive oil, patients with diabetes required nearly 13 percent less insulin.

"We think this is a plan that those with diabetes and their families could follow easily and enjoy, and it would be healthy," says lead researcher Abhimanyu Garg, M.D., associate professor of internal medicine at the Center for Human Nutrition. Other foods typically featured in Mediterranean cookery—whole grains, lots of fruits and vegetables, legumes like white beans and small amounts of meat—can be easily worked into meal plans, he notes.

"The beauty of the Mediterranean diet is that it contains lots of fiber and lots of complex carbohydrates, which are good choices, within bounds, for those with diabetes," Dr. Garg says. "The key to the whole thing is watching your calorie intake. Yes, you'll gain weight if you eat too much olive oil. So you have to be careful."

One mainstay of Mediterranean meals—wine—should remain off-limits if you have diabetes, cautions Dr. Garg. "Alcohol adds calories and can lead to obesity," he notes. "It increases triglyceride levels and can raise blood pressure. It's better to steer clear."

pick-me-up. At lunch, save bread or crackers and some low-fat cheese, yogurt or another piece of fruit for a nosh during the midafternoon slump. Carry dried fruit with you, says Thom. Hold off on that glass of milk at dinner and enjoy it at bedtime with a final carbohydrate food such as crackers or bread, suggests Franz.

Fit in the fiber. Nutrition experts no longer believe that fiber slows the absorption of sugar into the bloodstream, says Dr. Wishner. "You would need a huge amount, well beyond the 30 grams recommended for the American diet," she notes. "People with diabetes should eat fiber for the same reasons everyone else does—to stay regular, reduce the risk of colon cancer and maintain healthy cholesterol levels to fight heart disease."

Quench your thirst. "I have clients whose blood sugar seems to get higher when they don't get enough fluids," notes Thom. Her best advice? Consume two to three quarts of sugar-free fluids a day—water, diet soda and so forth—and only moderate amounts of coffee or tea.

Bypass salt. Salty foods can raise blood pressure, notes Thom, and women with diabetes are two to three times more likely to develop high blood pressure. "The combination of high blood pressure and high blood sugar is a time bomb," she says. To prevent problems, the American Diabetes Association recommends limiting sodium to no more than 3,000 milligrams a day—less if you already have diabetes and high blood pressure. When buying prepared foods, read labels—they give the sodium content in milligrams. When cooking, remember that 3,000 milligrams of sodium is equal to about 1½ teaspoons of salt.

Skip dessert. Some women with diabetes can tolerate a small sweet dessert such as a cookie or a small scoop of frozen yogurt, but others cannot, says Franz. Even desserts sweetened with fructose, which seems to raise blood sugar less dramatically than sucrose, can be a problem, says Dr. Wishner. "Desserts also tend to be high in fat," Dr. Wishner says. "They're often empty calories."

Walk off excess pounds. Losing just 10 to 20 pounds can substantially improve diabetes control. Exercise helps those with diabetes to lose weight, increases the body's ability to use blood sugar for energy and builds lean muscle that helps the body expend more calories, says Dr. Wishner. Together, weight control and exercise are powerful diabetes prevention tools for *any* woman, says diabetes educator Broatch Haig, R.D., director of outreach services at the International Diabetes Center in Minneapolis. "It's so simple: 30 to 40 minutes of exercise three to four times a week burns calories and reduces the risk."

17

FATIGUE

Help for when there's no get-up-and-go

Your days feel like a dawn-to-dusk dance marathon: Up with the sun, you marshal the troops out the door and grab some coffee and a quick doughnut to munch in the car. With a full afternoon of work ahead, a burger is all you can manage for lunch. After battling the 3 o'clock slump, suddenly it's time to race home, cook dinner and survive an evening of laundry, kids' homework and a batch of bills to pay.

Small wonder you're feeling irritable, frustrated and decidedly unamorous—as if your brain is grinding along in low gear. You're tired—and your diet may be the reason. If so, you're not alone.

"On any given day, one-quarter of the population is tired, and an estimated 2 to 3 percent of the entire U.S. population feel fatigue that's nearly disabling," says Richard Podell, M.D., clinical professor of family medicine at the Robert Wood Johnson Medical School in New Brunswick, New Jersey, and author of *Doctor, Why Am I So Tired?* "Of these people, more are women than men. And dietary changes help about one in four feel better."

WHY WOMEN CRASH AND BURN

Why is fatigue one of the top ten complaints that women report to doctors? Blame it on our hectic lifestyle: Women who juggle jobs, families and household responsibilities often get little sleep and less exercise. Instead of making sure we eat nutrition-packed, energy-boosting meals, we graze at salad bars and fast-food drive-throughs, thus missing out on essential vitamins and minerals—notably iron, B vitamins, magnesium and folate—that are needed to maintain energy.

Many women intentionally undereat in an attempt to lose weight, and they undernourish themselves in the process. Others feel drained of energy due to pregnancy, childbirth or menopause.

Some of us overeat and feel sluggish because our bodies are busy digesting and storing excess fat. That, says researcher R. James Barnard, Ph.D., professor of physiological science at the University of California at Los Angeles and consultant to the Pritikin Longevity Center in Santa Monica, actually slows blood circulation, reducing the delivery of oxygen to the body's cells. Or we choose the wrong foods at the wrong time and feel sluggish instead of energized.

By the way, smoking, drinking and recreational drugs can also tire you out, as will a variety of diseases, from anemia to diabetes to depression. If you're suddenly bone-tired for no obvious reason or have been barely able to function for a month or longer, it's time to see a doctor. Otherwise, you may simply need an oomph-restoring meal makeover.

FOOD FOR YOUR BRAIN

Firsthand experience has taught many women what research now reveals about food's power to boost—or flatten—energy levels.

"If I eat a big lunch," says Lydia W., a woman who responded to our *Food and You* survey, "I'm mentally sluggish all afternoon. A couple of light meals during the day work better."

"There have been times when I feel tired and realize I have not been eating well," says Alycia S., another respondent.

If mustering mental energy—to finish a report for an afternoon deadline or work late on your income tax—is your goal, did you know that eating small amounts of protein as part of a low-fat meal plan can actually help your brain manufacture more of the neurotransmitters that make you mentally alert?

By topping your morning toast with nonfat or low-fat ricotta cheese, choosing a turkey sandwich for lunch or having broiled fish for dinner, you can subtly override your natural body rhythms, fighting the built-in tendency to grow mentally tired as the day wanes and increasing your brain's high-energy time by up to three hours.

"When your mother said 'Eat fish, it's a brain food,' she wasn't that far off," says Judith Wurtman, Ph.D., nutrition research scientist at the Massachusetts Institute of Technology in Cambridge and author of *Managing Your Mind and Mood through Food*.

It's true that we need complex carbohydrates like pasta and wholewheat breads to fuel muscles. But according to Dr. Wurtman's research, carbohydrates eaten alone make more of the amino acid tryptophan available to your brain. Your brain uses the tryptophan to manufacture serotonin, a nerve-transmitting substance that leaves you feeling "less stressed, less anxious and more relaxed," says Dr. Wurtman.

In contrast, protein gives your brain cells more of the amino acid tyrosine, which is converted to dopamine and norepinephrine—the very chemicals that leap from nerve ending to nerve ending inside your brain when you're engaged in thought. "Sharp thinking skills, word retrieval and mental quickness depend on protein," she says. "If you don't eat much protein, you will probably find you're not as mentally alert."

The advice doesn't hold for everyone, Dr. Wurtman notes. A few of us may experience fatigue along with depression or tension, anger or anxiety if we don't satisfy our carbohydrate cravings. "For these people," she says, "eating carbohydrates does make them feel better and more focused."

CARBOHYDRATES FOR THE LONG HAUL

Carbohydrates are also the body's basic brain fuel, vital for sustaining body functions. While carbs can be found in everything from beans and rice and fruits and vegetables to candy bars and soft drinks, don't fall for a quick sugar hit—all carbohydrates are not created equal.

"Some carbohydrates like sugar, honey, candies and baked desserts give you a very quick fix, but you end up being hungry and tired and back at the refrigerator, eating, in a matter of hours," says nutritionist Elizabeth Somer, R.D., author of *Nutrition for Women and Food and Mood.*

In contrast, complex carbohydrates that are also high in fiber—like beans, vegetables and whole-grain products—may provide a steadier source of fuel for your body, says David Jenkins, M.D., Ph.D., professor of medicine and nutritional sciences at the University of Toronto. Why? Your body digests them more slowly. Meals and snacks that combine carbohydrates with small amounts of fat or protein may also provide an even release of energy, for the same reason.

For snacks that combine carbohydrates, low-fat protein and fiber, try a piece of fruit with crackers and peanut butter, rice cakes with low-fat cheese or yogurt, a baked potato with nonfat cottage cheese, three-bean salad, or an English muffin with all-fruit spread and nonfat cheese, suggests Somer.

Just as important, Somer notes, is giving your body a steady fuel source that begins promptly with the first meal of the day. "You are literally breaking a fast—your body hasn't had food for the past 8 or 10 or 12 hours. If they skip breakfast, some people never rebuild their energy stores for the day," she says.

Your best bet for steady energy may be smaller, more frequent meals—say, five a day, says Dr. Podell. "Eating a large amount of food, say more than 1,000 calories at a meal, will typically make many people tired within 30 to 60 minutes. This is due to neurochemical changes in the brain relating to the amino acid tryptophan. In addition, some people will experience a 'hypoglycemic' rebound three to four hours later, which could make them tired and irritable. These are two distinct reactions. Some people get one or the other, and some get both," he says.

MICRONUTRIENTS FOR MACRO-ENERGY

By nature, women have special vitamin and mineral needs. Menstruation and childbirth can drain our iron stores, leaving us fatigued and even anemic. So can diets bereft of rich and reliable sources of iron such as lean meats and iron-rich beans, dried fruit, shellfish and nuts.

Birth control pills can bring on deficiencies of vitamin B_6 and folate, causing a run-down feeling. If you're on the Pill, make sure you get plenty of B_6-rich foods such as wheat germ, bananas, avocados, cabbage and cauliflower as well as folate-rich foods such as apricots, pumpkins, carrots, beans and green leafy vegetables like spinach.

Taking diuretics and drinking too much alcohol can drain both potassium and magnesium, leaving you fatigued, with weak muscles and poor concentration. To correct this, turn to potassium-packed dried fruits, citrus fruits, bananas and green leafy vegetables and magnesium-rich nuts, seeds and green veggies, Dr. Podell suggests. And if you do take diuretics, ask your doctor about blood tests for potassium levels, as well as diuretics that don't drain this vital nutrient.

And don't forget to drink six to eight eight-ounce glasses of water a day, suggests Somer. "Fatigue is a sign of mild dehydration," she says. "We tend to go for coffee or tea to feel peppier, but the caffeine acts as a diuretic and takes water out of our bodies. Most women aren't getting enough water."

SLUGGISH? SKIP THE COFFEE CART

Speaking of caffeine, coffee may be an old standby for anyone needing a pick-me-up, but experts warn that it just might slam-dunk your energy levels, leaving you with less vim than before.

Coffee, experts say, is a two-edged sword: Research shows that caffeine improves alertness, but sipping too much—or enjoying your java too late in the day—could leave you tossing and turning on your pillow at night.

"A cup of coffee in the morning will get you going and

SPORTS DRINKS AND ENERGY BARS
Real Food Will Do

With their high-performance promises, neon-bright labels and fruit flavors, sports drinks are popping up everywhere these days. So are foil-wrapped sports energy bars. You can't miss them. But do you need them?

Probably not, if you work out for less than 90 minutes, says Edward Coyle, Ph.D., an exercise physiologist in the Department of Kinesiology at the University of Texas in Austin. Aerobics adherents, fitness walkers and joggers and others who work out to lose weight and stay fit can easily meet their energy and fluid needs with water and healthy snacks.

Drinks like Gatorade, All Sport and Powerade *do* work, notes Dr. Coyle. Some sports drinks contain scientifically engineered blends of carbohydrate, sodium and (of course) water, formulated to quickly replace fluids, minerals and calories lost during sweaty exercise. "But it's nothing magic," he says. The same ingredients are found in regular food.

"There's no evidence that a moderately active woman, who is exercising for one hour or less a day at below 85 percent of maximum heart rate, needs the extra carbohydrates or minerals for energy or rehydration," says Dr. Coyle, who has researched sports drinks extensively. "Unless she's an endurance athlete running hard for longer than one hour or playing back-to-back sets of tennis on a really hot day, all she needs is plenty of water, plus a snack or a meal within a few hours after exercising."

To stay hydrated: An hour or so before your workout, down 16 ounces of water. During your exercise routine, drink another 8 ounces every 20 minutes. Afterward, weigh yourself and drink enough water to replace the weight you've lost, says Michael Sawka, Ph.D., environmental physiologist in the thermal physiology and medicine division of the U.S. Army Research Institute of Environmental Medicine in Natick, Massachusetts. And here's why.

"You could easily lose a quart of water in an hour of

exercise," Dr. Sawka says. "That's two pounds. Even that small loss can raise your body temperature and heart rate, which will make it harder for you to perform well."

As for sports bars, you can get the same 200-calorie burst of energy with "four fig bars or a large banana or other similar snack," notes Nancy Clark, R.D., director of nutrition services at SportsMedicine Brookline in the Boston area. And those alternatives are less expensive.

sharpen your thinking," says Somer. "But drinking more than three five-ounce cups a day, and especially drinking coffee after midday, can interfere with sleep," she says. And poor sleep translates into below-par energy levels.

Skip the caffeine and you may recoup your zest. In a series of studies at Texas A&M University in College Station, Larry Christensen, Ph.D., now chairman of the Department of Psychology at the University of South Alabama in Mobile, found that depressed men and women who eliminated sugar and caffeine from their diets felt more energetic and less depressed.

"If you're depressed or have constant feelings of fatigue, then it's worth trying," says Dr. Christensen. "Though I should warn you," he adds, "people went through some withdrawal giving up both sugar and caffeine. They can be hard habits to break."

In a Yale University study, eight normal volunteers who sipped caffeine-containing sodas—the equivalent of two to three cups of drip-brewed coffee—experienced dizziness, trembling and other typical symptoms of hypoglycemia when their blood sugar was lowered to levels that are close to hypoglycemia but do not usually produce any symptoms.

Why? Researcher Pierre Fayad, M.D., assistant professor of neurology at the Yale University School of Medicine and co-director of the Yale Vascular Neurology Program, says the caffeine actually slowed blood flow to the brain, probably lowering the availability of sugar for the brain to use. Drinking less coffee, switching to decaf or eating food along with the coffee may help prevent low blood sugar, says Dr. Fayad.

Want to quit entirely? Don't go cold turkey. Pour yourself one-fourth less coffee than usual per cup and continue to cut down until you've weaned yourself entirely, suggests Wahida Karmally, R.D., director of nutrition at the Irving Center for Clinical Research at Columbia University in New York City.

Or switch gradually to decaf. Start out by mixing three-quarters of a cup of regular brew with one-quarter decaf. Every two or three days, replace a little more caffeinated with decaf until your cup's 100 percent decaf. "Go slowly," says Karmally, "weaning yourself off caffeine at your own pace."

FATIGUE-FIGHTING FOODS

To stay alert and energized for active days and busy evenings, plug into this high-energy meal plan, designed by nutritionist Elizabeth Somer, R.D., author of *Nutrition for Women* and *Food and Mood*.

Her guiding principles: Small meals or snacks every three to four hours. Complex, fiber-rich carbohydrates combined with low-fat protein. (Carbohydrates alone may make you sleepy, says Somer.) And, for women of childbearing age, an adequate supply of iron-rich foods, essential to fending off fatigue. At the same time, remember to limit the energy-robbers—fat, sugar and caffeine.

POWER BREAKFASTS

To power up in the morning, start your day with one of these breakfasts.

1. Toasted bagel topped with one tablespoon peanut butter; eight ounces skim milk; one banana.
2. Three-quarters cup oatmeal, cooked with skim milk and topped with two tablespoons wheat germ, one tablespoon honey or brown sugar, one tablespoon

chopped nuts and one tablespoon raisins. Serve with six ounces apple juice.

3. Egg substitute scrambled with green pepper and onion and topped with salsa. (Spray the pan with vegetable spray instead of using butter.) Serve with a fat-free flour tortilla and six ounces orange juice (add a twist of lime for extra flavor).

4. One or two slices french toast topped with a quarter-cup fat-free cottage cheese and a quarter-cup pineapple (fresh or canned in juice). Serve with eight ounces skim milk.

ENERGY-ROBBING BREAKFASTS

These are examples of the kind of starters that can bog you down or leave you hungry by midmorning.

1. Danish pastries topped with butter and coffee with cream.
2. Pancakes with butter and maple syrup and coffee.
3. Fast-food sausage-and-egg sandwich on a croissant.
4. Half-cup of fruit and tea.

REVITALIZING MIDMORNING SNACKS

For a midmorning pick-me-up, choose from these options.

1. Half a cantaloupe filled with six ounces low-fat lemon yogurt and topped with one tablespoon unsalted sunflower seeds.
2. Bran muffins with two tablespoons apple butter; eight ounces skim milk.
3. Fruit smoothie (a half-cup skim milk blended with six canned and drained apricots, four tablespoons orange juice concentrate, a quarter-cup pineapple chunks and a quarter-cup wheat germ).
4. Two slices thinly sliced, low-fat turkey luncheon meat with six whole-wheat, fat-free crackers. Serve with six ounces apple-cranberry juice.

LOW-ENERGY MIDMORNING SNACKS

The following make poor choices any time of the day, especially midmorning.

1. Candy bar or chocolate-covered granola bar.
2. Doughnut and coffee.
3. Can of cola and jelly beans.

LUNCHES FOR GET-UP-AND-GO

With hours of work ahead of you, these are the kinds of lunches you need to keep on going.

1. Small bowl canned, low-fat minestrone soup and two ounces turkey on whole-wheat bread with lettuce and mustard. Serve with eight ounces skim milk.
2. Tossed salad (two cups greens, a quarter-cup canned, drained kidney beans, one ounce low-fat cheese, cubed, three tablespoons low-fat dressing). Serve with two slices sourdough bread and lemon-flavored sparkling water.
3. Peanut butter crunch sandwich (two tablespoons peanut butter mixed with one tablespoon wheat germ and two teaspoons honey, spread on multigrain bread). Serve with eight ounces skim milk and one cup fresh strawberries.
4. Three ounces extra-lean roast beef on whole-wheat roll with tomato, lettuce and mustard. Serve with one piece fruit and one cup raw cauliflower florets, sliced carrots and broccoli.

ENERGY-ROBBING LUNCHES

The wrong choice at lunch can leave you dragging.

1. Double cheeseburger with sauce, large french fries and a soft drink.
2. Tossed green salad and spaghetti marinara.
3. Batter-dipped fried vegetables, fish or chicken.

SNACKS THAT BEAT MIDAFTERNOON SLUMP

To avoid the three o'clock slump, try one of these mini-meals.

1. Two cups baby carrots dipped in a quarter-cup fat-free cream cheese flavored with dill.
2. One whole-wheat pita bread, broken into pieces and dipped in a quarter-cup hummus. Serve with one apple.
3. One diced kiwi mixed with six ounces low-fat strawberry-kiwi yogurt. Serve with three graham crackers.
4. Six ounces vanilla low-fat yogurt sprinkled with one-third cup low-fat granola and two tablespoons dried cranberries, raisins, chopped dates or other dried fruit.
5. Corn muffin with jalapeño jelly; eight ounces skim milk.

LOW-ENERGY AFTERNOON SNACKS

Ignore the temptation to reach for junk food, and you'll breeze through the afternoon.

1. Bag of chocolate chip cookies.
2. Bag of potato chips.
3. Coffee and a candy bar.

DINNERS FOR EVENING ALERTNESS

So far, so good. Smart choices like these can give you a second wind after dinner.

1. Four to six ounces broiled salmon topped with dill and lemon; one baked potato topped with fat-free sour cream; one cup steamed broccoli; one cup tossed salad with two tablespoons low-fat dressing. For dessert, a quarter honeydew melon or a half-cup fresh blueberries.
2. Four to six ounces grilled chicken; three-quarters cup pasta salad with garlic and one teaspoon olive oil; ten asparagus spears; one cup spinach salad with two ta-

blespoons low-fat dressing. For dessert, one cup fresh
strawberries or one mango, cubed.

3. Two cups stir-fried tofu and vegetables served over
   three-quarters cup rice; three-bean salad in vinegar
   dressing. Serve with eight ounces skim milk.
4. Two cups tomato-based fish chowder with two slices
   French bread; one cup spinach salad with two tablespoons low-fat dressing; a half-cup carrot-raisin salad
   with low-fat mayonnaise. Serve with eight ounces skim
   milk.

LOW-ENERGY DINNERS

Nothing saps your energy faster than a heavy meal in the
evening. Avoid these energy sinkers.

1. Steak; baked potato topped with sour cream; buttered
   vegetables.
2. Pasta with cream sauce.
3. Turkey with stuffing, gravy and "the works."

EVENING SNACKS FOR WINDING DOWN

After a high-energy day, try one of these calming treats to
prepare for a good night's sleep and an energetic day tomorrow.

1. Almond milk (several drops of almond extract added
   to eight ounces warmed skim milk). Serve with two fig
   bars.
2. Two cups fruit such as strawberries or kiwi, banana or
   orange slices drizzled lightly with two tablespoons
   chocolate syrup.
3. Half a toasted English muffin topped with all-fruit jam.
4. One frozen whole-wheat waffle topped with half a
   banana and one tablespoon maple syrup.

SLEEP-ROBBING SNACKS

If it's a sound sleep you seek, never end the day with the
following.

1. Black or green tea, cola or hot chocolate.
2. Leftovers from the refrigerator (a full stomach interferes
   with sleep).

18

FOOD ALLERGIES

Sidestepping trouble without sacrificing nutrition

One woman's pounding headaches ease when she stops eating tomatoes, eggs and corn. Another quiets a ten-year history of coughing spells by giving up wheat. A girl's mood swings subside when doctors remove yeast and dairy products from her diet.

Food reactions? Definitely. Food allergies? Probably not.

What's going on? These true-life stories from a medical journal article on food reactions illustrate the puzzling, powerful connection between what we eat and how we feel—a connection so confusing that one-quarter of all American adults believe they have a food allergy, while just 1 in 100 really does.

"Plenty of people have adverse food reactions, and those reactions are real," says Paul A. Greenberger, M.D., an allergist-immunologist and professor of medicine at Northwestern University Medical School in Chicago. "But they are not the same as a true food allergy. With a food allergy, your body's immune system reacts to a protein in a particular food. Sometimes the reaction can be life-threatening."

THE FEMALE SIDE OF FOOD ALLERGY

While women and men seem equally disposed to food allergies, women may have stronger physical reactions to food during the second half of the menstrual cycle, speculates Janice Joneja, R.D., Ph.D., allergy nutrition consultant at the Allergy Nutrition Research Program at Vancouver Hospital and Health Sciences Centre in British Columbia and author of *Understanding Allergy, Sensitivity and Immunology.*

It's not just a menstrual phenomenon, says Dr. Joneja. "I've also seen women develop new food allergies and reactions after going on birth control pills or hormone replacement therapy," she adds, being careful to emphasize that this is her personal observation and not based on scientific studies. "No one knows quite why it happens," she says.

Yet for any woman with a food allergy or intolerance, giving up particular foods can have nutritional and emotional impacts. If you don't use any milk and dairy products because of a milk allergy, you miss out on a major source of calcium, for example, and if you avoid citrus, you lose an important source of vitamin C and folate.

If you have a severe fish allergy, it may mean that you can't go to a fish fry with your friends, even if they'll be disappointed and you'll feel left out, says William Ziering, M.D., an allergist and founder of the Ziering Allergy and Respiratory Medical Center in Fresno, California. "An ear, nose and throat specialist who was allergic to peanuts survived a close encounter with carrot cake. His keen sense of smell enabled him to detect a peanut aroma just as he was about to taste his favorite dessert. Detective work uncovered that the chef had baked the cake using peanut oil."

ALLERGY OR INTOLERANCE?

As mentioned, food allergies happen when the immune system mistakes a food protein for a dangerous invader. The first time the "invader" is encountered, an allergy-prone immune system manufactures antibodies to fight it off. The second time, it deploys the antibodies in an all-out biochemical attack that may cause swelling of the lips, mouth and throat; an upset stomach, gas or diarrhea; itching, rash or hives; or even a simple runny nose. In rare cases, the reaction is life-threatening anaphylaxis—chest pain, low blood pressure and difficulty breathing.

Eggs, cow's milk, nuts, wheat, soy products and shellfish are the most common foods that cause serious allergic reactions. But people have also reported anaphylactic reactions after eating barley, rice, wheat, citrus fruits, melons, bananas, tomatoes, spinach, corn, potatoes and soybeans.

The best defense? Stay away.

"If you have a bona fide food allergy, you have to avoid the foods in question," says Dean Metcalfe, M.D., head of the Allergic Diseases Section of the National Institute of Allergy and Infectious Diseases at the National Institutes of Health in Bethesda, Maryland. "If you know you just have a few hives after eating some rice, well, it may not be too bad an allergy. But peanuts causing hives may be a warning of a more severe reaction to come." And if you've ever had a serious reaction, you've got to be vigilant. Medication—injectable epinephrine—can squash a reaction immediately, but you need to carry your medication at all times and take it if you accidentally swallow a food to which you are allergic. Once you're allergic to a food, it's safest to assume you'll be allergic to it for the rest of your life.

In contrast, a food intolerance is rarely dangerous but often unpleasant. Typical symptoms include gas, diarrhea or bloating. The cause may not be obvious. Your body may lack enzymes that are necessary to digest milk—a condition called lactose intolerance, which is discussed in chapter 25. You may have trouble digesting the gluten found in wheat, oats, rye and barley—a condition called celiac disease. Or a food additive could be giving you a headache—as with monosodium glutamate, or MSG (Asian food, including soups) or nitrates (hot dogs and other cured meats).

FRUSTRATED? READ THIS

If you aren't sure whether you have a food allergy or intolerance (or some other problem) or need help deciding what to eat or not to eat, it might be worthwhile to get professional advice.

See an allergist. To sort out the allergy-or-intolerance question, consult an allergist who is certified by the American Board of Allergy and Immunology. She will take a detailed diet and medical history, probably do skin-prick or blood tests and possibly gauge your reaction to specific foods.

Recruit a food counselor. "People with vague symptoms who are convinced they are allergic to many foods and stop eating them can have serious nutritional deficiencies," says Dr. Joneja. "If you have a food allergy or suspect you do, you should see a registered dietitian/nutritionist, who will help you to determine the foods to which you react and make sure that you obtain adequate nutrition." She will help you to determine your food intolerances by elimination and challenge, Dr. Joneja says. (Elimination and challenge involve omitting all food allergy triggers, usually for five days, then reintroducing possible offenders to the diet one by one.)

A NUTRITIONAL BACKUP PLAN

Doctors emphasize that if adverse reactions force key foods out of your life, you may be shutting the door on important nutrients.

Allergic to milk? You'll need alternate sources of calcium—and vitamin D—to help protect against osteoporosis and possibly high blood pressure. Got a gluten intolerance or wheat allergy? The breads and pastas you cannot eat are good sources of B-complex vitamins that are essential for plenty of energy. Avoiding eggs? Quick breads, pancakes, muffins and other baked goods made with eggs may be problematic, depriving you of a convenient and favorite source of carbohydrate. Here are some other guidelines.

Be careful with soy. Women with soy allergies may have nutritional problems when they try to eliminate all foods that contain soy. "It's not that soy is a major contributor of nutrients in most American diets, but it's found in a huge array of foods that someone on a soy-restricted diet must avoid," says Celide Koerner, R.D., a nutrition research manager at Johns Hopkins Hospital in Baltimore who counsels families about allergies and nutrition. "There's soy flour in breads. And it shows up as flavoring in many foods because soy protein is a

POLLEN ALLERGY?
Watch What You Eat

Does ragweed season find you in a state of sneezy, stuffy, teary-eyed misery? Then watch your reaction to bananas, melons and even crunchy sunflower seeds and that soothing cup of chamomile tea.

Pollen allergies sensitize some people to specific foods—a phenomenon called cross-reactivity (also known as oral allergy syndrome.) The foods in question contain a substance that your body mistakes for allergens in pollen. Typical symptoms include itching or swelling of the lips, tongue, throat or roof of the mouth.

Women who are allergic to ragweed pollen may be allergic to bananas, watermelon, cantaloupe, honeydew melon, chamomile tea and sunflower seeds. A person who is allergic to birch pollen may cross-react with apples, carrots, hazelnuts or potatoes.

"It's a peculiar phenomenon," says Paul A. Greenberger, M.D., an allergist-immunologist and professor of medicine at Northwestern University Medical School in Chicago. Symptoms usually begin 5 to 30 minutes after eating the offending food and usually subside without treatment, rarely progressing to the life-threatening stages that are possible with other food allergies.

"Most of the time, cross-reactions are fairly minor," says Dean Metcalfe, M.D., head of the Allergic Diseases Section of the National Institute of Allergy and Infectious Diseases at the National Institutes of Health in Bethesda, Maryland. Taking antihistamines to treat minor allergic reactions to foods can help. But, says Dr. Metcalfe, the only safe course of action is to avoid the offending foods.

The first few times a cross-reaction occurs, it may be hard to tell a minor flare-up from a full-blown allergic reaction. If you experience symptoms and aren't certain what's happening, doctors advise treating any food reaction, including a cross-reaction, as potentially serious. Get to the doctor's office or emergency room. And, Dr. Metcalfe advises, if you carry epinephrine for other allergies, use it.

good way to disperse things like meat flavoring. Cooking from scratch is often the best advice here.''

THINK "SUBSTITUTIONS"

To cope with an allergy or intolerance, try making substitutions, says Koerner. Substitute carob for chocolate in baking; use corn or rice products if you have gluten intolerance and nonwheat flours such as those made from rice, rye, oats, soy, potatoes or corn for baking if your allergy is to wheat. Try corn or rice pasta instead of wheat pasta.

In restaurants, choose simple menu items, without sauces or lots of ingredients, suggests Dr. Greenberger. "You may have to ask the waitress or waiter—or even the manager and chef— what ingredients are used in a dish."

Enjoy the foods allowed. As for the frustration created by having to deal with food allergies, focus on what you *can* eat, not on what you have to give up. Go beyond substituting ingredients for troublesome items and "look for new food ideas," says Koerner. "Think variety," she says.

CARRY YOUR MEDICATION—JUST IN CASE

While avoidance is your first line of defense, vigilance may not be enough, says Dr. Ziering. Women with life-threatening allergies should be prepared for inadvertent exposure by carrying injectable epinephrine—also known as adrenaline—such as EpiPen or Ana-Kit (an anaphylaxis emergency kit) to halt anaphylaxis in the event of an allergic episode. It is available by prescription only.

Act fast. When it comes to treating an allergic reaction, "minutes may be too long, and hours are certainly too long," Dr. Ziering says. "But seconds could be life-saving. If you eat a peanut or a piece of shrimp by mistake, for example, you may not have time to get to the emergency room. If you're at risk, you need to keep this medication close at hand at all times."

Practice, practice, practice. Make sure you know how to use the medication ahead of time, says Dr. Ziering. "Get your doctor to show you what to do, then practice on an orange."

A SHORT COURSE FOR FOOD SLEUTHS

The challenge of coping with a food allergy is watching out for hidden ingredients.

"If you're allergic to peanuts or nuts, you may assume plain chocolate is safe but have a reaction and find out that your candy bar was flavored with peanuts or walnuts," notes Paul A. Greenberger, M.D., an allergist-immunologist and professor of medicine at Northwestern University Medical School in Chicago. So reading food label ingredient lists is vital, doctors say. If you can't eat eggs, for example, you need to watch out for ovalbumin—dried egg whites.

Below you'll find some of the ingredients to avoid if you're on certain kinds of diets. This is only a partial list, and it's continually being updated, but it will help you identify some of the most problematic ingredients when you're reading food labels.

Milk-fee diet: Avoid casein, caseinates, curds, ghee (clarified butter), hydrolysates, lactalbumin, lactoglobulin, nougat and whey—as well as dairy products like yogurt, cheese, butter and cream.

Note: Kosher symbols on product labels can help steer you to safe foods: The letter *D* denotes a dairy product; the word *pareve* usually (but not always) indicates that the product contains no milk or dairy products. Sometimes, says Dr. Greenberger, pareve foods contain the milk derivative casein. If in doubt, call the manufacturer; many provide a toll-free customer service number on the package.

Wheat-free diet: Avoid bran, bulgur, couscous, cereal extract, cracker meal, gluten, high-protein flour, semolina and spelt, as well as all foods with wheat-derived ingredients (such as white vinegar, coffee substitutes made with grains, instant beverages with malt, beer and some baking powder and soy sauces).

Peanut-free diet: Avoid peanuts, mixed nuts and cold-pressed peanut oil. Foods that may contain peanut protein include baked goods, candy, chili, chocolate, egg rolls, marzipan, nougat and foods with hydrolyzed plant or vegetable protein.

Egg-free diet: Avoid albumin, apovitellin, globulin, mayonnaise, ovalbumin, ovomucin and ovomuccoid.

Soy-free diet: Avoid miso, shoyu sauce, tamari, tempeh, textured vegetable protein and tofu.

Carry emergency antihistamines. For less-than-life-threatening food reactions, notes Dr. Ziering, over-the-counter antihistamine allergy pills (such as Actifed or Sudafed Plus) or an inhaler loaded with a relative of adrenaline may be enough. "If someone gets a headache or diarrhea—known as Chinese restaurant syndrome—after eating food prepared with MSG, that may be all she needs," he says.

19

GALLSTONES

A dietary defense against gallbladder trouble

One woman who responded to our *Food and You* survey learned that being overweight put her at risk for gallstones. In hopes of losing weight, Annabelle M. went on a low-calorie liquid diet. Guess what? She got gallstones.

"Excessive overweight increases the risk of gallstones," says Dominic J. Nompleggi, M.D., Ph.D., assistant professor of medicine and surgery and director of nutrition support services at the University of Massachusetts Medical Center in Worcester. "But, ironically, so do rapid-weight-loss diets," he adds.

That's not the only puzzling thing about gallstones. Researchers aren't sure why, but women between the ages of 20 and 60 are twice as likely to develop gallstones as men are. Pregnant women and those who've taken birth control pills or estrogen replacement therapy also get them more often. And by age 75, approximately one woman in three has gallstones, compared to one man in five. Native Americans—particularly members of the Pima tribe—and Mexican Americans are particularly prone to gallstones.

Here's another puzzler: If gallstone attacks lead to removal of the pear-shaped organ tucked beneath your liver, your body will get along just fine without it.

WHY ESKIMO WOMEN DON'T GET GALLSTONES

Researchers at Johns Hopkins Hospital in Baltimore are finding that omega-3 fatty acids—a type of dietary fat found in cold-water fish like Atlantic herring, anchovies, salmon and sardines—seem to put the brakes on gallbladder trouble.

In this study, 17 people scheduled for gallbladder surgery, the majority of whom were women, took fish-oil capsules. After 14 days, doctors found that the gallstone-forming crystals in their bile formed more slowly. Earlier studies had produced similar results.

"One of our clues was that Eskimos, who eat a lot of fish, get few gallstones, even though they are genetically similar to Native Americans in the Southwest who are prone to gallstones," says Henry A. Pitt, M.D., director of the Gallstone and Biliary Disease Center at Johns Hopkins University, who was one of the fish-oil researchers.

Dr. Pitt says it's too soon to make firm diet recommendations for women at risk for gallstones. "But my personal feeling is that fish oil is good for you," he says.

How much fish oil? People in Dr. Pitt's study took 960 milligrams of omega-3 fatty acids three times a day, or a total of 2,880 milligrams per day. "For people who typically take fish oil, that amount isn't unusual," says Dr. Pitt.

Eating fish would work just as well as taking fish oil, he says. Six ounces of salmon, for example, supplies 2,900 milligrams of omega-3's.

"The gallbladder concentrates and sends bile to the small intestine for digesting food," says Dr. Nompleggi. "But your liver also constantly secretes bile. It's usually plenty to meet digestive needs." If you're worried about gallstones, read on.

THE SILENCE OF THE STONES

As big as a golf ball or as small as the period at the end of this sentence, most gallstones are "silent," causing no pain and needing no treatment.

Most are made of cholesterol in the bile itself, growing from tiny cholesterol crystals much the same way pearls "grow" inside oysters, says James E. Everhart, M.D., of the Division of Digestive Diseases and Nutrition at the National Institute of Diabetes and Digestive and Kidney Diseases, part of the National Institutes of Health in Bethesda, Maryland. (About 20 percent of gallstones develop from conditions such as cirrhosis of the liver or hereditary blood cell disorders such as sickle cell anemia.)

When is a gallstone painful? When it lodges in the duct between the liver and the small intestine. Although pain sometimes occurs in the upper abdomen, it is often felt between the shoulder blades. Once pain is persistent, surgery is usually the only recourse.

Short of that, experts say there are steps you can take to lower the risk or avoid a painful attack.

A WEIGHT-LOSS PLAN YOUR GALLBLADDER WILL LOVE

So back to our original paradox: Being overweight puts you at risk for gallstones, but losing weight does, too. Here's what doctors suggest.

Don't starve yourself. "Studies show that people on very low calorie liquid diets, who get about 520 calories a day, have a 10 to 25 percent chance of developing gallstones," says Dr. Nompleggi. Keeping your daily intake above 1,000 or 1,200 calories helps lower the risk, he says.

Eat small, frequent meals. "People who don't eat anything from, say, dinner until lunch the next day are at higher risk for gallstones," says Dr. Everhart. "Not eating for 14 hours can be a problem." The solution? Have three well-spaced meals during the day or divide lunch into two mini-meals if you plan a late dinner.

Avoid yo-yo dieting. Once you've lost weight, keep it off. "Huge weight swings aren't good," says Henry Pitt, M.D., director of the Gallstone and Biliary Disease Center at Johns Hopkins University in Baltimore. "Gaining and losing weight, over and over again, is clearly a risk factor for gallstones."

Lower the fat. Following the same meal plan recommended to combat heart disease may help prevent gallbladder trouble, say doctors. ''I personally believe that high-calorie, high-fat diets do cause gallstones, and low-calorie, low-fat diets are part of the formula for prevention,'' says Dr. Pitt.

''People with high serum triglycerides (a measure of blood fats) seem to get more gallstones,'' notes Dr. Everhart. It's worth keeping fat to less than 30 percent of your daily calories. It's also good advice if you already have gallstones: A large, fatty meal could stimulate a gallbladder attack, notes Dr. Nompleggi.

Have a little oil. Notice that doctors don't advise eliminating every gram of fat. Your gallbladder needs about ten grams of fat—about the amount found in two teaspoons of olive oil—to contract after a meal, says Dr. Everhart. With less fat, bile may accumulate, creating the perfect growing conditions for gallstones. Consuming ten grams of fat per meal ensures that your gallbladder will keep working and adds only about 270 calories a day, notes Dr. Everhart.

But if you've had a gallstone attack and your doctor has scheduled surgery, you will most likely be advised to avoid all fat until after the operation, says Dr. Nompleggi. ''Fat causes the gallbladder to contract,'' he says. Those contractions could lead to another attack.

Focus on fiber. ''If there's one dietary factor that can prevent gallstones, evidence suggests it's fiber,'' says Dr. Everhart. Water-soluble fiber, the kind found in beans and fruit, has the most benefit. Increasing your daily dose of fiber to between 20 and 35 grams, the amount recommended by the American Dietetic Association, may help.

20

HEART DISEASE

An artery-clearing diet for women

Picture a woman at risk for heart disease, and you'd never picture Lois H., one of the women who responded to our *Food and You* survey.

She's slim and vibrant, her skin glows and her eyes sparkle. At 49, Lois looks more like 40. Yet five years ago, this executive assistant for a large media company learned her family's history of heart trouble was catching up with her.

"My mother had high blood pressure and clogged arteries, and my aunt had high blood pressure," Lois told us. "My father died of a massive heart attack at 51. When I found out I had outrageously high blood pressure and my cholesterol was over 200, it was time to make changes."

Out went butter, most red meat and whole-fat cheeses. "But I also managed to stick to the cuisines of my heritage," says Lois. "I started to cook with olive oil exclusively, plus low-fat mozzarella and low-fat ricotta cheese."

More fruit, vegetables and bean dishes appeared on Lois's dinner table. The results? Thanks to her new way of eating (and regular exercise), Lois's cholesterol and blood pressure are back within healthy limits.

PAY ATTENTION TO HEART HEALTH

Once women and their doctors thought only men had to worry about heart disease. But the truth is, cardiovascular disease kills ten times more women than breast cancer, making it the leading cause of death among adult women in the United States. Yet in one Gallup poll, 80 percent of women surveyed didn't know that. No wonder the American Heart Association (AHA) calls heart disease among women the "silent epidemic."

"Coronary heart disease does not discriminate against women," notes Marianne J. Legato, M.D., associate professor of clinical medicine at Columbia University in New York City. But certain risk factors make some women more susceptible.

Do you smoke? Half of all heart disease among women ages 30 to 55 is related to cigarette puffing. If you smoke *and* take oral contraceptives, your risk of a heart attack is 40 times higher. "Quitting is the best thing you can do for yourself," says Dr. Legato.

Are you overweight? Tipping the scales 30 percent or more above your ideal weight triples the risk of heart disease, says JoAnn E. Manson, M.D., associate professor of medicine at Harvard Medical School, co-director of women's health at Brigham and Women's Hospital in Boston and co-principal investigator of the cardiovascular component of the Harvard University Nurses' Health Study (an ongoing study of 115,000 women considered a landmark source of evidence regarding women's health). Generally, a weight gain of 20 or more pounds by the time you reach your middle years doubles your risk, she says. And researchers have concluded that carrying fat around your waist is more of a risk factor than wearing it on your hips.

Do you have high blood pressure? In one study, the risk of fatal heart disease was ten times higher among women who had high blood pressure than in women who did not.

Do you have high cholesterol? Total cholesterol readings over 200 and high-density lipoprotein (HDL, the "good" kind) levels under 45 are significant risk factors for heart disease in women, says Dr. Legato.

Do you have diabetes? This disorder raises a woman's risk of heart disease fivefold or more.

Did your mother or father have heart disease before age 60? If so, your risk of following in their footsteps is 2.8 times higher, according to research.

Have you reached menopause? Before menopause, estrogen bestows some protection from heart disease. It prevents clogging of the arteries—in part because circulating estrogen keeps "good" HDL levels high and "bad" low-density lipoproteins (LDL) low. Some studies have shown estrogen replacement therapy following menopause may lower the risk of heart attack by one-third to one-half.

"Waiting until you're at high risk to worry about heart disease is not a good idea," says Margo A. Denke, M.D., associate professor of internal medicine at the Center for Human Nutrition at the University of Texas Southwestern Medical Center at Dallas and a member of the AHA's Nutrition Committee. "Heart disease is a 40-year process. We have plenty of time to work on preventing it."

FIRST, FINESSE FAT

Butter on your toast. Grilled cheese for lunch. Pizza and a half-pint of premium ice cream for dinner. Ever wonder where all that excess fat goes?

Straight into your bloodstream.

For most women, high intake of dietary fat is an important cause of heart disease. Too much fat—especially saturated fat—tends to raise blood levels of cholesterol. The higher your total cholesterol, the more likely it is that fats will build up inside artery walls. Superimposed on an inherited tendency to overproduce cholesterol, a high-fat diet amplifies the risk.

So you should eliminate all fat, right? Well, not exactly.

"Women need some fat in their diets and should keep fat intake at 25 to 30 percent of calories," says Dr. Legato. "If you restrict fat more than that, levels of HDL cholesterol will fall along with total cholesterol."

This beneficial HDL may keep arteries clear by escorting fat to the liver, where it is then passed out of the body. That's why an HDL reading of 60 or better is considered protective, and a reading below 45 is a risk factor for heart disease, Dr. Denke says.

"You still have to watch total cholesterol," says Dr. Legato. "Readings over 200 can mean higher risk. But you also have to look at the HDL." Your best heart-health strategy?

Cut saturated fats. Animal fats—like fatty meats and butter, cheese or other whole-milk products, as well as palm and coconut oils, are very high in saturated fat. So minimizing your intake of foods high in saturated fats is the most important dietary step you can take, says Dr. Denke. Limiting saturated fat intake to no more than 7 percent of total daily calories reduces total cholesterol as well as the LDL cholesterol that tends to clog arteries.

"If you don't cut back on saturated fats, you cannot improve your cholesterol levels," says Dr. Denke.

Choose unsaturated fats. Meet as much as possible of your fat quotient with unsaturated varieties like olive oil, canola oil and corn oil, suggests Alice Lichtenstein, D.Sc., associate professor and research scientist at the Jean Mayer USDA Human Nutrition Research Center on Aging at Tufts University in Boston.

Researchers once thought that oils high in monounsaturated fats—like olive and canola oils—did a better job than oils high in polyunsaturated fats—like corn, sunflower and safflower oils—at protecting or enhancing HDL levels, says Dr. Lichtenstein. "But now it seems they all do about the same job," she says. "It's best to use a variety."

In a Tufts University study that compared the cholesterol levels of 15 older women and men who consumed moderate amounts of olive, canola or corn oil, researchers found almost no difference in the way the oil affected HDL cholesterol, notes. Dr. Lichtenstein, who was the lead researcher for the study.

Avoid stick margarine. Hydrogenation, the process that hardens vegetable oils into stick margarine or solid vegetable shortening, creates substances known as trans-fatty acids and changes unsaturated into saturated fatty acids. When compared to liquid oils, solid fats raise total cholesterol and LDL, according to a Tufts study. "The softer the fat, the better it is for you," says Dr. Lichtenstein, who also headed this study. "So avoid fried fast food and prepared baked goods—75 per-

FOODS YOUR HEART WILL LOVE

Here are 20 foods with the attributes doctors say are best for preventing heart disease. The reason these foods make the grade? Each one has no cholesterol and is:

- High in fiber—effective in lowering cholesterol.
- Low in fat—to reduce total cholesterol and "bad" LDL cholesterol.
- Packed with antioxidants—nutrients that intercept LDL cholesterol before it can build up in your arteries.

Note: Beta-carotene is usually expressed on food charts in units of vitamin A, the form it—and other carotenoids—takes after being digested. The beta-carotene values given below have been calculated from the vitamin A values for the foods.

1. **Blackberries:** One cup contains 7.2 grams of fiber, 0.6 gram of fat, 30.2 milligrams of vitamin C and 0.9 milligram of alpha-tocopherol vitamin E.
2. **Chick-peas:** A half-cup, canned, contains 7 grams of fiber, 1.4 grams of fat and 4.6 milligrams of vitamin C.
3. **Green peas:** A half-cup, boiled, contains 2.4 grams of fiber, 0.2 gram of fat and 11.4 milligrams of vitamin C.
4. **Passionfruit:** Five medium fruits (about 3½ ounces) contain 1.7 grams of fiber, 0.7 gram of fat, 30 milligrams of vitamin C and 233.1 international units of vitamin A (0.1 milligram of beta-carotene).
5. **Raspberries:** One cup contains 6 grams of fiber, 0.7 gram of fat and 30.7 milligrams of vitamin C.
6. **Apricots:** Three fresh fruits contain 2 grams of fiber, 0.4 gram of fat, 110.6 milligrams of vitamin C and 921.4 international units of vitamin A (0.6 milligram of beta-carotene).
7. **Apple:** One medium fruit (about 5 ounces) contains 3 grams of fiber, 0.5 gram of fat, 7.9 milligrams of vitamin C and 0.8 milligram of alpha-tocopherol vitamin E.

8. **Red bell peppers:** A half-cup, chopped, contains 0.8 gram of fiber, 0.1 gram of fat, 95 milligrams of vitamin C and 949.1 international units of vitamin A (0.6 milligram of beta-carotene).

9. **Papaya:** Half a fruit contains 2.6 grams of fiber, 0.2 gram of fat and 93.9 milligrams of vitamin C.

10. **Black currants:** One cup contains 4.4 grams of fiber, 0.5 gram of fat, 202.7 milligrams of vitamin C and 1.1 milligrams of alpha-tocopherol vitamin E.

11. **Cantaloupe:** One cup of cubes contains 1.3 grams of fiber, 0.5 gram of fat, 67.5 milligrams of vitamin C and 1,715.6 international units of vitamin A (1 milligram of beta-carotene).

12. **Broccoli:** A half-cup, chopped and cooked, contains 2 grams of fiber, 0.3 gram of fat, 58.2 milligrams of vitamin C and 361 international units of vitamin A (0.2 milligram of beta-carotene).

13. **Brussels sprouts:** A half-cup, boiled, contains 3.4 grams of fiber, 0.4 gram of fat, 48.4 grams vitamin C and 187.1 international units of vitamin A (0.1 milligram of beta-carotene).

14. **Grapefruit:** Half a pink or red grapefruit contains 0.7 gram of fiber, 0.1 gram of fat and 46.9 milligrams of vitamin C.

15. **Carrots:** 1 carrot (about 2½ ounces) contains 2.3 grams of fiber, 0.1 gram of fat, 6.7 milligrams of vitamin C and 6,744.6 international units of vitamin A (4 milligrams of beta-carotene).

16. **Spinach:** A half-cup, boiled, contains 2 grams of fiber, 0.2 gram of fat, 8.8 milligrams of vitamin C and 2,454.5 international units of vitamin A (1.5 milligrams of beta-carotene).

17. **Butternut squash:** A half-cup of baked cubes contains 2.9 grams of fiber, 0.1 gram of fat, 15 milligrams of vitamin C and 2,377.6 international units of vitamin A (1.4 milligrams of beta-carotene).

18. **Sweet potato:** One potato (about 4 ounces), baked, contains 3.4 grams of fiber, 0.1 gram of fat, 28 milligrams of vitamin C and 8,285 international units of vitamin A (5 milligrams of beta-carotene).

19. **Strawberries:** One cup contains 3.9 grams of fiber, 0.6 gram of fat and 84.5 milligrams of vitamin C.
20. **Wheat germ:** One-quarter cup, toasted, contains 3.7 grams of fiber, 3 grams of fat and 4 milligrams of alpha-tocopherol vitamin E.

cent of the trans-fatty acids in our diet comes from sources like this. Also, sauté in oil (not margarine), brush oil (not margarine) on your garlic bread and choose margarine in a squeeze bottle or tub (not stick form)."

Lose weight. For every ten pounds you lose, you can raise your good HDL levels by two to three points, says Dr. Denke.

Exercise. Aerobic activity four days a week for at least 40 minutes can increase HDL levels by two to four points, say Dr. Legato and Dr. Denke.

THE JOYS OF (SOLUBLE) FIBER

Soluble fiber, which is found in foods like oat bran, oatmeal, beans and pectin-rich fruit, can help lower blood cholesterol as part of a low-fat diet. Lowering your intake of saturated fat and cholesterol is the most powerful way to reduce blood cholesterol, but adding soluble fiber can help reduce it even further, says Linda Van Horn, R.D., Ph.D., professor of preventive medicine at Northwestern University Medical School in Chicago and an oat bran researcher. One study of people with high cholesterol, for example, found that eating as little as a quarter-cup to a half-cup of cooked beans daily cut total cholesterol by 15 to 23 percent in just three weeks.

"All fiber is not created equal," says Dr. Van Horn. "The insoluble fiber found in vegetables or grains (like wheat) does not seem to reduce cholesterol levels but is important for maintaining good health. Soluble fiber, found in oat bran, oatmeal, barley and beans, has been shown to be effective in lowering LDL cholesterol."

How does it work? It's not certain, but some researchers theorize that soluble fiber may simply sweep fat quickly out of the intestines, before it is absorbed. Or it may indirectly aid in the efficient production of bile, a cholesterol-laden digestive juice, so that your body does not produce extra cholesterol.

"On average, two to three servings of soluble fiber a day, as part of a low-fat diet, are really effective in lowering cholesterol," Dr. Van Horn says. Here are some of his suggestions for easy ways to up your soluble fiber quotient.

Try oatmeal with fruit and skim milk or a low-fat oat bran muffin for breakfast. Or enjoy Dr. Van Horn's oat-powered pancakes: Use low-fat pancake mix and substitute oatmeal for half the mix called for in the instructions, mix with egg whites (instead of whole eggs), skim milk and cinnamon, then cook in a nonstick griddle or pan. For extra fiber, top your pancakes with sliced pears, raisins or chopped prunes.

Extend with oat bran. Add oat bran or oatmeal to meat loaf, casseroles and other recipes that call for flour.

Baking? Substitute some oat flour for one-fourth to one-half of the wheat flour in muffins—but if you use one-half or more, you might want to add a small amount of gluten, available at health food stores. "Experiment with the amount," Dr. Van Horn says. "You need gluten for elasticity and to help the dough rise, since oat flour does not have that ability."

Choose chick-peas. At the salad bar, sprinkle chick-peas (garbanzo beans) liberally on your fixings. Or make hummus, a dip of mashed chick-peas and garlic that is very tasty as a spread on pita bread or nonfat crackers.

Keep cans on hand. Stock up on canned chick-peas and pinto, white, navy or black beans. Add a half-cup (drained) to soups.

Befriend barley. Add regular or quick-cooking barley to soups and stews, says Dr. Van Horn. This versatile but underutilized grain can also be used as a pilaf or mixed with rice as a side dish or salad.

Go meatless. At dinner, try low-fat bean dishes such as red lentil soup, vegetarian chili with kidney and white beans, black bean soup or red beans in spicy tomato sauce over brown rice, says Dr. Van Horn. Or substitute canned beans for beef in your favorite stew recipe. For a quick meal, spoon hot beans onto soft flour tortillas, top with salsa and a little shredded low-fat cheese and serve.

Snack on fruit. For midday or late-night snacks, grab an apple, pear, orange, grapefruit or a few prunes.

PROTECT YOUR ARTERIES WITH ANTIOXIDANTS

When Harvard University researchers compared the diets of 87,245 nurses, they saw that women who consumed the most vitamin E had a 34 percent lower risk of heart disease. Risk fell 22 percent for those who consumed the most beta-carotene, the substance that gives carrots, squash, broccoli, melons and spinach their rich orange or green hue. The risk dropped 20 percent among those whose diets contained the most vitamin C, found in citrus fruits, peppers, strawberries, tomatoes and cantaloupe. Nurses who ate the most of these antioxidant nutrients (and others) had a 46 percent lower risk of heart disease.

What is it about E, C and beta-carotene that makes them so protective for women? This trio of nutrients is among the most abundant dietary antioxidants—a family of natural substances that may protect LDL from damage by oxidation, which in turn can lead it to build up as fatty streaks in your arteries.

Getting antioxidants from foods like carrots, oranges, spinach and cereal grains is best, notes Michael Gaziano, M.D., director of cardiovascular epidemiology at Brigham and Women's Hospital in Boston. He suggests eating five servings a day.

"The data consistently shows that those who consume high amounts of fruits and vegetables have less heart disease," says Dr. Gaziano. "What's more, eating plenty of fruits and vegetables automatically supplies you with dozens of other antioxidants that show promise as protective nutrients."

Here's what researchers suggest to ensure you're getting enough of these antioxidants.

Make sure of vegetable oils, cereal grains, nuts and green vegetables. They're the best sources of vitamin E. Limit vegetable oils to less than three tablespoons a day, including what you use in cooking.

Load up on carrots, squash, melons, spinach and broccoli. Green, yellow and orange fruits and vegetables provide beta-carotene. And the darker or deeper the color, the better.

Seek out citrus fruit, cranberry juice, strawberries, guava, papaya, kiwifruit and black currants. They're tasty sources of vitamin C.

EDIBLE PROTECTION

Nutrition researchers in the Netherlands are discovering that some flavonoids—natural substances found in fruits and vegetables—may lower heart disease risk by a third. How? These antioxidant compounds may reduce the ''stickiness'' of blood platelets, making them less likely to clump together into clots and block blood flow to the heart. In laboratory studies, flavonoids scoop up free radicals—highly reactive forms of oxygen that attack LDL cholesterol and can lead to artery-clogging plaque. Fewer free radicals may mean less plaque buildup and less heart disease.

To reap the benefits of these protective flavonoids in foods, researchers offer these suggestions.

Lift a glass of grape juice. Both wine and grape juice contain flavonoids. University of Wisconsin researchers have found that drinking purple grape juice could have the same impact against clogged arteries as drinking red wine.

Crunch an apple, slice an onion, sip some tea. In the Netherlands study, those who drank or ate the most flavonoids, mostly from black tea, apples and onions, had a 32 percent lower risk of heart disease and heart attack. This benefit came from consuming about four cups of tea, an apple and about a one-eighth cup of onions each day.

OTHER HEART-HEALTHY FOODS

Some of the oldest and humblest foods known to woman (and man) offer surprising powers of protection against heart disease, according to researchers.

Take a garlic clove a day. Several studies on the impact of a daily dose of garlic on women and men with high cholesterol indicate that the equivalent of one-half to one clove of garlic can significantly lower total cholesterol by at least 9 percent.

Add a little soy. At the University of Illinois, a study of 26 volunteers with mildly high cholesterol levels found that those who ate baked goods fortified with soy protein, roughly a quarter-cup a day, lowered both their total cholesterol and LDL levels by about 12 percent. A plus: HDL did not drop.

Doctors and researchers agree: Loading your plate with fruits, vegetables and beans—plus trimming the fat and raising the fiber quotient at breakfast, lunch and dinner—are important heart-healthy changes that can cut a woman's risk of heart disease.

"A sensible low-fat diet with lots of fiber, plus aerobic exercise, can significantly improve cholesterol readings and cut a woman's chances of heart disease," says Dr. Legato. "The only thing more important is quitting smoking."

21

HEMORRHOIDS

Natural relief for straining and pain

Uh-oh. There's a scarlet splotch on the toilet paper and searing pain when you move your bowels.

You've joined the hemorrhoid club—and you have plenty of company. By age 50, about half of all Americans have hemorrhoids. And women often receive an early introduction to annoying hemorrhoidal troubles. Why? Pregnancy and childbirth put enormous pressure on the delicate webbing of blood vessels that cushion the anus. Pressure and hormonal changes make hemorrhoids happen.

"Usually hemorrhoids go away after childbirth because the pressure drops," says Amnon Sonnenberg, M.D., professor of medicine in the Division of Gastroenterology at the University of New Mexico in Albuquerque and a staff physician at the Veterans Affairs Medical Center there. "Meanwhile, about all you can do is try to make yourself comfortable."

Ice packs, warm baths or a film of petroleum jelly can help soothe the irritation.

NOT TO BE TAKEN LIGHTLY

Pregnancy aside, diet-related habits could contribute to hemorrhoids, although the exact mechanism that leads to their development still eludes researchers. They suspect that straining for a bowel movement, spending too much time sitting on the toilet and excessive overweight put stress on blood vessels inside the rectum and under the skin around the anus. When these vessels swell—much like varicose veins do in your legs—you have hemorrhoids. The swollen vessels may bleed, itch, hurt and even protrude.

Surprisingly, diarrhea can also induce hemorrhoids, according to a study conducted in Milwaukee. "When muscles contract in the anus, blood flow out of the hemorrhoidal cushions is restricted and blood vessels swell," says Dr. Sonnenberg, who was one of the researchers. "If you have hemorrhoids and frequent diarrhea, I would look at the cause of the diarrhea and try to correct it."

The biggest complaint with hemorrhoids? Bleeding. Next come itching and pain. "Rectal bleeding should be taken very seriously," Dr. Sonnenberg says. "It could be a sign of colon cancer, particularly in anyone older than 50."

See a doctor if you discover blood after a bowel movement. If you do in fact have hemorrhoids, a fiber-charged diet plan and some comfort measures can help (and may even avoid the need for surgery).

SOFTER STOOLS, THE NATURAL WAY

Once hemorrhoids appear, diet can play a role in easing the discomfort, for pregnant and nonpregnant women alike. Here's how.

Soften up. Hard stools and straining to relieve constipation can scratch, scrape and push against tender, swollen veins, says Dr. Sonnenberg. You can try to keep your hemorrhoids "quiet" by following an anticonstipation meal plan, he adds.

Choose fresh fruits, leafy vegetables and whole-grain breads and cereals, especially those containing bran, and aim to eat 25 to 35 grams of fiber a day. Reading food labels will help you tally your fiber total.

Wash it down with water. Hard, dry stools are the bane

HEMORRHOID HELPERS

By eating foods rich in soluble fiber at breakfast, lunch or dinner, you can add a cushion of comfort between hemorrhoids and painful bowel movements.

"There's no question that avoiding constipation is important if you have painful hemorrhoids," says Pittsburgh dietitian Pat H. Harper, R. D., spokeswoman for the American Dietetic Association. "Eating more insoluble fiber will help to avoid constipation. But insoluble fiber won't make your stools really soft or slippery. For that, you need soluble fiber (the kind found in oatmeal)."

How does it work?

"Think about the last time you cooked oatmeal," says Harper. "In water, it becomes gel-like. That's what it does in your body, too."

Most fiber-packed foods contain both soluble and insoluble fiber, but some have more soluble fiber than others. To conquer constipation and hard, scratchy stools at the same time, gradually increase your fiber intake to a total of 25 grams a day and include several helpings of rich sources of soluble fiber.

Nutrition labels list the fiber content of individual foods but do not list soluble and insoluble fiber separately. Here are the best stool-softening sources of predominantly soluble fiber.

- Quaker Oat Bran cereal: 3 grams of soluble fiber per 1¼ cup
- Cooked oatmeal: 2 grams per cup
- Cooked pearl barley: 1.8 grams in ¾ cup
- Canned baked beans: 2.6 grams in ½ cup
- Chick-peas: 1.3 grams per ½ cup

Oranges, kiwifruit, fresh and dried figs, prunes, strawberries, acorn squash and potatoes are also good sources of soluble fiber.

"Add fiber gradually, each week adding another one or two servings a day, to avoid gas pain and discomfort," says Harper. "There's no formula for how much soluble fiber an individual needs to correct her particular regularity problem. Experiment with the number of servings until you get results."

of anyone who has hemorrhoids. So remember to down six to eight glasses of fluid (but not alcohol or coffee) daily. Water helps "bulk up" all that fiber, creating soft, bulky stools that will slip easily from the body.

Think twice about spice. Love the way fiery foods excite your palate? Well, hot peppers and other spicy favorites may also burn irritated hemorrhoids—an experience you're guaranteed *not* to enjoy. If your nether parts are tender, go easy on hot stuff, suggests William Ruderman, M.D., chairperson of the Department of Gastroenterology at the Cleveland Clinic–Florida in Fort Lauderdale.

22

HIGH BLOOD PRESSURE

Minerals take the "hyper" out of hypertension

When Doretha B. was 12, her mother threw out the kitchen salt shaker.

"She'd just been hospitalized with high blood pressure, and she was only in her early forties," says Doretha, a 26-year-old receptionist in New York City who responded to our *Food and You* survey. "Her doctor advised cutting out salt to control her blood pressure. When my mother came home, the household went salt-free."

Today Doretha's doctor might prescribe a diet high in minerals—potassium, magnesium and calcium—in addition to (or possibly in place of) salt restriction.

Research indicates that this trio of minerals can relax blood vessels and play a crucial role in controlling—and preventing—high blood pressure, or hypertension, says David McCarron, M.D., head of the Division of Nephrology, Hypertension and Clinical Pharmacology and director of the Clinical Nutrition Research Unit (part of the National Institute of Diabetes and Digestive and Kidney Diseases) at Oregon Health Sciences University in Portland.

These three minerals help blood vessels relax and open up, giving your blood more space and thereby reducing the pressure, Dr. McCarron says. "If your blood vessels clamp down and won't open wider," he says, "blood pressure goes up.

"When mineral intake is balanced, salt becomes a nonissue," says Dr. McCarron. "In my view, compared to other nutritional factors, salt restriction is much less important than it was ten years ago."

So why have doctors told patients for decades to throw out their salt shakers? "We didn't know the whole story," says Dr. McCarron. The "whole story" involves genetics, hormones and diet.

EASILY PREVENTABLE

One out of ten women between 35 and 44 has high blood pressure. Genetics can predispose a woman to it: African American, Hispanic and Asian women are at higher risk than White women, says Dr. McCarron. Taking birth control pills leaves you more susceptible. But for all women, the risk rises after menopause, when levels of estrogen—a reproductive hormone that protects a woman's cardiovascular system—decline. By age 55, one in four of us has high blood pressure.

High blood pressure is nothing to be taken lightly. It makes your heart work harder delivering blood to muscles and vital organs from the top of your head to the tip of your toes. It's no surprise, then, that women with uncontrolled high blood pressure are 12 times more likely to suffer a stroke, 6 times more likely to have a heart attack and 5 times more likely to die of congestive heart failure. It also increases the risk of kidney failure.

The benefits of controlling your blood pressure, on the other hand, are pretty enticing. "Controlling these factors can save you from expensive blood pressure medication," says John M. Flack, M.D., medical director of the Hypertension Clinic at Bowman-Gray School of Medicine at Wake Forest University in Winston-Salem, North Carolina. "It can also preserve your quality of life. And you can do something about it."

KNOW YOUR NUMBERS

The problem is, you may have high blood pressure and not know it, says Dr. Flack. So it's a good idea to have your blood pressure checked regularly.

Measuring blood pressure is easy: The doctor or nurse slips a rubber cuff around your upper arm, inflates it to briefly cut off the blood flow to the artery and then deflates it while listening with a stethoscope and noting when your pulse starts again and when it can no longer be heard. The result? Two numerical readings, both measured in millimeters of mercury (abbreviated mm/Hg).

The first reading measures how hard your heart pumps to push blood through your arteries—the systolic pressure. The second reading measures the pressure of the blood on artery walls between heartbeats—the diastolic pressure. Together, the two readings quantify your blood pressure.

"In general, doctors have said that readings lower than 140 over 90 mm/Hg are healthy," says Dr. Flack. "But we're finding that a blood pressure reading closer to 120 or 130 over 80 or so is better." Also, at one time, doctors felt that of the two readings, the lower number was more critical. But further research indicates the systolic reading is probably more important.

If your blood pressure is high, don't panic. Paying attention to your mineral and alcohol intake, weight, exercise and diet can help, say physicians.

CLOSING THE MINERAL GAP

Where to start? First, close the mineral gap. "Most women are getting so much less than the recommended amounts of important minerals that just getting enough should help," says Dr. McCarron.

Indeed. Between age 30 and 50, women need 1,000 to 1,500 milligrams of calcium a day, but most women that age get only about 720 milligrams. We need 280 milligrams of magnesium but take in roughly 250 milligrams. As for potassium, we may need up to 3,500 milligrams daily, yet we get just 2,430.

Boosting your mineral quotient can be as easy as milk,

beans and greens. Here's how the experts say you can close the gap.

Consider calcium. In the Harvard University Nurses' Health Study (an ongoing study of 115,000 women considered a landmark source of evidence regarding women's health), researchers found that women who said they got 800 milligrams of calcium a day enjoyed a significantly lower risk of high blood pressure than women who reported an intake of 400 milligrams.

Another study showed that the risk of pregnancy-induced hypertension may be reduced 40 to 50 percent for mothers-to-be who take 1,500 to 2,000 milligrams of calcium a day.

By far, nonfat dairy products are the richest dietary source of calcium. Skim milk on your cereal. Nonfat yogurt at lunch. Low-fat cheese sprinkled on pasta. It's easy to keep the calorie count low and the calcium count high, says Dr. McCarron, and with a double benefit: You'll help prevent osteoporosis as well as high blood pressure.

If you drink coffee, make it café latte. "Women don't realize that a cup of latte from an espresso stand is mostly milk," says Dr. McCarron. "You could get a whole serving that way!"

Shop for magnesium-rich foods. A European study of 91 women with mild to moderate high blood pressure found that magnesium supplements lowered their blood pressure. It's best to get your magnesium from foods, says Dr. McCarron. Broccoli, a baked potato with the skin and lima beans are especially rich sources. Whole grains, green leafy vegetables, nuts, seeds and cooked dry beans are other reliable sources.

Add potassium. Potatoes and beans do double duty—they also contain potassium. According to the National Institutes of Health (NIH), getting enough potassium—along with cutting salt and losing weight—may be an optimal strategy for preventing high blood pressure.

While you're at it, have a banana, a honeydew or some prunes. Eating a potato or a half-cup of lima beans, a banana, a cup of nonfat yogurt and two cups of honeydew melon cubes and drinking an eight-ounce glass of prune juice would enable you to reach the optimal intake of 3,500 milligrams of potassium a day.

PRODUCE UP, BLOOD PRESSURE DOWN

From oranges and red peppers to brussels sprouts and cantaloupes, vitamin C-packed fruits and vegetables have the power to help keep your blood pressure in check.

Comparing the diets of 410 volunteers, researcher Paul F. Jacques, D.Sc., assistant professor of nutrition at Tufts University in Boston and an epidemiologist at the Jean Mayer USDA Human Nutrition Research Center on Aging at Tufts, found that those who consumed the least vitamin C had up to double the risk of high blood pressure. In contrast, those who consumed 60 to 120 milligrams a day—up to twice the Daily Value of 60 milligrams—had blood pressure readings 6 to 7 percent lower. Consuming more than 120 milligrams did not further improve blood pressure readings, says Dr. Jacques.

Researchers at the Medical College of Georgia in Augusta found a similar link when they measured blood levels of vitamin C in 168 women and men. The higher the vitamin C intake, the lower the blood pressure.

Fresh produce may be better for blood pressure than taking a vitamin C supplement, says Dr. Jacques. "More is better," he says. "The benefit to blood pressure could be coming from something else in a vitamin C-rich diet," he says. "It could be other nutrients such as potassium. Also, people who eat a lot of fruit and vegetables tend to eat less fat and less sodium and to increase the fiber and nutrient density of their food. That's why eating a variety of fruits and vegetables is the best idea."

Best sources of vitamin C include black currants, citrus fruits, strawberries, kiwifruit and broccoli. Dr. Jacques suggests eating at least five servings of fruit and vegetables a day.

Step up to the scale and away from the bar. In addition to these dietary strategies, experts advise people with high blood pressure to watch their weight, cut back on alcohol consumption and step up their physical activity levels. Losing as little as six to eight pounds, limiting yourself to two alcoholic beverages or less a day and getting regular exercise can all significantly reduce blood pressure.

THE PLACE FOR SALT CUTBACKS

Some experts say a low-sodium diet can lower systolic blood pressure by five to six points—a modest amount but often enough to return mildly elevated blood pressure to normal. And researchers in Australia offer evidence that women may be more sensitive to salt than men. In a study of 66 elderly women and men, the women's systolic blood pressure readings changed about six points when salt levels in their diet were altered, while the men averaged less than a one-point change.

Dr. McCarron says a mineral-poor diet makes women—particularly older women—salt-sensitive. "I would tell a woman with high blood pressure to control her weight, reduce her consumption of alcohol and be sure to eat mineral-rich foods," he says. "Only if the problem persisted for two to three months of using those measures would I look at salt."

Some experts say the best approach pairs low sodium intake with high potassium intake. A Dutch study of 97 women and men with mild to moderate high blood pressure found that those who consumed more potassium and magnesium—and less salt—saw a drop in blood pressure. Eating four times more potassium than sodium helps right the chemical balance in the body cells, says Richard D. Moore, M.D., Ph.D., professor emeritus of biophysics at the State University of New York in Plattsburgh and author of *The High Blood Pressure Solution*.

But a low-salt regimen needn't be bland.

"When you put away the salt shaker and high-salt foods like soy sauce, dill pickles, canned foods and most fast foods, train your taste buds to enjoy other flavors," says Calabasas, California, dietitian Bettye Nowlin, R.D., a spokesperson for the American Dietetic Association.

Substitute fresh for processed foods. If you're cutting down on the sodium (salt) in your diet, this may be all you have to do to cut your sodium intake, says Nowlin. Canned and processed foods contain more sodium than fresh alternatives, says Eva Obarzanek, R.D., Ph.D., a nutritionist at the National Heart, Lung and Blood Institute in Bethesda, Mary-

land. Take canned foods: A half-cup of chopped fresh tomatoes has less than 70 milligrams of salt, while three-quarters
of a cup of canned tomato juice has 660 milligrams. A half-
cup of home-cooked red kidney beans without salt has less
than 2 milligrams, but a half-cup of canned red kidney beans
has 436 milligrams.

As for soups, frozen dinners and other processed foods,
"they contain a large amount of sodium to prolong shelf life,"
says Nowlin. "But you don't need it. If you select fresh foods
and use herbs and spices instead of salt for flavor, your foods
will taste just as good."

Rinse what you can. Authorities at the NIH suggest rinsing
canned foods like beans and tuna to remove some of the salt.

Read every label. The sodium content of a particular type
of staple, like canned tomatoes, may vary widely from brand
to brand. To judge salt content in one serving of a food product, look for "Sodium" and "Percent Daily Value (% Daily
Value)" on the Nutrition Facts panel of the label. You can
also scan the ingredients list for monosodium glutamate and
disodium phosphate, two additional sources of sodium, Nowlin
suggests. Experts recommend a 2,400-milligram sodium limit
for the entire day, she says. Also check the label for phrases
like "no salt added," "sodium-free," and "low-sodium."

Spice it up. Lemon, onion, garlic and peppers, as well as
dried spices, add zing and zest. One caution: Choose onion
powder or garlic powder over sodium-packed seasoned salts,
Nowlin suggests.

Try a salt substitute. Some substitutes are sodium-free and
contain potassium chloride as the primary ingredient. But
products purporting to be "light salt" or "less salt" still have
lots of sodium—as much as 390 milligrams per quarter-
teaspoon.

Desalt the menu. Steer clear of restaurant foods prepared
in the following high-salt styles: pickled, smoked, teriyaki, au
jus, barbecue, in cocktail sauce or with a tomato base, says
Nowlin. "Baked, broiled or steamed foods are better choices,"
she says.

Watch your tap water. If you're counting every milligram
of sodium, you may want to call your local water company
and ask about sodium levels, as some areas may have amounts
exceeding 250 milligrams of sodium per quart. Most water

supplies, however, have less than 20 milligrams per quart. Sodium in water is not usually a big concern unless you use a water softener, which can really boost the sodium level in your water, Dr. Moore says. "If it's too high, consider distilled bottled water for drinking," says Nowlin.

23

HYPOGLYCEMIA

Emergency rations for low blood sugar

Celeste P., one of our *Food and You* survey respondents, told us that when she gets cranky, spacy or impatient, her husband hands her a granola bar or some cheese and crackers. Having a bite to eat seems to work wonders for her disposition.

"It's like taking medicine," says Celeste. "Within five minutes, I feel so much better—alert, even-tempered and able to concentrate."

At one time, Celeste thought she had hypoglycemia, or low blood sugar. But a fasting blood test measured her blood glucose at 90 milligrams per deciliter (mg/dl) of blood—normal, by medical standards—and also ruled out thyroid disease and other possible causes for her symptoms. Through trial and error, Celeste eventually learned to prevent feelings of weakness and light-headedness, which are often associated with low blood sugar.

"I may not have true hypoglycemia," says Celeste. "All I know is, as long as I don't skip meals—or eat a candy bar on an empty stomach—I'm fine."

IS IT REAL?

Lots of women think they have hypoglycemia. Like Celeste, many say they feel better when they follow dietary guidelines customarily prescribed for hypoglycemia—not going without eating for hours and not eating sweets on an empty stomach. Yet few are truly hypoglycemic, says endocrinologist Kay McFarland, M.D., professor of medicine at the University of South Carolina School of Medicine in Columbia.

"Real hypoglycemia is based on three criteria—symptoms like sweating, weakness, trembling and mental fuzziness; blood sugar levels below 50 mg/dl; and relief from the symptoms after eating, when blood sugar levels rise," says Dr. McFarland.

"A lot of times, stress or just feeling anxious can release the body's fight-or-flight hormones," she says. "When that happens, blood sugar can rise somewhat, then drop, making you feel shaky. But it isn't hypoglycemia."

Sometimes just missing a meal can have a similar effect, says John P. Bantle, M.D., associate professor in the Division of Diabetes, Endocrinology and Metabolism of the Department of Medicine at the University of Minnesota in Minneapolis–St. Paul. "I never used to believe this, until it happened to my daughter," says Dr. Bantle. "It's not a disease. It's not hypoglycemia. You just get cranky and irritable and when you eat, you feel better. It can happen to healthy women." But you shouldn't feel shaky every time you miss a meal: If you do, discuss it with your doctor.

Researchers are also discovering that downing the amount of caffeine in several cups of morning coffee or breaking a strict low-calorie diet with a big carbohydrate-rich meal could be associated with symptoms of hypoglycemia.

"For some people who feel hypoglycemic, drinking caffeine may be responsible," says David Kerr, M.D., a hypoglycemia researcher and staff physician at Royal Bournemouth Hospital in Dorset, England.

If your symptoms are bothersome, see a doctor. Thyroid problems, kidney disorders, diabetes, heart trouble, menopause and some antibiotics and drugs like lithium (used to treat manic depression), as well as insulin and birth control pills, can all mimic hypoglycemia.

SO EAT ALREADY

Among doctors, the consensus seems to be that unless you take a blood test and the results show levels below what doctors consider normal, you don't have hypoglycemia. But that doesn't mean you should ignore symptoms that mimic the disease. Some experts believe that wild swings in blood sugar can cause symptoms even in women whose blood glucose levels don't drop into the official hypoglycemia zone. Sometimes a meal plan that evens out the blood sugar highs and lows can bring relief. Here's what doctors recommend.

Mix complex carbs with protein. To help curb the fatigue, mood swings and headaches that can feel like hypoglycemia, doctors advise planning meals around complex carbohydrates like whole-grain breads and cereals and lean proteins like fish and skinless chicken.

"If carbohydrates are consumed along with protein, fiber and some fat in a meal, blood sugar will rise and fall more slowly," says Dr. Bantle. "In contrast, eating pure carbohydrates, like bread, potatoes or sweets, makes blood sugar rise and fall quickly."

Avoid high-sugar meals and snacks. Candy, cake, fruit juice or a sweet breakfast such as syrup-drenched pancakes can raise blood sugar levels, then set off a delayed insulin reaction as your body tries to metabolize all that sweet stuff, says Dr. McFarland. "The insulin helps your cells store the glucose, and then blood sugar levels fall sharply," she says. "For people who get these symptoms, the best thing is to avoid a lot of concentrated sweets on an empty stomach, or at least delay eating sweets until the end of the meal."

"If you have hypoglycemia, try to keep refined carbohydrates to less than 8 percent of your total calories," suggests Fred Hofeldt, M.D., professor of medicine at the University of Colorado Health Sciences Center and chief of endocrinology at Denver General Hospital, both in Denver. On a standard 2,000-calorie diet, that's 160 calories—the equivalent of one cola drink.

Graze. Eating four to six small meals a day can steady blood sugar levels. Eating frequently helps people with reactive hypoglycemia—a type of low blood sugar that occurs when the body reacts to a meal, says Dr. Hofeldt.

SHAKY?
Skip the Caffeine

Eight people at a Yale University research lab sipped caffeinated soda. Within an hour, they all felt dizzy, shaky and light-headed—classic symptoms of hypoglycemia. Yet their blood sugar levels were in the lower range of normal.

"What these people experienced felt just like low blood sugar," says Pierre Fayad, M.D., assistant professor of neurology at the Yale University School of Medicine and co-director of the Yale Vascular Neurology Program, who was a researcher on the study.

Though small, the study may begin to unlock the mystery of why some people feel decidedly hypoglycemic at times, despite normal blood sugar levels. It could also explain the midmorning slump some women feel a few hours after breakfast, says David Kerr, M.D., a hypoglycemia researcher and staff physician at Royal Bournemouth Hospital in Dorset, England, who was a co-investigator in this study.

How? The caffeine—equivalent to two or three cups of drip-brewed coffee—seemed to slow blood flow to the brain. Less blood meant less fuel, leaving the volunteers shaky, weak and mentally fuzzy.

"So if you don't feel so good, consider drinking less coffee, eating something with your coffee or switching to decaf," says Dr. Fayad.

Carry emergency rations. Missing meals, getting hungry and then downing a big lunch or dinner may perpetuate big blood sugar swings. So be prepared. Linda Z., one of the women who responded to our *Food and You* survey, packs a cooler with raw vegetables and sandwiches on whole-wheat bread for long car trips when meal stops are hard to plan. It's her strategy for coping with diagnosed hypoglycemia.

And Linda's strategy makes sense, says Dr. Hofeldt.

"The best approach to hypoglycemia is to try to prevent the symptoms," he says. "That means following a reasonable diet, shifting toward crude carbohydrates rather than refined carbohydrates and eating at least three meals a day."

Watch out for sugar splurges. Drastic calorie-cutting can alter your body's blood sugar regulation and could leave you more susceptible to episodes of hypoglycemia, according to researchers at the Harbor-UCLA Medical Center in Los Angeles. Tracking 13 women on 600-calorie-a-day meal plans, they found that blood sugar plummeted within hours after the women "splurged" on soda and cake with chocolate syrup.

Eat before you exercise. To avoid a slump in energy during your workout, snack on complex carbohydrates—like a bagel, a handful of crackers or a small bowl of sugar-free cereal—within an hour before exercising, suggests William J. Rutherford, Ph.D., assistant professor of physical education at Eastern Kentucky University in Richmond.

"Avoid candy bars, sweets and even fruit—such simple sugars metabolize very quickly and leave you feeling weak," says Dr. Rutherford. "But something like a bagel should give you a steady energy supply."

24

IRRITABLE BOWEL SYNDROME

Foods that soothe "gut feelings"

Talk about a stormy Monday! First your annual performance review, then a hurried lunch and then a bout of diarrhea. It got worse: Tuesday brought crampy gas pains, and Friday found you constipated.

If you are among the estimated 36 million American women who have irritable bowel syndrome (IBS), you know that your bowels can move in mysterious and inconvenient ways. IBS may be a chronic or a recurring disorder, and its symptoms may include bouts of diarrhea, with pain, gas and sometimes constipation. So far, no one knows what causes it.

Sometimes food and stress seem to spark the symptoms of IBS—so much so that some women avoid certain foods altogether, leaving them vulnerable to nutritional deficiencies. Yet there's reassuring news about diet and IBS—doctors say the right food choices can help to control your symptoms.

"IBS is not life-threatening, but it can be a nuisance for some women and a life-altering experience for others," says Roger Gebhard, M.D., professor of medicine at the University of Minnesota in Minneapolis–St. Paul and staff physician at the Minneapolis Veterans Administration Hospital. "No one really knows what causes these abnormal spasms in the small intestine and colon. It may seem that certain foods can set

RELAX AND ENJOY YOUR LUNCH

How, when and where you eat can be as important to a trouble-free bowel as what you eat, says Charlene Prather, M.D., a senior associate consultant in the Department of Internal Medicine, Division of Gastroenterology, at the Mayo Clinic in Rochester, Minnesota. "Mealtime stress can trigger bowel contractions and spasms that cause problems. Also, when people eat too quickly or are anxious while eating, it increases air swallowing—which can make you feel bloated and give you gas," adds Dr. Prather.

So don't mix mealtime with business.

"I always advise people with irritable bowel syndrome—and everyone else, for that matter—to devote their lunch break to lunch and nothing but lunch," notes Elizabeth Ward, R.D., nutrition counselor with the Harvard Community Health Plan in Boston. "Don't chow down on a sandwich and then run ten errands. You need time to relax."

The same goes for breakfast and dinner. *Slow down.* And save animated conversations for later. Talking a lot while eating may also cause excess air-swallowing, says Barry Jaffin, M.D., a specialist in gastrointestinal motility disorders at Mount Sinai Medical Center in New York City. "Bolting your food or talking at the same time can be long-standing habits that are hard to break," he says. "Changing may take a little time."

things off, and so can anxiety or tension or an important deadline at work."

We all get a touch of diarrhea, irregularity or a tummy ache once in a while. But you may have IBS—and should see a doctor—if you experience abdominal distress daily or intermittently for at least three months and your bowel movements seem to be an on-again, off-again affair at times. Pay attention to changes in stool frequency and consistency (from watery to hard, for example), excessive straining, passage of mucus and abdominal bloating.

"The first thing we look at is the relationship between a woman's diet and how she's feeling," says Charlene Prather,

M.D., senior associate consultant in the Department of Internal Medicine, Division of Gastroenterology, at the Mayo Clinic in Rochester, Minnesota. "Just removing certain foods, or adding others, can work wonders."

IBS is tough to "cure." If dietary strategies bring only limited relief, doctors sometimes recommend over-the-counter medications containing loperamide for diarrhea, dietary fiber supplements to relieve constipation and prescription spasm-stopping medicines to block the clutching aches that many people with IBS feel after eating. Relaxation exercises are often part of the treatment, too.

UNCOVER YOUR MEALTIME LAND MINES

Where to start? That depends on whether your biggest IBS complaint is diarrhea, pain or constipation, says Dr. Prather, so pay attention to your symptoms. At the first sense of pain or diarrhea, try to remember what you ate last. The usual culprits include (but aren't limited to) sugar-free candies and cookies containing sorbitol and antacids containing magnesium.

If you're lactose-intolerant (meaning that you lack the enzyme that digests milk sugars), milk products could cause a stir. Did you have a cappuccino? Caffeine and fat can stimulate your colon, making it move uncomfortably fast. Beer and tacos? Alcohol and spicy foods may rile things up, as may carbonated drinks.

For some people, certain carbohydrates seem to be problematic, says Dr. Prather. Beans, broccoli, cauliflower, apples and other fruits and vegetables—even salads and forms of bran—can cause cramping and diarrhea.

"There are about 20 different kinds of carbohydrates that some people digest poorly, leaving them with gas and loose stools, even if the food is natural. A patient of mine was drinking a gallon of apple juice a day, for example. Once she stopped, her symptoms cleared up. For other people, the problem food might be mushrooms or even lettuce. It's very individual."

If you're not absolutely certain you've nabbed a culprit, you may experiment with eating *more* of that food and note the results, Dr. Gebhard suggests. If it bothers you, you'll know it.

CALMING YOUR COLON

Obviously, if you've made a clear connection between IBS and certain foods, you should stop eating the foods that provoke symptoms, says Dr. Prather. Here's what else experts suggest.

Eat lean. Fat is the strongest dietary stimulant of intestinal contractions. Trim all visible fat from meat, switch to nonfat dairy products and use butter, margarine and oil sparingly. (For more specific tips, see chapters 46, 51 and 52.)

"Fat will stimulate a hormone that can cause contractions of the bowel," says Barry Jaffin, M.D., specialist in gastrointestinal motility disorders and clinical instructor in the Department of Gastroenterology at Mount Sinai Medical Center in New York City. "If you decrease fat intake, it may decrease the contracting hormones. I'll tell a patient with pain-predominant IBS to try that."

Introduce yourself to fiber—gingerly. If constipation's got you all clogged up, you may need more fiber and fluids in your diet, says Dr. Gebhard. One caveat: If you have IBS, you may have to add fiber more slowly, he says.

"Start with a small amount and build up," he suggests. "Fiber is a balancing act. Add too much, too fast, and you can get bloating, gas or pain. Increasing your intake slowly is less likely to make you uncomfortable."

How slowly? Dr. Prather suggests adding 5 grams a day (about the amount in a half-cup of high-fiber cereal) for one week. Every week, add another 5 grams a day until you're consuming 20 to 35 grams a day.

Drink lemonade—or other fluids. "I ask women to please make sure they get a minimum of eight, eight-ounce glasses a day of water, juice, lemonade, skim milk and herbal tea," adds Dr. Prather. "You need plenty of liquids so the fiber bulks up and moves stools more quickly through your bowels. Otherwise the fiber just sits there and makes matters worse." (For additional tips on adding more fruit, vegetables and whole grains to your menu, see chapter 15.)

Divide and conquer. Overeating stretches your lower gastrointestinal tract—and it's the stretching that causes pain, says Dr. Prather. "So skipping breakfast and lunch and eating a huge dinner is not a good idea. Spread your intake throughout the day," he suggests.

If even regular-size meals leave you in agony, try four or five mini-meals spaced throughout the day instead of three main meals, says Elizabeth Ward, R.D., nutrition counselor with the Harvard Community Health Plan in Boston. "Plan ahead, and include fruit, vegetables, whole grains and protein—everything you'd normally eat, redistributed. And focus on good nutrition—a doughnut and a cup of coffee won't do it," she adds.

25

LACTOSE INTOLERANCE

Coping when milk isn't kind

Remember that bouncy old television jingle that went "Milk's a natural"? If you're among the 30 to 50 million Americans— half of them women—who cannot digest a primary milk sugar called lactose, it just isn't so.

For the lactose-intolerant woman, a tall, frosty glass of moo juice or a bowl of ice cream can bring on nausea, cramps, bloating, gas and diarrhea within 30 minutes to two hours.

"It's genetic," says Louis N. Aurisicchio, M.D., a gastro-enterologist in the Department of Gastroenterology and Clinical Nutrition at Our Lady of Mercy Medical Center in the Bronx. "Over time, people with lactose intolerance produce less and less lactase, the enzyme that breaks down lactose in the small intestine. Problems with milk can begin in childhood or adolescence or as late as 20 or 30 years of age."

Lactose intolerance is particularly common among some ethnic and racial groups. Because up to 75 percent of African Americans and Native Americans and 90 percent of Asian Americans are lactose-intolerant, doctors don't necessarily consider lactose intolerance a medical condition. Despite that fact, however, it's an important consideration for women striving to prevent osteoporosis and high blood pressure by con-

YOGURT
Topping, Snack and Spread

Brimming with over 400 milligrams of calcium per cup, cool, creamy, low-fat yogurt is a bone-healthy treat that even women with lactose intolerance can enjoy, says Wahida Karmally, R.D., director of nutrition at the Irving Center for Clinical Research at Columbia University in New York City. But don't stop at snacking—plain yogurt is great in salad dressing and as a topping for baked potatoes or fruit.

Or make a quick batch of luscious, low-fat yogurt cheese, a favorite of Karmally's. Here's how: Spoon a cup or more of low-fat yogurt into a strainer or cheesecloth bag to drain overnight. Discard the liquid and keep the "cheese." Plain, it's a nice alternative to cream cheese on bagels or English muffins for breakfast, says Karmally. "Or spice it up with garlic, oregano and basil and spread it on bread topped with grilled peppers or eggplant as an elegant appetizer," Karmally suggests. "Sweetened with a little sugar, vanilla and nuts, it's delicious, like a whipped dessert."

suming calcium-rich foods, since many such foods are also high in lactose.

EASING INTO THE DAIRY

"The good news is, most patients I see can tolerate milk in small amounts, or with meals," notes Douglas B. McGill, M.D., professor of medicine at the Mayo Medical School and consultant in medicine and gastroenterology at the Mayo Clinic in Rochester, Minnesota. "Most people produce enough lactase for that. You may never have to give up dairy products or use special preparations. Of course, two glasses on an empty stomach is probably going to be too much for your body to handle."

If you want to drink milk—for the taste or the calcium— try a glassful with food, suggest doctors. Researchers say lactose digestion is three times better with a meal than alone. "Having milk with a meal slows the digestion of lactose," says Dr. McGill. "The milk moves into the intestines more slowly when food is present."

Look too for safe choices from the dairy case—yogurt, aged cheeses, buttermilk and lactose-reduced milk.

- Low-fat or nonfat yogurt with live yogurt cultures contains bacteria that produce beta-galactosidase, an enzyme that breaks down up to 40 percent of the lactose in yogurt. So be sure to choose brands that say "live cultures" or "active cultures" on the label—these enzymes continue to break down lactose during digestion. As a bonus, low-fat or nonfat yogurt generally supplies more calcium than whole-milk varieties and helps cut cholesterol. One caution: Frozen yogurt does not count, because freezing kills the active cultures.

- Naturally aged hard cheeses like Swiss, brick and Cheddar are generally low in lactose and high in calcium. "Most of the lactose is in the whey liquid, which is drained off when the cheese is made," explains Judith Jarvis, R.D., coordinator of technical services for the National Dairy Council. As with yogurt, choose low-fat or nonfat varieties to avoid adding cholesterol and calories to your diet.

- Buttermilk contains some milk sugars, notes Dr. McGill, but the fermentation process reduces lactose content and therefore leaves your body with less lactose to digest.

- Lactose-reduced milk is available two ways: 70 percent or 100 percent lactose-reduced. Sold under various brand names, it tastes sweeter than regular milk, and you can choose from whole, low-fat and skim, as well as calcium-fortified and even chocolate varieties. Also look for reduced-lactose cheese at the dairy counter.

MORE HELP FOR THE LACTOSE LEERY

There's even more you can do to cope with lactose intolerance.

Consider a supplement. Taken just before mealtime, lactase tablets or caplets help digest milk sugars. Three major brands include Lactrase, Lactaid and DairyEase. A study at Baylor College of Medicine in Houston found that all three work to varying degrees, although it appears that within the study group of eight women and two men, Lactrase outperformed Lactaid and DairyEase in relieving symptoms. Whichever brand you decide to try, remember to follow the manufacturer's directions—some tablets should be chewed, and some should be swallowed intact.

But even better may be liquid lactase drops that convert regular milk in the carton before you drink it. Five drops per quart can break down more than 70 percent of the lactose in 24 hours. To convert more milk sugar, add more liquid or let it stand up to 72 hours.

Count your calcium. Women concerned with boosting their calcium intake can consider nondairy sources: three ounces of canned sardines with bones, for example, contains 372 milligrams of calcium—more than one-third of the Daily Value recommended by the Food and Drug Administration. Other good choices: calcium-fortified orange juice, cooked collard greens, kale or broccoli.

"Still," says Dr. Aurisicchio. "It's kind of tough to get adequate calcium without dairy products. I usually advise my female patients to try a calcium supplement or chew a calcium-rich antacid tablet." (For more on calcium, see chapter 27.)

Look out for hidden lactose. There's lactose in the most unlikely foods, such as instant potatoes, powdered eggs, salad dressings, lunch meats (kosher varieties are dairy-free) and even some vitamin supplements, antacids, asthma medications and birth control pills. If you're sensitive to small amounts of lactose, scan product labels for lactose-rich milk derivatives like whey, curds, milk by-products, milk solids or nonfat dry milk powder.

Taken together, these simple strategies can help women consume the calcium they need without discomfort.

26

MIGRAINES AND OTHER HEADACHES

Tracking troublesome foods

Oven-fresh bread, aged Cheddar cheese and a goblet of red wine. A romantic picnic? Maybe. But for a migraine-prone woman, this classic repast could be a sure-fire recipe for agony.

"I'd been getting migraines for years," notes Sarah M., an accounting supervisor at a computer firm who responded to our *Food and You* survey. "When I stopped eating cheese and drinking red wine, I got far fewer painful headaches."

What's going on? From Brie to bologna, chocolate to coffee, lima beans to pickled herring, dozens of foods contain natural substances or added ingredients that can ignite headache pain. These substances alter brain chemistry and prompt blood vessels that service the brain on the outside of the skull to swell, pressing on sensitive nerves, explains Frederick Freitag, D.O., associate director of the Diamond Headache Clinic in Chicago.

"Whether you get migraines or tension headaches, the basic mechanism is the same—a central nervous system disorder," says Ninan T. Mathew, M.D., director of the Houston Headache Clinic. "The pain can be mild or severe, and it can be triggered by many things. Dietary factors can account for one attack out of five."

Women, who get migraines nearly three times more often

than men, can be especially sensitive to food. No one's sure why women are more migraine-prone, but doctors say reproductive hormones are often the culprits. Half of all women with migraines report the most attacks around the time of menstruation. In one study, 50 percent of women with migraines said they had more severe or frequent headaches while taking birth control pills.

For many, food becomes a powerful player in the headache equation at particular times, such as on the days just before and at the start of a menstrual period, says Dr. Freitag. Plus, the consequences of a busy lifestyle—notably missed meals, irregular sleep habits and stress—can not only cause a pounding headache or a migraine but may also leave you extravulnerable to one triggered by food.

WAS IT SOMETHING YOU ATE?

At times the food/headache connection can be downright puzzling. On Monday you devour an entire chocolate bar and feel no ill effects; on Friday one bite makes your cranium feel like it's about to explode.

"There are well-established connections between certain foods and headaches, but people usually report it only happens sometimes," notes Dr. Freitag. One reason, he says, is that the amount of headache-causing chemicals can vary dramatically in different brands of the same food due to differences in processing, preparation or storage.

The best way to identify your own food triggers is to keep a diary, says Joel Saper, M.D., clinical professor of neurology at Michigan State University and director of the Michigan Head Pain and Neurological Institute, both in Ann Arbor.

In your diary, note the date, time and severity of the headache, as well as medication you're taking, food you've eaten and any emotional or physical factors—from arguments to strenuous exercise. Also, to spot a trend or pattern, note whether the headache occurs on a weekday or a weekend, before or during your menstrual period or on a day when the weather is bad.

"Eliminating foods that hurt your head won't cure the reason you get headaches, but it could make you more treatable or less likely to experience an attack," says Dr. Saper. "The tendency for headaches will still remain.

"Look for the obvious foods initially, then expand if you don't come up with anything at first," suggests Dr. Saper.

FOOD TRIGGERS TO WATCH OUT FOR

Certain foods contain vasoactive substances—chemicals that prompt your blood vessels to either constrict or swell, causing pain. If you're sensitive to such substances, eating foods that contain them can trigger a headache. Here's what to watch out for, say migraine specialists.

Tyramine. This naturally occurring substance—found in strong aged cheese, pickled herring, chicken livers and the pods of lima, fava and other broadbeans—acts on brain chemistry and makes blood vessels swell, causing pain. Women sensitive to tyramine may lack an enzyme that breaks this substance down, so it keeps circulating in the body, says Dr. Freitag.

Similar, though less common, headache reactions can be caused by phenylethylamine (found in chocolate) and synephrine (found in citrus fruit and juices).

Histamine. When researchers from the University of Vienna in Austria asked 45 headache-prone women and men to stop consuming histamine-containing foods such as cheese, sausage, pickled cabbage and wine for four weeks, nearly three out of four reported fewer headaches. Vinegar (except white vinegar), fresh-baked yeast products, onions, bananas, figs, bacon, avocados and soy sauce all contain similar vasoactive amines that create headaches in the same way.

Nitrates, nitrites and monosodium glutamate. A hot dog at the ballpark or the lunch special at a Chinese restaurant could leave you with a splitting headache, too.

How? Nitrates and nitrites (used to preserve the color of cured meats like bacon, ham, salami and hot dogs) can alter brain chemistry and dilate blood vessels. So can monosodium glutamate (MSG), found in some restaurant food as well as packaged items from party dip to TV dinners.

Aspartame. Diet drinks and sugar-free foods—from yogurt to desserts—that contain the artificial sweetener aspartame *may* cause headaches in patients prone to migraines, says Dr. Mathew. "It's a controversial issue, but we strongly believe aspartame can cause headaches in migraine sufferers," he says. "Many patients report it to us."

Caffeine withdrawal. Caffeine in coffee, tea and cola drinks actually makes blood vessels narrow, but hours after the last cup, you may develop a rebound headache as vessels expand. Doctors think caffeine withdrawal explains why some people get headaches on weekends or holidays, when routines vary and the office—or kitchen—coffeepot isn't constantly beckoning.

ENJOY LIFE—AND FOOD—WITHOUT HEADACHES

Start a diary to zero in on likely culprits, says Dr. Saper. Then try the following tips.

Stick to small helpings. "For some, a small amount of a problem food is okay," Dr. Mathew says. "Experiment to see if you can tolerate small amounts."

Avoid and conquer. If as little as a sip of red wine or a bite of Brie, navy beans or anything else brings on a headache every time, write it off. "If your headaches are triggered primarily by foods, you can make a very big change by removing the offenders," says Dr. Freitag.

Switch brands. If one brand of cheese leads to a migraine, try another. The same goes for other tyramine-rich foods. "You may find you may not necessarily have to write off a food entirely," says Dr. Freitag. "There's a wide variance in the amount of tyramine by brand," he notes. "Many of my patients find they can tolerate a different one just fine."

Explore substitutes. Love chocolate, hate the headache? Try substituting carob, suggests Dr. Saper. Fresh-cooked roast beef and turkey are delicious substitutes for processed lunch meats, although he recommends avoiding meat whenever possible.

Looking for a "safe" cheese? Stick with processed types, such as American and loaf cheeses like Velveeta, as well as farmer's cheese, cottage cheese and cream cheese, which are usually low in tyramine, says Dr. Mathew. Mozzarella, Havarti and other mild, soft varieties generally contain less ty-

FOOD CRAVINGS CAN PREDICT MIGRAINES

Yesterday you had a powerful longing for chocolate. Not content to stop at one bite, you needed (and consumed) *lots* of it. Today a migraine's got you down for the count.

Cause and effect? Not necessarily, say experts.

"In some women, the earliest phases of a migraine may trigger food cravings for certain types of foods or tastes," says Joel Saper, M.D., clinical professor of neurology at Michigan State University and director of the Michigan Head Pain and Neurological Institute, both in Ann Arbor. "Most often it's for chocolate, pizza or something salty like potato chips. And the craving may hit up to three days before their head starts pounding," he says.

In other words, the suspect is not necessarily the culprit, just an early warning signal—part of what doctors call the prodrome. Besides cravings, the constellation of premigraine symptoms can include depression or euphoria, a stiff neck, a chilly feeling, yawning, constipation or diarrhea and water retention. All are possible tipoffs that the shifts in brain chemistry responsible for migraines have begun.

Not all migraines are preceded by powerful food cravings, Dr. Saper notes. But if you notice a pattern, take whatever measures you can to reduce stress, relax or have migraine medication handy. And whatever you do, don't give in to the craving. "Doing so could make matters worse," he says.

ramine than hard, crumbly, strong-tasting cheeses. For overall health reasons, look for low-fat varieties.

Read the label. Scan the ingredients list of any prepared product you plan to eat for nitrites or nitrates and MSG, suggests Dr. Mathew. But beware. "Nitrites, nitrates and MSG may be listed only as hydrolized protein or natural flavor on a label," he says. "That could be the only clue you get."

Make it fresh. All food—particularly meat, fish and poultry products—should be prepared and eaten fresh. Tyramine levels build quickly as food sits, even when refrigerated, so don't consume leftovers held for more than one day.

Talk food with your party host. Sizing up party finger foods can break the conversational ice. "Ask about the food in a nice, nonoffensive, neutral way," suggests Dr. Freitag. "Comment on the cheeses and find out what they are. If you see a dip that may be safe to eat, make a simple inquiry like 'Boy, where'd you get the dip?' If the answer is the local convenience store, it probably has MSG in it. If the answer is 'Well, I whipped it up myself,' it's probably fine."

Try calcium. At Mount Sinai Hospital in New York City, two women whose migraines were related to their menstrual cycles felt significantly better after taking calcium and vitamin D supplements for two to three months. One found she could stop oncoming migraine attacks by taking 1,200 to 1,600 milligrams of calcium (in chewable form).

Think twice about alcohol. If you opt to enjoy an occasional glass of wine with a meal, consider white wines. Red wines like Chianti and sherry, as well as beer, burgundy and vermouth, contain more headache-promoting substances like esters, tannins and acids than do white wines.

As for hard liquor, well, if you're headache-prone, you may find you're better off without it, says Dr. Freitag. Instead, try an alcohol-free "mock" cocktail or a white-wine spritzer, which is white wine mixed with club soda.

Consider the herbal route. The herb feverfew has proven abilities to reduce migraine pain and lengthen the period of time between migraines—provided it's taken daily, says Varro Tyler, Ph.D., professor of pharmacognosy at the Purdue University School of Pharmacy in West Lafayette, Indiana. "The usual dose is a capsule or tablet with 380 milligrams of feverfew in it, but make sure the label says it contains two-tenths of 1 percent of parthenolide, the active ingredient," Dr. Tyler says. "It only works when taken regularly."

If you find that you can avoid headaches only by limiting yourself to a very narrow selection of foods, see a doctor. Severely restricting your food choices can leave you deficient in key nutrients, says Dr. Saper. Also see your doctor if, after trial and error, you can't detect any link between your headaches and food. Other nondrug tactics—like stress reduction or meditation—may offer help.

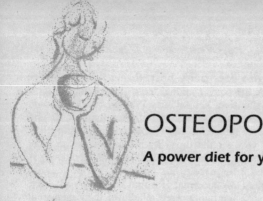

OSTEOPOROSIS

A power diet for your bones

When asked about their health goals, several women who responded to our *Food and You* survey expressed an earnest desire to prevent osteoporosis. One was Kathryn B., a woman in her midforties who told us, "My grandmother has the typical dowager's hump and stooped posture of osteoporosis. I want to do whatever I can to avoid it."

Kathryn exercises regularly, eats a healthy, low-fat diet and takes a daily calcium supplement. Still, she wonders if she's doing enough.

Kathryn's concern is warranted: Osteoporosis, the disease responsible for that little-old-lady look, affects up to half of all American women (and one in five American men). Sometimes known as brittle-bone disease, osteoporosis weakens the bones, leaving them fragile and susceptible to breaking.

In fact, osteoporosis accounts for 1.5 million fractures a year in this country, mostly of the hip, wrist and spine. One in every three women over the age of 65 will suffer from a vertebral fracture of the spine. Some doctors call it an epidemic.

PREVENTION BEGINS EARLY

The right diet, with lots of calcium, is crucial to preventing osteoporosis, whether you're 25 or 65.

Why calcium? Your body takes the calcium you consume—whether from food or supplements—and stores nearly all of it in the skeleton. If the body doesn't get enough calcium from outside sources, it draws calcium out of the bones, which gradually weakens them. The bones are already at a disadvantage because they slowly weaken with age: Women reach their peak bone mass at about the age of 30 and thereafter lose up to 1 percent every year until menopause. Once lost, this bone density cannot be replaced.

''The first two decades of life are the most significant in forming strong, healthy bones,'' notes Richard S. Bockman, M.D., Ph.D., professor of medicine at Cornell University Medical College and co-director of the Osteoporosis Prevention Center at the Hospital for Special Surgery, both in New York City. So while you're paying attention to your own bone health, don't forget to enlighten your daughters.

Estrogen also contributes to bone health. Thus, an added challenge for women is that when they go through menopause and the supply of estrogen in their bodies declines, bone loss accelerates, putting them at further risk for osteoporosis.

Fewer than 50 percent of American women get the 1,000 milligrams of calcium the average adult needs daily to bank bone mass and head off fractures. Here's what you can do to ensure you get all you need.

FOOD THAT FENDS OFF FRACTURES

As much as possible, calcium should come from food, because the ratio of calcium to other needed ingredients is more naturally balanced in food than in a supplement, according to Yvonne Sherrer, M.D., director of clinical research with Rheumatology Associates of South Florida in Pompano Beach and author of *A Woman Doctor's Guide to Osteoporosis*.

Eat three or four servings a day of the calcium champs. A save-your-bones diet should include dairy foods that supply a minimum of 300 milligrams of calcium per serving, according to Robert A. Heaney, M.D., professor of medicine at

YOUR DAILY CALCIUM INTAKE GUIDE

Of all the nutrients critical to a woman's health, the needs for calcium vary the most widely, depending on your age, sex and estrogen status. To hammer out specific guidelines, the National Institutes of Health in Bethesda, Maryland, convened the Optimal Calcium Intake Consensus Conference. Their guidelines, given here, can help you assess your individual need for this mineral.

Adolescent and young adult women (ages 11 to 24):
   1,200 to 1,500 milligrams

Pregnant or nursing teens: 1,500 milligrams

Adult women (ages 25 to 50): 1,000 milligrams

Pregnant or nursing women: 1,200 to 1,500 milligrams

Postmenopausal women on estrogen replacement
   therapy: 1,000 milligrams

Postmenopausal women not on estrogen replacement
   therapy: 1,500 milligrams

Postmenopausal women over age 65: 1,500 milligrams

Creighton University in Omaha, Nebraska, and chairperson of the Science Advisory Panel on Osteoporosis of the U.S. Congress Office of Technology Assessment. An eight-ounce glass of skim milk contains 300 milligrams of calcium. Drink four glasses a day, and you'll get all you need. If you don't like to drink that much milk, you can get the rest of your calcium through such rich sources as plain nonfat yogurt (452 milligrams per 8 ounces), Swiss cheese (408 milligrams per 1½ ounces), calcium-fortified orange juice (300 milligrams per cup) and calcium-enriched bread (300 milligrams in two slices). Dark green vegetables, tofu, salmon and plain or fruit-flavored low-fat yogurt are also excellent sources of calcium.

Consider lactose-reduced options. If you are lactose-intolerant (a condition in which you don't digest milk well), you can still have a calcium-rich diet by including calcium-fortified foods—such as juices, cereals and breads—and yogurt, cheese, soy milk or lactose-reduced or lactose-free milk. (For other tips on ensuring adequate calcium intake if you're lactose-intolerant, see chapter 25.)

Give fat the boot. Contrary to many women's concerns, a calcium-rich diet doesn't have to be high in fat. Nor should it be. A study conducted by Grace Wyshak, Ph.D., professor at Harvard University School of Public Health, suggests that the risk of bone fractures for women over 50 who average more than 25 grams of animal fat daily is five times greater than for women who consume fewer than 25 grams. So Dr. Wyshak recommends that women control the animal fat in their diets.

Keep a lid on coffee consumption. Studies indicate a link between heavy caffeine consumption and hip fractures. Moderate consumption—no more than two cups per day of coffee or two soft drinks with caffeine—appears to pose no risk, say Dr. Bonnick and other researchers.

Limit cola drinks to one a day. A preliminary study of adolescent girls done by Dr. Wyshak suggests that high cola consumption may be related to higher rates of bone fracture. Some experts think the real problem may be the low-calcium diets that result if sodas replace milk. So don't go overboard on colas.

Curb alcohol intake. Alcohol abuse is considered a risk factor for osteoporosis. Alcohol is a bone burglar—it can have direct toxic effects on bone cells. What's more, heavy drinkers, say doctors, tend to eat fewer calcium-rich foods. As a result, drinking more than two glasses of wine or four ounces of hard liquor per day results in drinkers having less bone mass than nondrinkers of the same age and sex, according to Dr. Bockman.

Seek out vitamin D from dairy and sunlight. Calcium doesn't operate alone; it needs vitamin D to work its way to your bones. Vitamin D is also found in milk, and breakfast cereals are fortified with it. Your goal should be 400 international units of vitamin D a day, according to Dr. Sherrer. She is a proponent of getting vitamins naturally in food, but a supplement would work as well. We also get vitamin D naturally through sunlight, although sunscreen blocks its absorp-

A SAMPLE BONE-SAVING MENU

Working calcium into your diet isn't nearly as tough as many women think. This sample menu shows how easy it can be to do it, without loading up on calories or saturated fat.

MEAL	CALICUM (mg.)
Breakfast	
1 cup whole-wheat flakes	40
1 cup 1 percent milk	300
1 medium peach	5
Morning Snack	
1 cup calcium-fortified orange juice	300
1 large popcorn cake	—
1 tablespoon peanut butter	5
Lunch	
1 cup bean soup	80
3 pieces sesame-rye crispbread	—
2 one-ounce slices reduced-fat Cheddar cheese	300
Afternoon Snack	
1 blueberry muffin	14
Dinner	
1½ cups steamed Chinese vegetable mix	86
1½ cups cooked brown rice	30
13 medium cashews	9
2 tablespoons sweet-and-sour sauce	—
Bedtime Snack	
1 cup raspberry low-fat yogurt	350

Nutritional analysis: Supplies 1,799 calories, 1,519 mg. calcium and 48 g. fat (24 percent of calories).

tion. And older people may have some problems with absorption, according to Dr. Sherrer. For older women (especially those who spend little time involved in outdoor activities), Dr. Sherrer recommends talking to your doctor about vitamin D supplements. Because high doses of vitamin D can be toxic, supplements should be taken only under a doctor's supervision. As a rule, 400 international units a day is considered the safe limit, say experts.

WHEN A SUPPLEMENT MAKES SENSE

Even if you enjoy a calcium-rich diet, experts say you should also consider taking a daily calcium supplement as added insurance. But with dozens on the market, which one is right for you? Here's what's recommended.

Go for calcium carbonate. Sydney Lou Bonnick, M.D., director of osteoporosis services at Texas Woman's University in Denton and author of *The Osteoporosis Handbook*, advises women under age 65 to select a calcium carbonate supplement and to take it with food. Most women do fine with calcium carbonate. If it causes gas or constipation, you are taking medication to reduce stomach acid or are over 65 or have a history of kidney stones, however, take calcium citrate instead, and take it on an empty stomach, says Dr. Bonnick.

Calcium carbonate contains the highest percentage of calcium, and when taken properly, it is well-absorbed. (Calcium carbonate needs hydrochloric acid, released in the stomach in the presence of food, to be absorbed.)

OTHER BONE HELPERS

Diet alone can't fight osteoporosis. A woman owes it to her bones to stay physically fit.

Maintain an ideal weight. When it comes to bone health, carrying a few extra pounds may give you a slight edge over thin, small-framed women, who run a greater risk of brittle bones. The best strategy for overall health is to strive for a middle ground, according to Dr. Sherrer.

Work out to save your bones. Weight-bearing exercises like walking, biking, jogging or aerobics and strength-training or workouts with light weights can improve muscle mass and overall bone fitness. According to Dr. Sherrer exercise needs to become a permanent way of life, and your program must be personalized to your needs.

Exercise not only increases bone density but also improves your dexterity and reflexes according to Susan Allen, M.D.,

Ph.D., assistant professor of internal medicine at the University of Missouri—Columbia School of Medicine. Brisk walking, jogging and dancing actually stimulate bone cells to build more bone, particularly in your back and hips. Be sure to get your doctor's approval and a trainer's advice on the safest routine for you.

Stick with it. Once you've found the weight-bearing exercises you like, keep at them for 30 minutes to an hour three to four times a week, Dr. Allen says. The bones most vulnerable to osteoporosis are those in the hips and the spinal vertebrae in the mid to lower back. Walking, jogging and aerobic dancing are particularly helpful for your back and hips, according to Dr. Allen.

Consider ERT. Since estrogen conserves bone mass in women past menopause, women who are approaching menopause and are concerned about osteoporosis should discuss estrogen replacement therapy (ERT) with their physicians. Dr. Sherrer (among other experts) recommends that women at risk for osteoporosis take both estrogen and calcium following menopause. (Caucasian and Asian women, for example, get this disease in greater numbers than African-American women.) Dr. Bockman says that if there is low bone mass and no potential risk factors from using ERT, he would probably recommend both.

Don't smoke. Smoking invalidates your body's warranty on your bones. According to the National Osteoporosis Foundation, smoking has been shown to interfere with the body's utilization of estrogen and therefore contribute to bone loss. So if you smoke, quit.

28

OVARIAN CANCER

Less fat, more fiber help beat the odds

Cut the risk of ovarian cancer with skim milk and sugar snap peas? It sounds farfetched. Yet in a joint study from Yale University School of Medicine and the University of Toronto, researchers found that eating less saturated fat and more vegetable fiber may cut the risk of ovarian cancer substantially. The study compared the diets of 450 Canadian women with ovarian cancer to those of 564 women who were cancer-free.

"It appears possible to cut your risk of ovarian cancer in half by an aggressive modification of the diet," says Harvey A. Risch, M.D., Ph.D., associate professor of epidemiology and public health at Yale University School of Medicine.

Dr. Risch and the other researchers found that for every ten grams of saturated fat women put on their plates—and into their mouths—daily, the risk of ovarian cancer rose 20 percent. No relationship was found between unsaturated fat and the cancer.

Risk fell as vegetable consumption rose: For every ten grams of vegetable fiber eaten every day, the chance of ovarian cancer dropped by 37 percent. In contrast, cereal and fruit fiber didn't seem to make a difference.

OF FOOD AND HORMONES

How could diet have an impact on ovarian cancer, which regrettably is one of the more life-threatening forms of cancer? There is evidence that hormones play a role in its development, note the study authors. In fact, women who bear children reduce their risk by 15 to 20 percent for each full-term pregnancy, and women who take oral contraceptives seem to decrease their risk by 5 to 10 percent for each year on the Pill.

The fiber in the vegetables may grab estrogen and escort it from the body. Vegetable consumption then may lessen the net presence of estrogen.

How can you take advantage of the high-fiber/low-fat link?

Reduce animal fat. Most women consume around 20 to 25 grams of saturated fat a day, and most saturated fat is animal fat. If you substitute olive oil (1.8 grams per tablespoon) for butter (4.8 grams in two tablespoons), you'll save 3 grams of saturated fat. Chicken is a much better meat choice than beef: Three ounces of skinless breast has 0.9 gram of saturated fat, while the same amount of lean, broiled rib-eye steak has 4 grams.

"The point isn't that people should never eat hamburgers," Dr. Risch says. "But things that are eaten regularly that are high in saturated fat should be cut back. People don't realize how little meat protein they need per day to live perfectly well. Four to five ounces of meat a day is probably sufficient for most women."

Trim down dairy. You could trim ten grams of saturated fat simply by drinking two glasses of skim milk instead of two glasses of whole milk. You could save nearly five grams by switching from whole-milk yogurt to a nonfat variety, and you could shave off four grams by cooking with part-skim ricotta cheese instead of whole-milk ricotta.

Up the vegetable fiber. Experts say we should have 20 to 35 grams of fiber in our diet daily—about twice as much as most women consume. The richest vegetable sources include lima beans, with 6.8 grams per half-cup; succotash, with 5.2 grams per half-cup; chopped chicory, 3.6 grams per half-cup; artichoke hearts, with 4.4 grams per half-cup; parsnips, with

3.8 grams per half-cup; canned pumpkin, with 3.4 grams per half-cup; and sweet potato, with 3.4 grams in one baked potato. And oh, yes—sugar snap peas. A half-cup serving supplies 2.6 grams of fiber.

29

OVERWEIGHT

Why weight control is a top health priority

One memorable summer, Joyce S. looked in a mirror and asked herself point-blank "What would it take to like myself better?" She knew the answer, and four months later she was 45 pounds lighter.

In June, Joyce was 65 pounds overweight. Her cholesterol reading was 293—so high that her doctor was ready to prescribe medication. "I was depressed," recalls this 44-year-old mom and office manager who responded to our *Food and You* survey. "My self-image was poor—I couldn't stand looking at myself."

By September, Joyce was wearing new blue jeans and a broad grin. Friends and relations complimented her new shape. Joyce had shed 45 pounds; moreover, her cholesterol level dropped 84 points. How did she do it?

"I started walking 10 minutes a day, then 20 minutes, and eventually 40 minutes," she says. "As I walked, I started thinking about eating healthier food. No more fried chicken and french fries for me! My body started to change noticeably—I lost weight, and I have more endurance."

BENEFITS BEYOND APPEARANCE

Across the country, women like Joyce are discovering something doctors have known for a while: Paring off pounds can exert a powerful and positive impact on your health while boosting self-esteem.

Sensible weight loss—or sensibly maintaining a healthy weight—may be the most dramatic step you can take to improve the quality of your life now and in the future, says Susan Zelitch Yanovski, M.D., an obesity expert with the National Institute of Diabetes and Digestive and Kidney Diseases at the National Institutes of Health in Bethesda, Maryland.

Sure, shedding flab puts to rest everyday annoyances like zippers that won't zip or thighs that jiggle when (and if) you walk down the beach. But by giving excess weight the heave-ho, you can also enjoy lower blood pressure and better cholesterol readings, which will reduce your chances of heart disease and stroke. And you'll also reduce the risk of diabetes.

"Even modest weight loss—shedding just five or ten pounds—can produce significant health benefits," says Dr. Yanovski. "It's important for women to realize that they don't necessarily need to get down to an ideal weight to see results." By bringing your weight closer to the ideal range for your height and age, you'll probably feel more energetic and cut your chances of developing pesky gallstones and osteoarthritis, the painful wear-and-tear erosion of joints

When it comes to weight control, the benefits are legion. And small losses *are* helpful. Consider these facts.

- If you are moderately heavy, paring just 10 to 15 pounds will improve your body's response to your own insulin and may reduce the risk of diabetes, says Broatch Haig, R.D., a certified diabetes educator and director of outreach services at the International Diabetes Center in Minneapolis. "You don't have to become a skinny Minnie to reduce your chances of diabetes," she notes.
- In one noteworthy study, women who lost 10 to 15 pounds and shed abdominal fat cut their risk of breast cancer by 45 percent. "Losing the weight that accumulates around the waist seems to do the most good," says David V. Schapira, M.D., chief of hematology/oncology and professor of med-

icine at Louisiana State University Medical Center in New Orleans and director of the Stanley S. Scott Cancer Center there, who led the study. "And for many women, abdominal body fat seems to come off the fastest."

- Shedding just 11 pounds could cut your risk of developing osteoarthritis of the knee in half, says David T. Felson, M.D., professor of medicine and public health at Boston University School of Medicine. "Even a small weight loss reduces the amount of force pounding on your joints," he says.

AND IF YOU *DON'T* LOSE WEIGHT . . .

News on the other side of the ledger is sobering. Women who remain overweight—particularly those whose waistlines are padded fat—may run a greater risk of heart disease, as well as cancer of the breast, endometrium (the inner lining of the uterus), cervix, ovaries and gallbladder. They may also develop varicose veins or carpal tunnel syndrome or face complications should they become pregnant. Among postmenopausal women, overweight is a significant risk factor for urinary incontinence.

And like it or not, evidence indicates that this is a society quick to demean overweight people, so being "big" can unfairly limit your social horizons and shrink the size of your paycheck.

"One of the reasons people are so obsessed with losing weight is that it's terribly painful to be fat in America," says Richard Atkinson, M.D., professor of medicine and nutritional sciences at the University of Wisconsin in Madison and president of the American Society for Clinical Nutrition. "There is enormous discrimination."

We should mention that overweight women *do* enjoy one health advantage: stronger bones. In a University of California study of 895 women, higher body weight meant denser bones. Why? Researchers offer two possible explanations: Extra body fat produces extra estrogen, which helps bones retain calcium. Also, in the normal course of moving around, heavier women exert more force on their joints, and this natural weight-bearing activity stimulates bone mineralization.

But in the balance, too much extra weight is a liability, not an asset.

BORN TO BE FAT?

Genetics. Gender. Hormones. Lifestyle. Age. These are the primary reasons women gain weight, say doctors.

A family history of obesity ups your chances of ending up with the same chubby shape by 25 to 30 percent. Evidence for why obese people may be born that way is mounting. Genetic studies conducted at Rockefeller University in New York City have isolated an "obesity gene" that, if faulty, fails to produce a special hormone called leptin. One theory is that leptin works as a gauge of body fat, the same way a thermostat gauges room temperature. High levels of leptin tell the body that it has too much fat, so the body adjusts by increasing metabolism and decreasing appetite, causing weight loss. Low levels of leptin tell the body that it doesn't have enough fat, so metabolism decreases and appetite increases, leading to weight gain. This may explain why, for some people, weight seems to drift back to a set point, or predetermined weight.

Gender is a powerful factor, too. Because men have more muscle while women have more body fat, men burn 10 to 20 percent more energy than women even at rest.

Of course, a sedentary "sit and snack" lifestyle—one in which you get little exercise and nosh on high-calorie foods—is a sure-fire way to pack on the extra pounds. Coupled with the slight but still significant tendency for metabolism to slow somewhat during adulthood, the net effect, for many women, is an extra 10 to 15 pounds (or maybe one-size-larger jeans) by middle age.

HOW FAT IS TOO FAT?

Researchers know that if you're within your ideal weight range (described in chapter 44), you stand a good chance of being healthy. If you're very overweight—say, 50 to 100 pounds or more—you're clearly skating on thin ice. But at what point in between does weight gain reach dangerous levels? No one is sure yet. Here's what they do know.

QUIT SMOKING NOW, DIET LATER

Susan P. smokes. Like other *Food and You* survey respondents, Susan knows she should quit cigarettes. But she worries that if she does, she'll gain weight. Won't that trade one health risk for another, she wonders?

Not quite. True, being overweight poses dramatic health risks for women. But doctors say smoking to maintain a low weight is much, much riskier. And despite common fears, most former smokers don't gain enough weight to create problems, says Edward Anselm, M.D., an internist and medical director of New York City's EHG National Health Services.

"Generally, smokers tend to be an average of 6 to 10 pounds underweight," says Dr. Anselm. "So you have to put the weight gain in perspective. Quitting adds an average of 5 to 10 pounds and may simply bring a woman up to a normal weight. You don't really increase your health risks until you're closer to 20 or 30 pounds overweight."

Moreover, studies show that women who quit smoking enjoy strong health advantages over those who do not: After ten years they reduce their risk of lung cancer by up to half, and after one year the risk of heart disease is cut in half as well. They suffer fewer colds and episodes of bronchitis and take fewer sick days. Potential for becoming pregnant improves, and the risk of delivering a low birthweight baby drops. Quitters also cut their chances for cervical and bladder cancer, ulcers and stroke.

In fact, doctors who treat women who are overweight often suggest they stop smoking first and lose weight later. The health gains attributed to snuffing out cigarettes are *that* important.

"Smoking is by far the greater health risk," says Susan Zelitch Yanovski, M.D., an obesity expert with the National Institute of Diabetes and Digestive and Kidney Diseases at the National Institutes of Health in Bethesda, Maryland. "I tell my patients, gaining five pounds is a small price to pay for the health benefits of quitting tobacco."

Tipping the scales at 20 percent above your desirable weight is an acknowledged health risk, says JoAnn E. Manson, M.D., associate professor of medicine at Harvard Medical School, co-director of women's health at Brigham and Women's Hospital in Boston, and co-principal investigator for the cardiovascular component of the Harvard University Nurses' Health Study (an ongoing study of 115,000 women considered a landmark source of evidence regarding women's health).

Beyond that, risk soars as pounds add up. "At 30 percent or more above their ideal weight, women run three times the risk of heart disease," Dr. Manson notes. "But even average weight in the United States is too much weight sometimes. I really think that being on the lean side is best for preventing heart disease."

So much for gaining 30 or 40 pounds. What about smaller gains that accumulate at the rate of, say, a pound a year for so many women between high school graduation and their twentieth reunion? Even this "normal" weight gain can be risky, says Dr. Manson.

Looking at the medical histories of the women in the Nurses' Health Study, Dr. Manson and other researchers discovered that women who gained just 11 to 17 pounds between their late teens and middle years had a 25 percent higher risk of incurring—or dying from—a heart attack.

In their study, Dr. Manson and her Harvard colleagues say that so-called middle-age spread is unhealthy, and weight charts that say otherwise provide "false reassurance" to women who've moved up a dress size or two since reaching adulthood.

Their best advice?

"A good rule of thumb is that gaining more than 20 pounds between early and middle adulthood about doubles the risk for heart disease," says Dr. Manson. "And even average weights are probably about 15 percent higher than what's considered to be desirable from a health standpoint."

(Two other measures—body mass index, or BMI, and waist/hip ratio—may be better gauges of health than absolute weight. See chapter 44 for details.)

YOUR WEIGHT AND YOUR HEALTH

Where should you draw the line on unhealthy weight? It depends. Researchers have come to realize that the problem with fat goes beyond sheer poundage. So to find out where you stand weight-wise, you need to ask yourself the following questions.

Does my weight accumulate on my hips or my abdomen? "We used to think fat was just an inert mass on the body," says Dr. Schapira. "Well, it doesn't appear to be inert at all. And fat on the abdomen is the most metabolically active."

Packed around your internal organs, shoulders and neck, central body fat is stored in big cells—in contrast to the smaller, more numerous fat cells on your hips. "This isn't 'quiet' fat like the fat on your hips," says Jeanine Albu, M.D., an endocrinologist and obesity researcher at the Obesity Research Center at St. Luke's—Roosevelt Hospital Center in New York City. "Fat is made up of triglycerides that are constantly being broken down and rebuilt. Central body fat in big cells does this more often, sending more fatty acids into the bloodstream."

This onslaught of fatty acids seems to change the chemistry of the blood. Extra fatty acids can mean higher triglycerides and lower levels of "good" high-density lipoprotein (HDL) cholesterol, Dr. Albu says.

After menopause, heavier women and women with more abdominal fat have more estrogens, notes Rachel Ballard-Barbash, M.D., research epidemiologist at the National Cancer Institute in Bethesda, Maryland. Estrogens (especially certain forms) promote the growth of breast and endometrial cancer cells.

In addition, excess abdominal fat may cause a woman's body to process insulin (the hormone that allows cells to break down blood sugar for energy) inefficiently. This causes insulin resistance, which is one cause of diabetes. The extra insulin may also promote cancer growth, although researchers don't yet know how.

"Abdominal body fat increases as women age," says Dr. Ballard-Barbash. "Gains in abdominal fat can have an adverse effect on metabolism. Women with more abdominal fat are more likely to develop endometrial and other forms of cancer, especially after menopause.

A pair of scientists sees the problem with body fat differently. According to Paul R. Abernathy, Ph.D., professor in the Department of Foods and Nutrition at Purdue University in West Lafayette, Indiana, and David R. Black, Ph.D., professor in the Department of Health, Kinesiology and Leisure Studies at Purdue, overloaded fat cells may no longer protect the body because they cannot filter excess sugars, insulin and fats from the bloodstream. Writing in the *Journal of the American Dietetic Association*, the two suggest that eating a low-fat, low-sugar diet and exercising will help restore the buffering activity of fat cells. (For details on how to cut back on dietary fat and sugar, see chapters 46 and 47.)

Do I have high blood pressure, high cholesterol or other risk factors for heart disease? In poring over the medical histories of women in the Nurses' Health Study, researchers looked for links between overweight and heart disease. The question was vital, because heart disease is the leading cause of death among women. And it was overdue, because for decades most studies focused on men only.

The link was obvious: Compared to their lean counterparts, women who weighed just 10 to 14 percent more than their ideal weight were 30 percent more likely to suffer a heart attack, fatal or not. At higher levels—15 to 29 percent above ideal weight—the risk jumped by 80 percent. At 30 percent overweight, the risk was three times higher.

"Even mild to moderate overweight increased the risk of coronary disease in middle-aged women," notes Dr. Manson. Forty percent of coronary problems among the nurses were due to excess body fat. Among the heaviest women, 70 percent of coronary heart disease was caused by obesity.

There was more. While 1 in 4 of the heaviest nurses had high blood pressure, just 1 in 12 of the lean nurses did. High blood pressure not only strains the heart, it creates a buildup of fatty acids in blood vessels that can block arteries, leading to a heart attack or stroke. Weighing 20 percent more than your ideal can increase your risk of high blood pressure at least fourfold.

Cholesterol readings, which predict heart disease risk, were twice as high among the most overweight nurses in the Harvard study.

Obesity seems to pack a one-two punch for the heart, eroding some vital protection. At the University of Texas Southwestern Medical Center at Dallas, researchers noticed that women's levels of HDL—the "good" cholesterol that prevents clogged arteries—fall with weight gain.

So if your weight, blood pressure and cholesterol levels are all high, and especially if you tend to accumulate weight in the abdomen, it would be wise to consult parts four and five of this book for corrective actions.

Do I have diabetes (or a family history of it)? The longer you are overweight—and the more overweight you are—the greater your risk of diabetes, according to the American Diabetes Association. Combined with other factors listed above— or a sedentary lifestyle—carrying extra pounds becomes an even more potent force, says Dr. Albu.

"If someone has a genetic predisposition, like a mother or aunt or grandfather with diabetes, the longer she is overweight and the more central body fat she has, the greater the chances of diabetes," Dr. Albu says. "But not every overweight woman is at higher risk. It depends in part on where you put the fat on." Most people who develop diabetes later in life have extra abdominal fat. (For more information about preventing and controlling diabetes, see chapter 16.)

One woman who cut her risk creatively is Marilyn K. "A year ago, I tipped the scales at 180 pounds," she told us in the *Food and You* survey. "Today, I'm 137 pounds." Marilyn, who lost her mother and younger sister to diabetes, says, "I want to see my grandkids, so I decided to do something about my weight." Her secret? Cutting fat and daily walks with her golden retriever, Dusty, whom she adopted from the local dog pound. "He saved my life," says Marilyn, "and I saved his."

Am I at increased risk for breast cancer? Although overall obesity may not cause cancer, the distribution of body fat may increase your risk for it, says Dr. Schapira. He compared 216 women with breast cancer to 432 cancer-free women and drew a surprising conclusion: Women with bigger waists were at significantly higher risk of breast cancer. "Women with a waist-to-hip ratio over 0.8 had a six times greater risk of breast cancer," says Dr. Schapira, who led the study team.

Dr. Schapira found a similar link to endometrial cancer among obese women: In a study of 80 women, those with high waist-to-hip ratios over 1.14 had a 15 times greater risk of developing this cancer of the lining of the uterus.

"The point is, it's not a good idea to be overweight and it's not a good idea at all to be shaped like an apple, with lots of upper-body fat," Dr. Schapira says. "But the good news is, women seem to lose this kind of fat the fastest. That's where you'll get the most bang for your buck if you diet or exercise to lose weight."

YOUR WEIGHT-LOSS INCENTIVE PLAN

Whatever your current weight or personal health history, the tactics in parts four and five can help you get your weight back to an ideal range. Part four details strategies that work best for permanent weight loss, and part five provides expert tips on meal planning, shopping, cooking, snacking and dining out.

"If I had a relative with diabetes or breast cancer, I would be very vigilant about exercise and diet and try to stay lean," Dr. Yanovski says. "I would take the same route if my weight were located around my waist and if I had existing health conditions that needed to be under better control."

30

SKIN PROBLEMS

Nutrients your skin will love

Back in the days of courtiers and kings, European noblewomen made a habit of dabbing their faces with old wine, convinced that this would keep their skin looking young.

As it turns out, scientific studies suggest that substances called alpha-hydroxy acids—naturally present in grapes, apples, citrus fruits and even milk—can help keep their fine lines at bay when applied to the skin. And alpha-hydroxy acids are the active ingredient in many moisturizers and foundation creams.

Research suggests that eating apples, citrus fruits and other nutritious foods may do your face some good, too. Eating the right foods may not eradicate wrinkles, but it can help protect against nasty annoyances like acne, canker sores and hives. And the benefits are more than cosmetic: Studies also suggest that a diet rich in fruits and vegetables may lower your risk of skin cancer.

A DIET FOR YOUNGER-LOOKING SKIN

Without a doubt, the single biggest favor you can do your skin is to protect it against overexposure to the sun, thus avoiding damage that can lead to skin cancer and wrinkles, says Qingyi

Wei, M.D., Ph.D., assistant professor of epidemiology at the M.D. Anderson Cancer Center at the University of Texas in Houston. Beyond that, a few dietary strategies can offer added insurance.

Order a tuna on wheat. Whole grains, fish, broccoli, cabbage, onions, garlic, radishes and mushrooms are all good sources of selenium.

Researchers at Texas Tech University Health Sciences Center in Lubbock found that mice who got a hefty dose of selenium in their diets were less likely to develop skin tumors than those who got little or none of the antioxidant.

Have a carrot salad. When scientists at Lawrence Berkeley Laboratory in California exposed mice to ultraviolet rays, they made an important discovery. The light appeared to deplete the animals' skin of vitamins C and E—antioxidants that normally protect cells from damage caused by radiation, pollution and other toxins. Fortunately, say researchers, there are ways to restock your skin's antioxidant supply and lower the risk of such damage.

In 1992 Australian scientists who compared men who had skin cancer with others who were cancer-free found that the latter ate significantly more antioxidant-dense produce—especially carrots, pumpkin and cabbage, which are rich in beta-carotene and vitamin C. The healthy men also ate more beans, peas, lentils and fish.

Consider a supplement. Do you eat at least five servings of fruit and vegetables daily? If not, it might be wise to take a vitamin supplement for antioxidant insurance, says Hasan Mukhtar, Ph.D., professor of dermatology at Case Western Reserve University and co-director of the Skin Disease Research Center, both in Cleveland. Other experts agree. Jeffrey Blumberg, Ph.D., associate director of the Jean Mayer USDA Human Nutrition Research Center on Aging at Tufts University in Boston, recommends taking a multivitamin, or a combination of a multivitamin and individual supplements, which supplies 25 to 70 micrograms of selenium, 10 to 20 milligrams of beta-carotene, 100 to 400 international units of vitamin E and 250 to 1,000 milligrams of vitamin C every day.

Drink green tea. In a study at Case Western Reserve University, researchers found that mice who drank green tea showed lower skin cancer rates than their nondrinking coun-

DIETARY TACTICS AGAINST THINNING HAIR

In the 1970 film *Ryan's Daughter*, the heroine is punished for an adulterous affair by having her hair shorn—a punishment guaranteed to humiliate her.

For women, hair is a sign of sexuality, youth and vitality, says Marietta Lynn Baba, Ph.D., professor of anthropology at Wayne State University in Detroit, so it's no wonder that any degree of hair loss is so traumatic.

Although women don't go bald the way some men do, a good 25 percent of us have a problem with thinning during our thirties, forties or fifties, says D'Anne Kleinsmith, M.D., a dermatologist and affiliate with William Beaumont Hospital in West Bloomfield, Michigan. Many forms of hair loss are usually temporary, she says.

If hair loss continues for more than a couple of months, see a doctor, says Farah Shah, M.D., assistant professor of dermatology and pediatrics at Texas Tech University Health Sciences Center in Lubbock. It may be a symptom of an underlying problem, such as a malfunctioning thyroid.

Severe dieting can cause temporary hair loss, as can iron-deficiency anemia. Fever, stress and hormonal changes—during pregnancy, for instance—are other common causes. Here's how to lessen the likelihood of temporary loss.

Get enough iron. The Daily Value (DV) for iron is 18 milligrams. If you're not eating three two- to three-ounce servings of red meat a week, you may be running short of this essential mineral. Your best bet is to include more iron-rich foods—such as enriched cereal grains, dark green vegetables and legumes—in your daily diet, says Mary Frances Picciano, Ph.D., professor of nutrition at Pennsylvania State University in University Park. If that still does not add up to the DV, many doctors recommend that you turn to supplements for some extra daily iron.

Ditch crash diets. Rapid weight-loss diets and the poor nutrition that accompanies them can also lead to hair loss. "If you go on a diet, don't eat so little that you lose more than two pounds a week," Dr. Shah says.

terparts. The mice were given the equivalent of four cups of green tea daily—and they were also examined for cancer growths every day, says Dr. Mukhtar.

Dr. Mukhtar, who headed the study, credits the anti-cancer effect to naturally occurring components called polyphenols in the tea, which, like vitamin C, beta-carotene and selenium, act as antioxidants.

Unlike black tea, green tea is obtained by chopping harvested tea and steaming it quickly. With this type of preparation, more polyphenols remain active than in black tea. Look for green tea at health-food stores and Chinese grocery stores. Conveniently, green tea has started showing up in supermarkets, too.

Eat skinny for good skin. Scientists at the Veterans Affairs Medical Center and Baylor College of Medicine in Houston put a group of volunteers with a history of cancerous skin growths on a low-fat diet for two years. Compared with similar individuals who ate a diet with twice as much fat, the low-fat eaters had fewer growths over the two-year period. Why? Certain components of fats may encourage harmful mutations in skin cells, explains Dr. Mukhtar.

Trash crash diets. Rapid weight loss can lead to thinning and wrinkling of the skin, says David M. Stoll, M.D. a Beverly Hills dermatologist and author of *A Woman's Skin*. Shoot for a weight loss of one to two pounds a week—at most.

TIPS FOR CLEARER SKIN

Acne isn't just for kids. Blemishes can persist into your thirties—or show up for the first time in adulthood.

A second kind of acne, called adult acne or rosacea (pronounced *ro-ZAY-shuh*), also affects grown-ups. Trademark blemishes in rosacea are pustules and enlarged blood vessels around the nose, cheeks and forehead. Here's what the experts have to say about diet and acne.

Cut back on fatty foods and chocolate. "Every now and then I run across a patient who swears that she breaks out if she eats chocolate or fries," says D'Anne Kleinsmith, M.D., a dermatologist and affiliate with William Beaumont Hospital in West Bloomfield, Michigan. "Those aren't the most healthy foods anyway, so I say, 'Well, don't eat those, then.' "

While it's rare, these foods can contribute to acne in some people, Dr. Stoll says.

Go easy on coffee, booze and the hot stuff. Caffeine and alcohol can aggravate rosacea. So can spicy foods, says Farah Shah, M.D., assistant professor of dermatology and pediatrics at the Texas Tech Health Sciences Center. So avoid them—but don't avoid your doctor. Prescription medications can make a significant difference, Dr. Shah adds, so see a dermatologist.

HELP FOR HIVES AND CANKER SORES

Your skin is your largest organ, but it's not the toughest. In fact, skin can be downright sensitive, irritated by all sorts of things you eat. Hives (itchy bumps resembling mosquito bites) and canker sores (sore spots inside your mouth) are signs that your skin has been offended. You can help placate it with these approaches.

Eliminate known culprits. Do itchy hives seem to appear after you eat certain foods? One helpful clue is timing. Hives due to food sensitivities usually show up within 30 minutes after the offending morsel has passed your lips, explains Nelson Lee Novick, M.D., associate clinical professor of dermatology at Mount Sinai School of Medicine in New York City and author of *You Can Look Younger at Any Age*. Common food triggers are eggs, milk, peanuts, wheat, seafood, strawberries and mints.

Say good-bye to sharp foods. When you break the soft protective mucous membrane inside your mouth, a canker sore may develop. For this reason, "hard or raw-edged foods, like nuts and potato chips, can sometimes trigger canker sores," according to Dr. Kleinsmith.

In the balance, eating foods that are kind to your skin—and avoiding those that seem to rile it—makes sense.

SIMPLE STEPS FOR PRETTIER NAILS

Nutritional shortfalls can do a number on your nails, leaving them misshapen or brittle. For stronger, more beautiful nails, follow this expert advice.

Beautify with iron. Spoon-shaped nails are a sign of anemia, explains David Stoll, M.D., a Beverly Hills dermatologist and author of *A Woman's Skin*. Eating a small (three-ounce) serving of red meat three times a week or taking a daily multivitamin with iron can straighten them out. (Of course, it's a good idea to consult your doctor to remedy the underlying condition.)

Feed your nails. Low-calorie diets and rapid weight loss can riddle your nails with horizontal ridges, Dr. Stoll explains. If you're trying to lose weight, don't consistently eat so little that you drop more than two pounds a week.

Ask your doctor about biotin supplements. Biotin, a B vitamin, can help strengthen both hair and nails, says Nelson Lee Novick, M.D., associate clinical professor of dermatology at Mount Sinai School of Medicine in New York City and author of *You Can Look Younger at Any Age*.

When Swiss researchers gave volunteers with brittle nails 2,500 micrograms of biotin daily, the volunteers' nails grew considerably less brittle and prone to splitting.

Milk, vegetables, nuts, whole grains, brewer's yeast and tuna are some foods that contain biotin. The Daily Value for biotin is 300 micrograms, but you should check with your doctor before taking biotin supplements to treat brittle nails.

Some simple topical measures can also help brittle nails, says Nicholas Lowe, M.D., clinical professor of dermatology at the University of California at Los Angeles School of Medicine. "Moisturizers such as petroleum jelly or urea-based creams and lotions such as Ultra Mide 25 lotion, used around and over the nails, will reduce brittleness by helping nail hydration," he says.

31

TOOTH AND GUM PROBLEMS

Safeguard your pearly whites

It's your first appointment with a new dentist. You're zipping through the pre-exam questionnaire when suddenly one question stops you abruptly: *"Do you expect to keep your natural teeth all your life?"*

"Of course," you answer automatically. "I assume I will." Then you think a moment. "I never thought about it before. Does this mean there's a chance I might not?"

Your teeth—those elegant, essential, multipurpose tools so necessary for crunching an apple or smiling at a loved one—need special care and feeding for optimal, long-term health.

We're talking about more than cavity prevention. True, the battle against tooth decay—which plagues 85 percent of us by age 17—never ends, no matter how old you are. But by the time you're 30 or 40, other concerns warrant attention: gum disease, called gingivitis, and the more destructive periodontitis, an infection of tissues that help anchor the tooth. Gingivitis can leave your gums red, swollen and even bleeding after a brushing. Periodontitis can ultimately lead to tooth loss. As your gums recede slightly with age, you also face a greater risk of root caries—cavities that attack the vulnerable foundations of your teeth.

HORMONES AND DENTAL HEALTH

Three out of four adults over the age of 35 can expect to experience some degree of gum disease at some point. And while cavities and gum woes bother both sexes, women have some unique dental concerns, says William H. Bowen, D.D.S., Ph.D., chairman of the Department of Dental Research and director of the Cariology Center at the University of Rochester School of Medicine and Dentistry in New York.

During pregnancy, hormonal changes exaggerate the gums' response to plaque, the sticky film of microscopic food particles, bacteria and saliva that lodges at the gumline. Up to 60 percent of pregnant women have some experience with red, bleeding or tender gums.

"During pregnancy, particular attention should be paid to oral hygiene," says Dr. Bowen. "This can be difficult for a pregnant woman who's snacking more to meet her caloric requirements."

Women who use diuretics to control premenstrual water retention, as well as those who take antidepressants, antihistamines or medication for high blood pressure, may find their mouths are dry. This is more than an annoyance, because not having enough saliva leaves you vulnerable to cavities and gum infections.

"Saliva is one of the most precious fluids we have, but it doesn't get the respect it deserves," says Dr. Bowen. "It washes away bacteria and food particles, helps neutralize acids and can even kill bacteria. Saliva also helps replace minerals that are eroded away in early cavities."

Eating disorders can also wreak dental havoc. Women with bulimia, who binge and then purge by vomiting, may find their tooth enamel worn away by stomach acids. Women with anorexia may have more trouble with gum disease due to nutritional deficiencies, says Carole Palmer, R.D., Ed.D., co-head of the Division of Nutrition and Preventive Dentistry at the Tufts University School of Dental Medicine in Boston.

Later in life, tooth loss can be a warning sign of osteoporosis—the leaching of calcium from your bones. In a study of 329 postmenopausal women, researchers at the Jean Mayer USDA Human Nutrition Research Center on Aging at Tufts found that bone loss correlated with tooth loss: the more teeth that were missing, the less dense the bones in the women's spines, wrists and hips—three areas most prone to fractures from osteoporosis.

CHOW FOR YOUR CHOPPERS

A few lucky women are naturally blessed with strong, gleaming, attractive teeth that are resistant to decay and gum disease. Most of us need to be ever-vigilant, though. Experts say we can keep our teeth and gums in tip-top shape by removing and starving the bacteria that are responsible for dental calamities— and feeding the structures supporting the teeth with enough vitamin C, folate and other nutrients vital for warding off infection, as well as the calcium that's necessary for jaw strength and patching early, microscopic cavities.

Food left in the nooks and crannies of your teeth—even for the few hours between lunch and dinner—provides ready fuel for the bacteria that release enamel-melting, cavity-causing acids.

"The bacteria convert carbohydrate—and that could be carbohydrate in candy or bread or fruit or a vegetable—into acids in a matter of minutes," says John D. Featherstone, Ph.D., chairman of the Department of Oral Sciences at the Eastman Dental Center in Rochester, New York. "Within seconds, the acid is diffusing into the tooth, dissolving minerals."

Brushing twice a day with a fluoride toothpaste, plus a once-a-day flossing, are the first lines of defense against bacteria and plaque, says Dr. Featherstone. If you can't get to a toothbrush right away, swishing water in your mouth will help, and so will chewing a piece of artificially sweetened gum, he says. But there's more you can do.

End a meal with cheese, tea or peanuts. Eating a small slice of cheese—particularly Swiss or Cheddar—can neutralize mouth acids, slow bacterial growth and contribute calcium to aid in rebuilding those beginning cavities.

What about the fat? "Low-fat cheese is just as effective, and you only need a small piece," says Dr. Palmer.

Nuts, such as peanuts and sunflower seeds, are among the few foods that do not cause cavities and are good after-meal choices because they promote saliva flow, says Dr. Bowen.

Unsweetened green tea and oolong tea both seem to have preventive powers. "The evidence is very new, but tea may work two ways, by killing bacteria and inhibiting the enzymes that form plaque," Dr. Bowen says.

Avoid sticky carbohydrates. Foods that stick readily to your teeth—such as oatmeal cookies, sugary breakfast cereals and granola bars—may do more damage than a hot-fudge sundae, which contains sugars that dissolve easily in the mouth and can be swept away by saliva, says Dr. Featherstone. "Sticky foods are potentially more damaging," he says.

Don't snack around the clock. Snacking delivers more sugar and carbohydrate fuels to the bacteria in your mouth. In a study from the Netherlands, eight women and men who consumed 12 to 15 sugary or high-carbohydrate snacks during the day had more loss of tooth enamel than a group that did not snack.

"It's important to have long periods of time when your mouth is free of sugars, so that saliva can repair the teeth," Dr. Bowen says. "Snacking, particularly on something like raisins that release sugar as you chew, only allows more cavity-causing acids to build up in your mouth."

Sip water, unsweetened drinks or sugar-free beverages. From orange and cranberry juice to your favorite cola, fruit drinks and sugary soft drinks fuel bacteria the same way snacking does, says Dr. Featherstone. "Sipping one of those big sodas from a convenience store, or sipping any sugar drink for long periods of time, is really not a good idea," he says.

Satisfy your calcium needs. Bone up on low-fat sources of calcium and consider adding a supplement to meet your daily needs for bone and tooth strength, says Dr. Featherstone. Optimal calcium intake for women under 65 is 1,000 milligrams a day; for pregnant women, it's 1,200 to 1,500 milligrams; and for women over 65, it's 1,500 milligrams a day.

NURTURE YOUR GUMS

When it comes to gum disease, food plays a starring role by readying your gums to fight infection, says Dr. Palmer. "Nutrition is part of the defense," she says. "But you have to

THE BEST AND WORST FOODS FOR HEALTHY TEETH AND GUMS

Doctors say that certain foods promote good dental health in women. Others get a big "thumbs-down." Here are dental experts' top picks and pans and how they work.

BEST FOODS

- Cheese: Neutralizes acid, contains calcium for tooth rebuilding.
- Nuts: Stimulate saliva.
- Unsweetened tea: Green and oolong teas may kill bacteria or stop plaque.
- Red peppers: Have lots of vitamin C for healthy gums.
- Beans: Contain folate for healthy gums.
- Steamed clams: Offer iron for healthy gums.

WORST FOODS

- Granola bars, sugary cereals, oatmeal cookies: Sticky carbohydrates stay on teeth.
- Sweetened drinks: Fuel bacteria that cause cavities.

ward off the attacks as well, by brushing and flossing to remove the bacteria that cause gum disease.''

According to both human and animal studies, deficits of vitamin C, folate, zinc and iron lower the gum's defenses against bacterial invaders. Your best response? "Eat at least five fruits and vegetables a day," says Dr. Palmer. "And if you're the kind of person whose diet really isn't up to par, consider a multivitamin." Here's what you need, plus some good ways to get the minimum requirements for key nutrients.

Eat foods high in vitamin C. The Daily Value (DV) for C is 60 milligrams. Best sources include green and red peppers, tomatoes, broccoli, collard greens, spinach and citrus fruits. (*Note*: According to a study reported in the journal *General Dentistry*, taking 500 milligrams of vitamin C three times a day after a tooth extraction may speed healing.)

Fixate on folate. The DV is 400 micrograms; good sources include beans and leafy vegetables.

Ensure yourself of adequate iron. The DV for women is 18 milligrams, but pregnant women should be getting 30 milligrams. Best sources include cream of wheat cereal, pumpkin seeds, cooked soybeans, tofu, steamed clams and mussels.

Zoom in on zinc. For women, the DV for zinc is 15 milligrams. Beef, lamb, Eastern oysters, toasted wheat germ and miso (a soybean paste used for soup) are the best sources of this mineral.

Be mindful of how you nurture your teeth and gums, and your smile will last a lifetime.

32

UNDERWEIGHT

Tipping the scales in your favor

Friends envy your sleek-as-a-greyhound physique. You slip effortlessly into size five jeans, with room to spare. You get great buys on dresses that few women over the age of 11 can fit into.

Yet in a world that loves the lean-and-leggy look, you feel downright scrawny. In private, you identify more with gawky Olive Oyl than with a svelte young Lauren Bacall or sexy Demi Moore.

Compared to the approximately one-third of American women who are overweight, less than 10 percent are considered underweight. Some are just slightly leaner than average, while others weigh in at 10 percent or more below their ideal weight.

SO WHAT'S THE PROBLEM?

Statistics say that slightly below-average weight may lower a woman's risk of high cholesterol, heart disease and diabetes, says JoAnn E. Manson, M.D., associate professor of medicine at Harvard Medical School, co-director of women's health at Brigham and Women's Hospital in Boston and co-principal investigator of the cardiac component of the Harvard University Nurses' Health Study (an ongoing study of 115,000 women considered a landmark source of evidence regarding women's health). But excessive thinness is another story. Very low body weight may leave you more vulnerable to colds and flu and hamper recovery if you do get sick, says Michael Steelman, M.D., president of the American Society of Bariatric Physicians and founder of the Steelman Clinic in Oklahoma City.

"Thin women may be more drained by an illness than women with more fat reserves," Dr. Steelman says. "They'll have less body fat to draw on if they get sick and start losing weight."

When a woman doesn't eat enough to meet her energy needs, her reproductive system may shut down. Estrogen levels drop, ovulation ceases and menstrual periods may also vanish, a condition called amenorrhea, which jeopardizes fertility. Even if she eventually regains weight, it may take longer than usual to conceive. Over time, low estrogen levels also erode bone density, contributing to osteoporosis.

"It takes a while for the bones to be affected," says Michelle P. Warren, M.D., head of the Division of Reproductive Endocrinology at St. Luke's–Roosevelt Hospital Center in New York City, who has studied the fertility and bone strength of professional dancers from the New York City Ballet and other companies. She adds, "There's evidence that this kind of infertility is higher than we thought among the general population of women."

A woman's body fat is usually 25 to 30 percent of body weight. In underweight women it can drop to 15 percent or less, setting the stage for infertility and bone trouble.

"Extreme weight loss can compromise the health of any woman who is experiencing an energy drain in her life," says Christine L. Wells, Ph.D., professor of exercise science and physical education at Arizona State University in Tempe and author of *Women, Sport, and Performance*. "We're seeing young women athletes with the fragile bones of a 60- or 70-year-old. They're getting a lot of fractures."

Dr. Wells suggests that an underweight woman ask herself three questions to assess her risk of bone loss: If you're premenopausal, are you menstruating? If so, are there signs that you are also ovulating, such as thickening of vaginal discharge around the midpoint of your menstrual cycle? If not, your estrogen levels are probably too low. Can you pinch a little flesh over your pelvic bone? If the answer is no, your body fat may be in dangerously short supply.

So much for the old saying, "You can never be too rich or too thin."

NOT NECESSARILY AN EATING DISORDER

Why are some women thin? It depends. For some, it's no mystery—they intentionally eat small portions to stay slim. Of these, a few are dancers or elite athletes—such as gymnasts and runners—who combine strenuous workouts with body-slimming diets. Others can't eat much—they feel full quickly or simply don't enjoy food. Still others consume plenty of calories but seem to burn food energy so quickly that there's little left to store as body fat. Occasionally, weight loss is the result of digestive problems like diarrhea or hormonal imbalances like hyperthyroidism (an overactive thyroid).

Being thin does not automatically suggest you have a medical problem or an eating disorder, says Kim Edward Le Blanc, M.D., clinical assistant professor of medicine at Louisiana State University Medical Center in Baton Rouge and director of the Le Blanc Clinic in Breaux Bridge. Women with eating disorders, he says, fear weight gain even though they are already thin and will refuse food or purge themselves to become even thinner. (The causes and treatment of eating disorders are discussed in chapter 9.)

"Disordered eating patterns like skipping meals, cutting down portions or avoiding certain foods like meats and dairy products just to maintain a low weight are not the same as eating disorders," says Dr. Le Blanc. "But it's still not healthy. Sometimes these women do not get enough iron or calcium in their diets."

ADD CURVES, NOT FLAB

You say you'd welcome a few pounds—and a few curves? Sounds good. But hold the french fries—nutritionists say suc-

A SHAPE-UP SHAKE FOR THE CALORICALLY DISADVANTAGED

For women who find weight gain a challenge (or even a chore), doctors, nurses and nutritionists sometimes suggest nutritionally supplemented beverages such as Ensure, Carnation Instant Breakfast or other flavored nutritional shakes. Available in serving-size cans, these shakes are high in carbohydrates and low in fat, and they supply generous amounts of vitamins and minerals. Plus, they come in vanilla and chocolate.

The advantage? Automatic portion control.

"A woman who undereats may think a food portion is bigger than it is," says Michael Steelman, M.D., president of the American Society of Bariatric Physicians and founder of the Steelman Clinic in Oklahoma City. "But when you drink a whole can of nutritional supplement, you get a full eight ounces." No measuring, no guessing, no calorie-counting.

cessful weight gain is a lot like successful weight loss: For best results, follow a nutritionally dense diet and plan on slow, steady change. Aim for a gain of a half-pound to a pound a week, say nutritional counselors, and keep fat intake between 25 and 30 percent of daily calories.

"Underweight is an unusual problem, but it has a solution," says Dr. Steelman. First of all, if you smoke, stop. Smoking one to two packs a day raises metabolism about 7 to 10 percent. Stopping smoking is often the simplest and most important way to gain weight and improve health, he says. And if stress—at home or at work—keeps you from eating regular meals, make some changes. And of course, increase your intake of healthy foods.

"Add 250 to 500 calories a day to what you already eat," suggests nutrition consultant Neva Cochran, R.D., spokesperson for the American Dietetic Association. "And keep it low-fat. You don't want to risk the nutritional integrity of your diet or risk healthy problems like high cholesterol levels in your quest to gain weight."

How should you add those extra calories? First, eat three meals a day, says Dr. Le Blanc. And supercharge breakfast, lunch or dinner with nutritious, easy-to-eat "secret ingredients," says Cochran. Here are some suggestions on how to supercharge your meals.

- Having a bowl of cereal? Top it with sliced strawberries, bananas or other fresh fruit. Fruit is also a tasty addition to low-fat yogurt or frozen yogurt.
- Concocting a casserole or stew? Mix two to four tablespoons of non-fat dry milk into the sauce. "It adds calories and calcium, but no bulk," says Cochran.
- Building a sandwich? Slip in a slice of low-fat cheese. "It won't increase the number of bites it takes to finish your lunch, but it will add about 70 calories and some extra calcium," notes Cochran. Or toss grated low-fat cheese on a salad.
- Top potatoes, rice or vegetables with margarine and add a teaspoon of olive oil to pasta. "Don't load your food with fat," Cochran says. "But a little adds calories and flavor."

Here are some other calorie- and appetite-boosting tips from nutritionists.

Don't fill up on water or other beverages before mealtime. They'll leave you feeling too full to eat.

Tackle the main dish first. When faced with a food-laden table, reverse the usual order of courses. First dig into nutrient-dense foods, such as meats, casseroles or other main dishes. Then help yourself to lower-calorie side dishes, like soup or salad.

Dine with a friend. "People who eat with others tend to eat more—it makes eating more enjoyable and fun," says Cochran. It's true: In a study of 120 women students at the University of Toronto, those who had a meal or cookie with friends consumed almost twice as much as those who dined solo.

Think snacks. Reach for a pick-me-up snack at midmorning, midafternoon or before bed—but go for one with complex carbohydrate, suggests Dr. Le Blanc. Good choices include a cup of skim milk, with 90 calories; four fig bars, at 200 calories; a cup of fruit-flavored low-fat yogurt, for 225 calories;

or an ounce of low-fat cheese and four to six crackers, for a total of about 140 calories. Also, don't overlook fruits, says Dr. Le Blanc. A medium-size apple, for example, supplies 80 calories; a banana has 105.

Dried fruit and nuts are also good, portable, energy-dense snacks. So are supplemental nutritional drinks. In contrast, diet soft drinks, coffee and tea contain virtually no calories or nutrients.

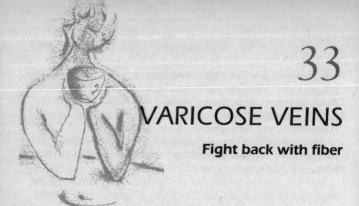

33

VARICOSE VEINS

Fight back with fiber

You expect internal body parts to keep a low profile, do their job and not draw attention. But it doesn't always work that way.

Veins, for instance, will make a spectacle of themselves if they become varicose. They'll protrude and appear blue or green—even purple. If that doesn't get your attention, they'll leave your legs feeling tired and achy.

A good 40 to 50 percent of women have a few such veins on their legs by their fortieth birthdays. You inherit a predisposition to varicose veins, but as is often the case with these dubious birthrights, you can lessen your odds of running afoul of these unsightly veins.

ANATOMY OF A VARICOSE VEIN

What makes a perfectly healthy-looking vein turn blue and ropy? The trouble starts with the tiny valves lining the walls of blood vessels, says Luis Navarro, M.D., senior clinical instructor of surgery at Mount Sinai School of Medicine and director of The Vein Treatment Center, both in New York City, and co-author of *No More Varicose Veins*. Normally the valves open, then close tightly to keep blood moving through the vein, in much the same way that canal locks open and close to control water levels. When the valves start leaking, though, the blood pools in the vein and distends it, says Dr. Navarro.

More often than not, varicose veins appear in the legs—although you can also get them in the groin, arms and hands—because that's where the most blood collects.

Valves can start leaking for two reasons. The vein walls can weaken and stretch, so the valves don't close tightly anymore. Or the valves themselves can weaken and fail, says Robert Weiss, M.D., assistant professor of dermatology at Johns Hopkins University School of Medicine in Baltimore.

Women seem especially prone to inheriting weak vein walls or valves, and with them a tendency to get varicose veins. According to a study conducted in France, if both parents had varicose veins, you have a 90 percent chance of getting them, too. If only one parent did, you have a 62 percent chance if you're a woman and a 25 percent chance if you're a man.

Why the higher incidence in women? Female sex hormones prevent the valves in our veins from working well, so blood flows less easily, causing the vein to bulge, says Dr. Navarro. That is why some women may notice that their varicose veins get worse just before their periods.

The tendency to get varicose veins is only partly inherited. Other factors play a part as well. Research suggests that pregnancy and the Pill can foster varicose veins. So can overweight, a low-fiber diet and inactivity—especially a lot of uninterrupted standing or sitting, says Mitchel Goldman, M.D., assistant clinical professor of medicine and dermatology at the University of California, San Diego, Medical Center.

So it makes sense that the right diet, regular leg-powered exercise and other good health habits can delay the appearance of varicose veins and possibly lessen their severity. If varicose veins run in your family, here's what experts say you should (and shouldn't) do.

If you spend hours standing or sitting, get moving. Leg-powered exercise—like walking or cycling—leaves varicose veins in the dust. The muscles in your legs help keep the blood moving through your veins, explains Dr. Navarro. Each time you move your muscles, they squeeze the veins nearby and push the blood in those vessels onward. Dr. Weiss suggests at least 30 minutes of exercise at least three times a week.

Wiggle your toes. If you sit or stand still for long periods of time, blood can start pooling in your legs and feet. If you don't have time for a walk around the block, flexing your toes or feet will help move blood through the veins in your legs. Raising your legs above the level of your heart will also help. Do one or the other at least every 15 minutes, Dr. Weiss suggests.

Slip on some fancy support. Special compression stockings, designed to hold the veins in your legs snug but not too tight, keep veins from stretching out of shape. Ask about them at your local pharmacy. These days, compression stockings come in several fashion colors, so you don't necessarily have to sacrifice appearance for relief. For best results, wear them daily, say doctors.

Eat more fiber-rich plant foods. Regular, soft bowel movements can lower your risk of varicose veins, Dr. Navarro explains. Straining to relieve your bowels puts pressure on your veins, and that pressure can also cause swelling and distention, Dr. Weiss says. Eating a high-fiber diet makes you far less likely to fall victim to constipation and end up straining in the bathroom, so build your diet around high-fiber fruits and vegetables, beans and whole-grain breads and pastas. The American Dietetic Association suggests you shoot for 20 to 35 grams of fiber a day.

If necessary, supplement. If, despite your best efforts, you're not getting enough fiber in your diet, consider taking a fiber supplement such as Metamucil or Citrucel, suggests Barry Jaffin, M.D., specialist in gastrointestinal motility disorders and clinical instructor in the Department of Gastroenterology at Mount Sinai Medical Center. A fiber supplement can help keep you regular, says Dr. Navarro.

Chase with H$_2$O. Without water, all the fiber in the world can't do its job, says Dr. Weiss. In fact, eating extra fiber while drinking too little water can make you more constipated. ''To keep your digestive system working right, you need both,'' says Dr. Weiss. So quaff at least eight eight-ounce glasses of water or other nonalcoholic fluids a day.

Lose the extra pounds. Doctors agree that people who are very overweight run a higher risk of varicose veins, but the reasons are not entirely clear. One theory is that being over-weight makes it more difficult for blood to be pumped from the legs back to the heart, says Dr. Goldman. Another theory is that overweight people have more blood circulating through their veins than their thinner counterparts, says Dr. Navarro, and more blood means more pressure on vein walls.

To lose weight, cut calories. To cut calories, cut fat—it's loaded with calories (nine per gram) compared to protein or carbohydrate (four per gram). For people prone to varicose veins, that makes low-fat foods like pasta with fresh tomatoes and basil a darn sight better choice than cream-laden fettuc-cine, for example. Twenty-five to 30 percent of your daily calories should come from fat. (For tips on how to reduce your fat intake, see chapter 46.)

Make sweets a treat. If you're faithful about avoiding fat but go whole hog on sweets, you won't lose weight. Limit your sugar intake to 10 percent of the day's calories, advises nutritionist Elizabeth Somer, R.D., in her book *Nutrition for Women*.

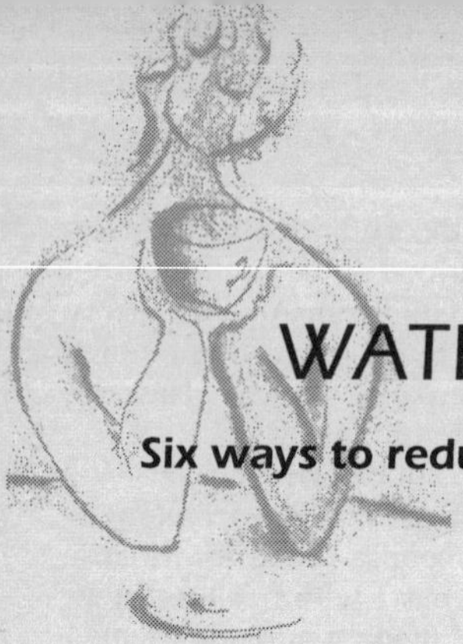

34

WATER RETENTION

Six ways to reduce premenstrual bloating

Live in a woman's body long enough, and you know that sometimes it can seem downright intractable. Like the week or so before your period, when you're too bloated to fit into anything but sweatpants. And what's with the craving for potato chips? By now you'd think your body would have learned that salty stuff like potato chips will only make you retain more water and feel more bloated.

What's going on? And what can you do about it?

"When you take in more salt, your body hangs on to more water by producing less urine," explains Eileen Hoffman, M.D., associate director for education for the Mount Sinai Women's Health Program in New York City and author of *Our Health, Our Lives*.

You're most likely to feel bloated midway through your menstrual cycle, says Dr. Hoffman. Although the exact mechanism is unclear, ten days or so before your period the kidneys hold on to more water than usual. "It happens even if you're going easy on salt," she says. "If you use a lot of salt, though, it is more pronounced."

"Premenstrual hormonal changes alter the kidneys' function," Dr. Hoffman explains. "Instead of letting out all the extra water, they hang on to it."

WHY YOU CRAVE CHIPS (OR OTHER SALTY FOODS)

Though it may seem vexing, there's a certain logic to the pre-menstrual salt cravings many women report. Your kidneys are preparing for pregnancy, a time when your body needs extra water to produce extra blood for a growing fetus, Dr. Hoffman says. In fact, your craving for chips and other salty foods may be your body's way of increasing salt intake so it can retain even more water, she suggests.

If you don't get pregnant during the cycle, the bloating should subside. If bloating persists throughout your cycle, see a doctor, Dr. Hoffman advises. Chronic water retention could signal kidney problems or other conditions that require treatment.

WHAT YOU CAN DO

More often, premenstrual water retention is temporary and nothing to worry about, says Lila A. Wallis, M.D., clinical professor of medicine and director of Update Your Medicine, a program of continuing education for physicians at Cornell University Medical College in New York City. A number of strategies will help keep the bloating at a minimum.

Ease up on the salt shaker. Or skip salt entirely before your period, says Peggy Gerlock, R.D., a spokesperson for the Washington Dietetic Association in Seattle.

"A high salt intake is going to make you retain more water," says Gerlock. "Use less salt, and you'll have less trouble with water retention."

The Daily Value for sodium is 2,400 milligrams. But before your period, says Gerlock, you should aim for less—2,000 milligrams, or the equivalent of about one teaspoon, a day, tops.

Use salt substitutes sparingly. Occasionally, using a salt substitute is okay, says Gerlock. But you really need to accustom your palate to a less salty taste, she says. If you rely on salt substitutes, it won't happen.

Rely on herbs, not salt, for cooking. Flavor dishes with seasoning mixes like Mrs. Dash, fresh herbs, savory spices and lemon juice, says Gerlock.

Cut down on prepared foods. Boxed macaroni and

FOODS TO BATTLE BLOATING

Dietitians advise women who experience premenstrual water retention to select less salty versions of everyday food choices. This list can help simplify your diet—and minimize bloating.

CHOOSE THESE FOODS	INSTEAD OF THESE
Whole-grain bread	Commercial muffins, rolls, biscuits
Cooked oatmeal	Instant hot cereals
Fresh poultry, fish, lean meat, tofu, cooked dried beans	Sausage, luncheon meats, hot dogs, canned pork and beans, bacon, canned meat and fish, corned beef, ham
Fresh and frozen vegetables	Canned vegetables
Fresh fruit	Potato chips, pickles or olives
Mozzarella, Monterey Jack or ricotta cheese	Parmesan or Cheddar cheese
Low-sodium canned soup	Canned soup
Unsalted nuts	Salted nuts

cheese entrées, canned soups and other prepared foods contain significant amounts of salt. If you must rely on prepared foods for convenience, look for low-sodium versions that have less than 140 milligrams of sodium per serving according to the labels.

Make milk your ally. Research suggests that women who get roughly 1,500 milligrams of calcium daily have less trouble with premenstrual symptoms, including water retention, than those who get 500 to 600 milligrams—the average day's intake for many women, says James Penland, Ph.D., a research psychologist at the U.S. Department of Agriculture's Human Nutrition Research Center in Grand Forks, North Dakota.

If you don't get 1,500 milligrams from calcium-rich foods like low-fat or nonfat milk, yogurt and cheese; collard and dandelion greens; or canned salmon with the bones, says Dr. Penland, a calcium supplement can help you reach your quota.

Exercise until you break a sweat. Perspiration flushes out excess water, says Dr. Hoffman. So working out hard enough to perspire is yet another simple way to get rid of retained water.

35

YEAST INFECTIONS

Get rid of the maddening itch

Want to steer clear of itchy, burning yeast infections? Then take a look at your diet. The yeast responsible for most of these all-too-common vaginal infections is *Candida albicans*, a naturally occurring type of fungus.

Avoiding this yeast is difficult. It's everywhere. In your bathroom. On your skin. Even in your mouth, digestive tract and vagina, says Gretchen Lentz, M.D., assistant professor of obstetrics and gynecology at the University of Washington in Seattle.

And while it hasn't been scientifically proven, one researcher claims that if you're sensitive to yeasts, even yeasty foods like bread can set you up for repeat infestations.

The vagina provides the kind of warm, moist conditions that yeasts love, says Joseph K. Hurd, M.D., chairman of the gynecology department at the Lahey Clinic in Burlington, Massachusetts. In the hospitable environment of the vagina, the yeasts can multiply and make you miserable: Primary symptoms are itching, burning and a cottage-cheese-like discharge. But yeasts flourish only under certain conditions.

If you're taking birth control pills, are pregnant or are receiving menopausal estrogen replacement therapy, the accompanying hormonal changes can make you more susceptible to a yeast infection. You're most vulnerable during the ovulation phase of your menstrual cycle. The hormonal changes that occur at those times suppress the growth of helpful bacteria known as lactobacillus, which are normally present in your digestive tract and vagina. Lactobacillus keeps candida in check. When lactobacillus dies off, the yeast takes over.

THE FOOD CONNECTION

The good news is that by making some simple dietary changes, you can stem yeast growth and help prevent infection.

Eat your yogurt. When researchers at Long Island Jewish Medical Center in New York fed 13 women eight ounces of lactobacillus-containing yogurt every day for six months, the incidence of yeast infections among the group dropped nearly 74 percent.

"It may be that the lactobacillus, while in the intestinal tract, limited the concentration of yeast there," Dr. Lentz says. That in turn may have limited the number of yeasts that made their way from the intestine to the vagina.

One caveat: Not all yogurt contains live lactobacillus bacteria. Dr. Lentz recommends you look for labels that state "with active yogurt cultures," "with living yogurt cultures" or "contains active cultures." The National Yogurt Association has established a seal that appears on some brands of refrigerated yogurt as well as on hard and soft frozen yogurt. When you see the seal, you can be sure that the yogurt contains significant amounts of live and active cultures. The seal says LAC (which stands for "live and active cultures").

Cut out the sweets. Yeasts feed on sugar, says Marjorie Crandall, Ph.D., a microbiologist and candida researcher in Torrance, California. So she advises cutting back on jam, jelly, candy and other foods that are high in sugar.

Sidestep yeasty foods. Chronic yeast infections may be a sign of possible yeast allergy, says Dr. Crandall. If you test positive for yeast allergy, your doctor may advise you to avoid food and beverages containing yeast and molds (a related organism) for six months or so. Possible troublemakers include bread, pizza, English muffins, bagels, croissants, raised dough-nuts, beer, wine, liquor, apple cider, moldy cheese (like Brie), wine vinegar, pickles, grapes, berries, cantaloupe, fruit juices, brown sugar, sprouts, mushrooms, yeast extract, vitamins derived from yeast, smoked meats and fish.

Manage your blood sugar. If you're diabetic and don't moderate your blood sugar (glucose) levels, you will have excess sugar in your bloodstream. Along with warmth and moisture, sugar is one of the things yeasts like most, and this can encourage yeast overpopulation, Dr. Lentz explains. (For more details on dietary control of diabetes, see chapter 16.)

Eat well and get enough sleep. Doctors observe that yeasts flourish when your immune system is too down-and-out to keep them in check. To prevent a yeasty population explosion, experts say it's a good idea to pay attention to good nutrition and get enough rest—both essential to a sound immune system. (For more details on getting adequate nutrition, see chapter 42.)

Go easy on antibiotics. Antibiotics are strong stuff—they kill whatever "bad" bacteria ails you, but they can also kill off good bacteria like lactobacillus, giving yeasts an opportunity to thrive. If you're prescribed antibiotics for, say, acne or a urinary tract infection, your odds of a yeast infection jump, says Dr. Hurd. So if at any time you have a condition for which your doctor needs to prescribe antibiotics, ask her to give you an antifungal medication to prevent yeast infection.

Ask about acidophilus. Eating yogurt, drinking acidophilus milk or taking acidophilus tablets may be helpful for a few days after completing the course of antibiotics, according to Jane Miller, M.D., assistant professor of urology at the University of Washington in Seattle.

Know when to call the doc. If you develop what feel like symptoms of a yeast infection and have never had one before, see a doctor, advises Dr. Hurd. Other disorders, including herpes, have similar symptoms and need to be ruled out. If you do indeed have a yeast infection, your physician will likely prescribe an oral or topical antifungal medication that kills yeast. If, after seeing your doctor for the first infection, you recognize the symptoms and feel that the infection is recurring, the doctor likely will suggest that you buy an over-the-counter antifungal medication such as Monistat or Gyne-Lotrimin.

PART 3

FOOD AND YOUR FEMALE BODY

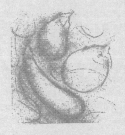

36

BODY SHAPE

Working with, not against, your destiny

One day back in the Stone Age, when human survival was a dicey proposition, a sculptor grabbed a rock and chiseled out a female figure. Today, in the Museum of Natural History in Vienna, there is a stone woman with bulging breasts, chunky hips and a big, wide, no-apologies behind—his timeless tribute to the female form.

When art historians unearthed the statue about 100 years ago, they named it the Venus of Willendorf after the Roman goddess of beauty and the village along the Danube where the statue was found. In its own primitive way, it is very beautiful.

In carving those chunky hips and breasts, art historians realized, the sculptor was glorifying the woman's physical attributes—attributes that guaranteed the survival of men and women as a species. Without the fat stored in her hips and bosom, a woman couldn't carry a child through pregnancy or breast-feed in times of famine, which were fairly common 22,000 years ago.

It's been a long time since Stone Age artists paid due respect to hippy women, but their shape remains a female legacy. Today we tend to carry proportionately more body fat than men do. And while men pack extra fat around their middles, we tend to wear it around our hips.

Though we're all shaped more or less like our guitar-shaped Stone Age ancestors, genetic deviations have introduced variety over the millennia.

Some of us are hippier than others and add inches to our hips when we gain weight. Favoring fruit metaphors over musical ones, researchers call such women pear-shaped. Others among us store a larger proportion of excess fat around our waists, the way men do. In researcher lingo, we're apple-shaped. Genes dictate where the weight will go (and in what proportion), and hormones carry out the marching orders.

Most of us aren't purely pear- or apple-shaped. We resemble one shape with a bit of the other thrown in, explains Christine L. Wells, Ph.D., professor of exercise science and physiology at Arizona State University in Tempe and author of *Women, Sport and Performance*. Maybe you're an Anjou with a little Mcintosh here and there, or a Granny Smith with some Bartlett curves. You may take after your father, a Red Delicious, or your mother, a nice Bosc, or both.

SEX, CURVES AND MEASURING TAPE

Unlike the Venus of Willendorf, your body shape isn't carved in stone. At 20 you may look exactly like your mother did at that age, yet at 60 you may end up looking very different than she did at 60. Not only your genes but your eating and exercise habits and hormones determine the shape your figure takes. Over the course of your life, your shape will change, depending largely on how you live.

Low-fat eating and exercise will give you a slimmer figure and cut your risk of chronic illness. But they won't transform you into an apple if you're a pear or a pear if you're an apple. Apples who lose (or gain) weight will still be apples, but slimmer (or less round) ones, Dr. Wells says. And for the most part, pears who lose weight will stay pear-shaped.

Pears who smoke are a noteworthy exception. According to a study by the National Institutes on Aging (NIA) in Baltimore, pears who take up smoking will add extra pounds to their middles rather than their hips. Why? Smoking may alter production of the hormones that normally make pears gain around the hips, explains Reubin Andres, M.D., clinical director and chief of the Laboratory of Clinical Physiology at the NIA.

Even if they've never smoked, most pears become more apple-shaped after menopause, packing proportionally more weight around their waists when they gain, says Melinda Manore, Ph.D., associate professor of nutrition at Arizona State University. Once again, sex hormones play a role. After menopause, women produce less of the female hormones progesterone and estrogen, so extra weight starts piling up on our waistlines.

At the same time, our breasts begin to sag because of the reduced production of estrogen (which once kept them from atrophying). Those of us with children often see our breasts sag even more. During pregnancy the milk-secreting glands around our nipples develop, adding bulk to our breasts. Past menopause, when the tissue begins to atrophy, the added bulk makes the breasts droop further.

SHAPE-SHIFTING AND YOUR HEALTH

All this is more than a matter of cosmetics, because your shape influences your health. For years researchers have warned that the heavier you are, the higher your risk of chronic illnesses like diabetes and heart disease. But *where* you carry the extra pounds also seems to influence health.

If you're born an apple or just start looking more like one as you age, it's particularly important for you to stay trim, says Dr. Wells. Excess fat anywhere on your body raises your risk of diabetes, heart disease and joint problems. But extra weight around your stomach further increases those risks.

Studies show that heavy apple-shaped women are more likely to develop high blood pressure, diabetes and breast and endometrial cancer than equally heavy pears. The sex hormone estrogen seems to be the culprit here. Studies show that these women have lots of free estrogen circulating in their bodies— more than pears do, explains David V. Schapira, M.D., chief of hematology/oncology and professor of medicine at Louisiana State University Medical Center in New Orleans and director of the medical center's Stanley S. Scott Cancer Center.

Fortunately, research suggests that apples can lower their

WINTER FLAB?
It's Nature's Way

If you accumulate a little extra body fat here or there—on your hips, thighs, waist or rear—over the winter, don't sweat it. Even the most diligent tend to add fat during the fall and winter, according to researchers at Tufts University School of Medicine in Boston. Come spring, chances are your body will revert to its preautumnal figure.

The researchers found that women tend to have more lean tissue during spring and summer and less in the fall and winter.

"Even taking into account the tendency for people to be more active in the spring and summer, we still saw the effect," says Bess Dawson-Hughes, M.D., associate professor of endocrinology at Tufts.

The changes may be due to seasonal shifts in hormone levels, Dr. Dawson-Hughes says. Animal studies suggest that hormone levels fluctuate in such a way that in the winter they trigger conservation of fat needed to bear young in the spring.

circulating estrogen levels by losing weight. And when it comes to losing weight, apples seem to have the advantage over pears.

"There's some evidence that women who carry fat at the waistline lose weight more easily than women who carry it on their hips," says Eric Poehlman, Ph.D., associate professor of medicine at the University of Maryland in Baltimore. "That's because the fat in the stomach is bio-chemically different from the fat in the hips. It seems to be more amenable to being lost."

A YOUNGER, SHAPELIER BOD—WITHOUT STARVING

Whether you're an apple or a pear, there's a right way and a wrong way to lose weight and slim down. The right way is to eat smart and exercise. Eating smart means just that: Eating, not starving. The wrong way to slim down is to go on a starvation diet, Dr. Poehlman says, because once you start eating normally again, you often eventually end up looking heavier than ever. Here's why.

When it's starved, your body does everything it can to conserve the energy stored in your body fat and keep you from withering away. It doesn't know that you intend to start eating again once you can fit into a smaller dress size. For all your body knows, you've found yourself in the midst of a long famine.

On a very low-calorie diet, you *can* lose weight and slim down. Along with body fat, though, you lose muscle. And since muscle burns calories faster than other tissue, muscle loss virtually guarantees that you'll quickly regain weight when you start eating normally again. When you regain, however, you add fat, not muscle. So you end up with proportionately more body fat and less muscle than you started with.

That's the problem. Fat isn't as dense as muscle, so a pound of fat occupies more cubic space than a pound of muscle. Thus, with more body fat and less muscle, you look heavier than you used to, even if you weigh no more than you did before the diet.

"If you lose very gradually, you're probably not relying a lot on body protein stores to make up the difference," Dr. Wells explains. "But if you lose weight fast, then you can lose a large amount of muscle."

Will repeatedly losing and regaining weight make you progressively less muscular and more fat? No one's certain. Some studies suggest it won't, but others suggest it might. Researchers also disagree over the effect pregnancy has on body shape. While a few studies suggest that obese women may get hippier after pregnancy, others suggest otherwise.

To be on the safe side, don't starve to slim down. And although you'll learn in this book that counting calories isn't all that important to your weight, you still need a certain number to maintain good health. So eat at least 1,200 calories a day, says Linn Goldberg, M.D., professor of medicine and head of the health promotion and sports medicine section at Oregon Health Sciences University in Portland. And exercise. Your best bet is a regimen that combines aerobic exercise and weight training.

"A combination of resistance training and aerobics produces a better lean-to-fat ratio,'' says George L. Blackburn, M.D., Ph.D., associate professor of surgery at Harvard Medical School and chief of the Nutrition/Metabolism Laboratory at Deaconess Hospital in Boston. ''The combination will give you a better shape than either aerobics or weight training alone.'' (And you'll learn in chapter 37 that it also steps up your metabolism.)

Aerobic exercises, like brisk walking, running and swimming, work because they burn lots of calories. You don't have to run marathons, though. Consider the results of a Japanese study that compared two groups of middle-aged women. Both groups went on the same moderate-calorie diet. But one group got 45 to 60 minutes of aerobic exercise three or four days a week, while the other lounged. After 12 weeks, the exercisers had lost an average of nearly ten pounds, while the nonexercisers had lost just two pounds.

Aerobic exercise will slim you all over, but it won't help you lose inches in specific spots. There's no way to do that. Neither exercise nor dieting will help you spot-reduce, says nutritionist Linda Eck, R.D. Ed.D., assistant professor of psychology at the University of Memphis.

Still, weight training will help you look both slimmer and younger. Remember: A pound of muscle is more compact than a pound of fat. If you're five feet four inches tall and weigh 120 pounds with 25 percent body fat, you'll look lots slimmer than a woman of the same height and weight who has 40 percent body fat.

''With exercise, a woman can have nearly as much muscle at 60 as she had at 20,'' Dr. Schapira says.

WHAT THE EXPERTS HAVE TO SAY

Here's the wrap-up on getting and keeping the shape you want.

Eat lean. Eat—but eat low-fat. Your body does less work and burns fewer calories when digesting fat than when digesting either complex carbohydrate or protein. That means there are more leftover calories adding inches to your waist after a high-fat meal than after a high-carbohydrate meal.

''Eating more fat in your diet puts more fat on your body,'' Dr. Schapira says. Make sure no more than 25 to 30 percent of the calories you eat each day come from fat. Another 12 to 15 percent should come from protein, like meat, fish, poultry and cheese. Get the rest from complex carbohydrates like rice, oatmeal, pasta, fruits and vegetables. Shoot for at least five servings of fruits and vegetables daily.

Eating low-fat is so core to your successful relationship with food that we've devoted a whole chapter to it (see chapter 46).

Ration the sugar. The rationale for a low-sugar diet is similar to the rationale for a low-fat one. A study at Indiana University in Bloomington suggests that your body does less work and burns fewer calories when digesting sugar than when digesting complex carbohydrates.

"In our study, we found obese people were eating more refined sugars than lean ones were," says Wayne Miller, Ph.D., professor of exercise physiology at the university and author of the study.

Say "Just one, barkeep." Alcohol adds calories and inches. And if you think you eat less when you imbibe, consider the results of a study at Laval University in Quebec, Canada. Researchers there found that people who drank with their meal ate just as much food as those who abstained at the table. All told, drinkers consumed more calories than teetotalers.

Lose slowly. To be sure you don't trick your body into conserving calories, you need to slim down slowly, advises Dr. Goldberg. That means eating enough food and calories— a minimum of 1,200 calories per day.

Don't overeat at one sitting. Eat often, but remember to eat small. Never eat more than 1,000 calories at a time. (That's *conservative* portions of turkey, mashed potatoes, stuffing and pumpkin pie, by the way—*without* buttered vegetables or creamed onions.) "The body can't use more than that amount at any one time," Dr. Goldberg says. It'll store the excess as fat.

Stop smoking. Next time you want to light up, ponder the results of the Institute on Aging's study of smoking and fat distribution. Lighting up, it suggests, may cause potbellies.

Mix aerobics and weight training. "The best way to change your shape is to increase muscle mass and decrease body fat," says Barbara McClanahan, Ed.D., director of the Metabolic Laboratory at the Universities Prevention Center at

STILL NO MIRACLE DIETS FOR CELLULITE

Cellulite is none other than regular, ordinary fat—fat that looks dimpled because it's caught in the web of connective fibers holding your tissues together, says David V. Schapira, M.D., chief of hematology/oncology and professor of medicine at Louisiana State University Medical Center in New Orleans and director of the medical center's Stanley S. Scott Cancer Center, who specializes in the study of body fat.

Either you inherit a tendency to have it, or you don't. It's more prominent on an overweight body, but thin women get cellulite, too.

Here's how the various options shake out.

BEST BETS

- Losing weight with a low-fat diet and exercise.
- Improving underlying muscle tone with resistance training.

MAY WORK

- Liposuction. This works best for small, localized accumulations of cellulite—saddlebags or a tummy bulge, for example, says Geoffrey Tobias, M.D., instructor in facial plastic surgery at Mount Sinai School of Medicine in New York City. "If you have cellulite everywhere, the effect won't be that appreciable," says Dr. Tobias.

UNPROVEN

- Over-the-counter thigh creams.

So when all is said and done, the only safe and sensible way to minimize cellulite is overall weight control and toning.

the University of Memphis. "You need to lift weights and perform some sort of aerobic exercise." Here are the basics.

- Start walking, even if it's just around the block at first, suggests Michael Yessis, Ph.D., founder of Sports Training, a fitness center in Escondido, California.
- Build up to 20 to 60 minutes of aerobic exercise three to five times a week.
- Get intense. Results from a study at Laval University suggest that a high-intensity workout can make you leaner than a moderate one. With intense exercise, your body needs so much energy, it seems to access and burn more stored fat than it burns during a moderate workout.

  The study's authors suggest incorporating brief periods of intense exercise into your aerobic workout. From 10 to 15 ten-second sprints with breaks of a couple of minutes in between should do the trick, says Jean-Aime Simoneau, Ph.D., professor of exercise physiology at the university.
- Learn weight-training basics from a trainer certified by either the American College of Sports Medicine, the U.S. Weight Lifting Federation or the Certified Strength and Conditioning Specialist Agency, suggests Dr. Goldberg. And start out light—a few repetitions with two to three pounds.
- Work each muscle group—upper body, trunk and lower body, Dr. McClanahan advises.

Above all, give your body-shaping regimen time. It may be a couple of months before you see a change, says Dr. Yessis, but the improvement will be worth the wait.

37

METABOLISM

Seven ways to rev up your calorie-burning potential

Why can some of us spend romantic evenings with beef burgundy or Dijon chicken, cozy lunches with pasta primavera or grilled polenta and moonlit nights with dark chocolate biscotti and never gain a pound, while others among us have just a few, guilty assignations with the foods we love and end up on the outs with our clothes practically the next morning?

No doubt you've asked yourself this question hundreds of times (and anguished over the unfairness it represents).

The truth is, some of us have higher metabolic rates than others. Simply put, certain people, by virtue of their genetic makeup, burn a higher-than-average number of calories—the energy units a body burns in the course of sleeping, breathing, working, playing and yes, eating—day in and day out.

This isn't fair, of course. But neither is it absolute. While you can't change your genes, they aren't the only factor that determines how fast you burn calories. When it comes to setting your metabolic rate, genes cast only 10 percent of the votes, says Michael Jensen, M.D., a consultant in endocrinology, metabolism and nutrition at the Mayo Clinic in Rochester, Minnesota.

Your age; hormones; how much fat and muscle you carry; what, how much and how often you eat; and when, how long

242

and how intensely you exercise cast the other 90 percent of the ballots, Dr. Jensen says. Whatever your genetic legacy or age, you can change your eating and exercise habits and shift your metabolism into higher gear.

A BLESSING, NOT A CURSE

This is good news for women, since we have slower metabolic rates than men do. According to a study by researchers at the Baltimore Veterans Affairs Medical Center, a man who's just as tall and just as heavy and has just as much muscle and fat on his frame as you do will burn an average of 50 more calories each day.

This sounds like a disadvantage for women. But in the overall scheme of things, a slower metabolic rate historically has been a real plus for us. A reliable and abundant food supply is a relatively modern development. In bygone eras, a woman's extra fuel efficiency probably increased the odds that she'd be able to deliver and care for a baby even in times of famine, says Eric Poehlman, Ph.D., associate professor of medicine at the University of Maryland at Baltimore and co-author of the study.

Over the ages, the women with fuel-efficient bodies were probably the ones who survived famines, delivered children who made it past infancy and passed down their energy-efficient genes. For the same reason that we have bigger hips, we have slower metabolic rates than guys do.

Your metabolism picks up some speed during pregnancy. It accelerates because your body is doing all that extra work, building a new person from scratch and toting it around for those nine months, Dr. Jensen explains. Once the baby is born, though, your metabolism returns to normal.

Overall, we see our metabolic rates drop as we age. After 30, the average woman can expect her metabolism to slow anywhere from 2 to 4 percent every ten years. Some decline in metabolic rate is an inevitable consequence of aging. But the slowdown is most pronounced in those of us who stop exercising and lose calorie-hungry muscle tissue.

And after menopause, we all see our metabolic rates slow a bit further. Past menopause, we're producing less of the sex hormone progesterone, and when progesterone levels drop, body temperature tends to drop, too, Dr. Jensen says. Since our bodies need less fuel to maintain a lower temperature— the same way a furnace needs less fuel to maintain a lower temperature—we burn fewer calories.

If you don't do anything to rev up your metabolism, you have to eat 2 to 4 percent fewer calories just to maintain your weight and not gain. And if you're trying to reduce, you have to eat even less. Either way, you lose out on lots of important nutrients and delicious calories.

WHY EATING LESS IS COUNTERPRODUCTIVE

The thing is, you don't have to make the sacrifice. By exercising and cutting back on fat, not food, you can offset some of the effects of aging and hormonal change and keep your metabolism revving higher.

Let's take eating first. You have to keep eating. The worst thing you can do to your metabolism is to do a lot less eating, says Linn Goldberg, M.D., professor of medicine and head of the health promotion and sports medicine section at Oregon Health Sciences University in Portland.

Here's why: If you feed your body just a couple of hundred calories a day, it's programmed to interpret this food shortage as a sign of impending famine. To save you from starvation, it automatically turns down the idle on your metabolism and starts conserving fuel. Consequently, you start burning fewer calories.

You may lose weight quickly at the start of a very low calorie diet. But as your body puts the brakes on your metabolism, the pounds get harder to drop. Even worse, months after you've ended the diet, your metabolism continues to plod along at its new, lower speed. Since you've probably lost calorie-hungry muscle tissue on the diet, your metabolism is even slower. This sets you up for a real fall. Even if you're eating no more than you used to eat to maintain your weight, you'll gain pounds when you start eating normally, because your metabolism will be dragging for months, Dr. Goldberg warns.

In fact, researchers at the University of Geneva found that

HOT NEWS FLASH
Chiles Boost Metabolism

Carry a torch for tamales? Swoon over salsa?

If it's spicy food that inflames your passions, you're in luck. Research suggests it'll inflame your metabolism as well.

According to scientists at England's Oxford-Brooks University, eating spicy food can boost your metabolic rate significantly. The warming effect seems to last a good three hours after the last blistering mouthful has passed your lips.

Researchers at the university's Department of Biological and Molecular Sciences studied the effects that two different meals had on metabolism. One meal was bland; the other was spiked with hot mustard and chili sauce.

Both meals boosted metabolic rate. (Remember, your body has to expend energy to digest all types of food.) But the spicy meal raised metabolism 25 percent higher than the bland one.

You don't have to feast on the hot stuff morning, noon and night to reap the benefits. In fact, you shouldn't try to make *every* meal super-spicy.

"It seems that if you eat spices regularly, that may blunt the effect," says Jeya Henry, Ph.D., professor of Biological and molecular science at the university, who headed the study. "What might be sensible is spicy foods maybe two or three times a week."

So go ahead—make yourself some mouth-tingling Caribbean jerk chicken, some black bean chili or some Chinese vegetable dumplings with hot, hot mustard sauce. Your metabolism will love you for it.

the metabolic rates of underfed rats ran 15 percent slower than the rates of well-fed rats in a control group. This effect seemed to persist for several months after the rodents went off their very low-calorie diets. And the same appears to occur in people on restricted-calorie diets.

"Say you're a person who goes on these modified fasts and loses a bunch of weight," says Dr. Goldberg. "Afterward, you say 'I'm going to feed myself again.' But your metabolic rate doesn't jump up. You've reset your metabolic rate to such a low level it doesn't come back for a long time. We've studied people for a couple of months and it didn't come back." A good rule of thumb, says Dr. Goldberg, is to eat no fewer than 1,200 calories a day.

THE EXERCISE FACTOR

While eating the proper combination of foods can help keep your metabolism purring, the very best way to crank up your fuel efficiency is with exercise—specifically, a combination of aerobic exercise and resistance training.

Aerobic exercises—like running, walking and swimming—raise your metabolic rate during and just after your workout. You continue to burn extra calories 30 to 90 minutes after your workout is done, Dr. Goldberg says. It adds up. While a very active 125-pound woman can easily burn 2,200 calories a day, for instance, a sedentary 125-pound woman may burn barely 1,750. That's a difference of 450 calories (about as much as supplied by three slices of pizza).

With weight training, you won't burn as many calories during a workout, but you will build muscle. That's not an insignificant thing—the virtue of muscle tissue is that it burns more calories than fat tissue does, all day long. When you carry proportionally more muscle—and less fat—your metabolism runs higher. Say you weigh 130 pounds and 20 percent of your body is fat. And say you have a twin sister who also weighs 130, but she has 30 percent body fat. By Dr. Jensen's calculation, you'll burn at least 120 calories more than she does every day.

"If you develop more muscle, you will increase your metabolic rate," states Dr. Goldberg. "The muscle is your engine. When you build a bigger engine, you burn more calories."

One of the main reasons our metabolic rate drops as we get older, in fact, is that we tend to get more sedentary and lose muscle. Aerobic exercise and weight training won't guarantee you'll have the same metabolic rate at 60 that you had at 20, but they will narrow the gap between the two, says Dr. Poehlman.

WHAT YOU CAN (AND CAN'T) CHANGE

Some disorders—especially thyroid gland abnormalities—can play havoc with your metabolism. An underactive thyroid will slow it down; an overactive one will speed it up. So if you notice an unexplained change in your weight, ask your doctor about a thyroid test. These problems can be managed medically.

Otherwise, you can pep up your sluggish metabolic rate yourself. Here's how.

Never crash diet. Go on a very low-calorie diet and you're begging your metabolism to stage a slowdown, Dr. Goldberg warns. No matter how badly you want to lose weight, be sure to eat at least 1,200 calories a day. If you exercise as well, you'll gradually lose weight. But the lost weight will be more likely to stay lost.

Always eat breakfast. You may plan to eat lunch, but your body doesn't know that. If you skip breakfast, all your body knows is that its food supply has been interrupted—maybe for a long, long time. So it starts burning calories more slowly to keep you from starving during an impending famine. To reassure your metabolism that there's plenty of food to be had—and keep it purring along—eat something when you wake up.

Nibble and nosh your way through the day. Grazing is the way to continue to reassure your metabolism that famine isn't at hand, says Dr. Goldberg. So eat small meals all day long.

Pick carbohydrates, pass on fat. Your body burns energy while digesting all kinds of food. But it may burn more calories digesting complex carbohydrates than it burns digesting protein or fat. So make sure you get no more than 25 to 30 percent of those calories from fat and get no more than 15 percent from proteins like meats, fish, poultry and cheese. Get the rest from complex carbohydrates like fruits, vegetables, whole-wheat pasta, breads and rice.

"Evidence indicates that eating lots of these foods can boost your metabolic rate," says Dr. Poehlman. He and his colleagues have found that vegetarians have higher metabolic rates than meat-eaters and speculate that the latter's high-carbohydrate diets may account for the difference.

Turn your back on TV. According to a Memphis State Uni-

YOUR PERSONAL METABOLISM CHECKLIST

Frustrated by fruitless efforts to lose weight and keep it off? Put your metabolism to work for you, not against you. Use this checklist to zero in on untapped ways to improve your fuel efficiency.

METABOLISM BOOSTERS

- ✓ High-carbohydrate foods like baked potatoes (supplying 65 percent of calories)
- ✓ Frequent, small meals (including breakfast)
- ✓ Aerobic exercise (30 minutes a day, at least three times a week)
- ✓ Resistance training (three times a week)
- ✓ More muscle, less body fat (for women, roughly 18 to 24 percent body fat)

METABOLISM HINDERERS

- ✓ Low-calorie diets (fewer than 800 calories per day)
- ✓ Skipping breakfast
- ✓ Missing meals
- ✓ Fatty foods like french fries (supplying more than 25 to 30 percent of daily calories)
- ✓ Lack of exercise
- ✓ Watching television
- ✓ Loss of lean muscle tissue

versity study, watching television can temporarily but significantly lower children's metabolic rates. University researchers studied 36 girls who watched an hour of *The Wonder Years*. The kids' metabolic rates dropped an average of 14 percent during the program. Researchers speculate the show, a warm-hearted kiddie drama, lulled the watchers into a sort of stupor.

For us big kids, too much TV may be equally fattening. Turn it off.

Get your metabolism running—with running, swimming, hiking or cycling. When researchers at the University of Vermont compared women who exercised regularly with their sedentary peers, they found the first group had significantly faster metabolic rates. More than ten hours after they'd finished exercising, the exercisers were burning calories 6 percent faster than the nonexercisers.

Experts recommend at least 30 minutes of aerobic exercise, at between 50 and 90 percent of your maximum heart rate, three times a week. The exercisers in the University of Vermont study swam, ran and cycled three or more times weekly.

Add weights. Aerobic exercise should always be a part of weight-loss plan, but when you add resistance training such as weight lifting, you'll keep your weight down with the help of "hungry muscles. Muscle tissue needs more calories," says Janet Walberg-Rankin, Ph.D., associate professor in the exercise science program in the Division of Health and Physical Education at Virginia Polytechnic Institute and State University in Blacksburg.

You don't have to pump iron like Arnold Schwarzenegger to get results from resistance training. A U.S. Department of Agriculture study found that adults who did two dozen repetitions of four basic resistance exercises three times a week boosted their metabolic rates by 15 percent after just 12 weeks.

We'll be honest: You may never be able to eat huge tubs of double-fudge ice cream with impunity. No amount of tinkering with diet and exercise can perform that kind of miracle metabolism makeover. But taken together, these strategies can go a long way toward balancing the scales of fairness between you and your beef burgundy–loving sisters.

38

APPETITE, CRAVINGS AND HORMONES

Decoding your body's dietary signals

A long time ago, scholars thought appetite was ruled by a dictator, namely your stomach. It grumbled vague orders for food, and it didn't stop until you filled it up.

As it turns out, though, not only your stomach but your brain, eyes, nose, taste buds, intestines, assorted other organs, nerves, neurochemicals and hormones all have a say in when, how much and even what you eat. They shout out dietary suggestions in a sort of rowdy democracy.

Sometimes you get the same message from all sources. Other times, your stomach, brain chemicals (known as neurotransmitters) and hormones propose one thing, like "Have a piece of fruit," while your eyes, nose and taste buds lobby for chocolate cake.

The first group is the more prudent, of course, encouraging you to eat when and what you really need to. It's the first group that you should listen to.

Take your stomach. A sort of Speaker of the House, it "growls" to tell you that it's empty, that you're hungry and in need of food, says Adam Drewnowski, Ph.D., professor and director of the Human Nutrition Program at the University of Michigan in Ann Arbor.

It's also worth paying attention to more specific but subtler messages that appear to come from your brain chemicals and hormones. A growing body of research suggests that they're the civic-minded legislators in the pack, responding to changes in the levels of nutrients in your bloodstream, the amount of fat that's stored on your body, the time of day and other variables. They'll lay low if there's no need for a meal or turn out to urge you to eat certain foods if you're lacking nutrients and calories.

After periods of starvation (including the self-imposed version typified by crash dieting), appetite regulators turn out in force and demand lots of food. That's one reason it's so hard to eat moderately after a starvation diet, explains C. Wayne Callaway, M.D., an obesity expert at George Washington University in Washington, D.C.

Specific brain chemicals also seem to trigger appetites for specific foods, such as carbohydrates rather than proteins or fats.

STRESS + MIXED SIGNALS = OVEREATING

Once you've started eating, chemical signals released from your gastrointestinal tract eventually tell you to stop, says Nori Geary, Ph.D., associate research professor in the psychiatry department at Cornell University Medical College in White Plains, New York.

But your eyes, nose and taste buds, like lobbyists promoting their cause, can mislead. "Veto the 'I'm too full for another bite' proposal," they plead, having caught sight of a chocolate eclair. "Have some dessert."

Following external eating cues from your eyes, nose and taste buds and ignoring internal ones from your brain transmitters, stomach and hormones can cause trouble, though. What you eat affects how well your internal appetite regulators do their job. And eating the wrong things can throw them off track.

Since the same brain chemicals and hormones that govern your appetite also help modulate your mood, a derailment can leave you both stuffed and feeling low. In turn, the blues can make you feel more like overeating.

"The problem is, because of erratic eating habits, emotional eating, stress, anything that upsets their normal routine, the neurotransmitters that regulate appetite get out of balance and end up fueling improper eating habits,'' says Elizabeth Somer, R.D., nutritionist and author of *Nutrition for Women* and *Food and Mood*. ''It becomes a vicious cycle.''

WHAT'S YOUR PLEASURE?

Certain internal eating cues are easier to recognize than others. Every four hours or so your stomach empties and begins to ''rumble,'' announcing that you're hungry, Dr. Drewnowski says. So what's to eat? Apparently your brain chemicals and hormones help decide.

Evidence suggests that levels of certain neurotransmitters peak early in the morning, stimulating an appetite for carbohydrates. Working with rats at Rockefeller University in New York City, behavioral neurobiologist Sarah Leibowitz, Ph.D., found that a high-carbohydrate meal seems to trigger production of other neurotransmitters and hormones that then shut down appetite.

This might explain why many of us prefer carbohydrates in the morning and feel better after a high-carbohydrate breakfast, Dr. Leibowitz says. The ''eat carbohydrates'' message makes sense at the start of the day. Waking after a seven- to eight-hour fast, we need the kind of quick energy carbohydrates provide.

In other experiments, Dr. Leibowitz has found that rats prefer proteins and fats when levels of yet another group of brain chemicals peaks. These levels usually start to rise in the afternoon and continue rising through evening.

Here too, the ''eat protein; have some fat'' message may serve a purpose. The body could be storing up calories in preparation for sleep, the seven- or eight-hour stretch when we won't be eating.

Additional research suggests that not only appetites but certain cravings—intense yens for specific foods—may be your body's way of tipping you off that it needs something.

Thomas Wadden, Ph.D., professor of psychology and director of the Weight and Eating Disorders Program at the University of Pennsylvania in Philadelphia, has found that people crave high-protein foods when they're put on restricted diets.

"On the low-calorie diet, it seems their bodies started to crave food of functional value," Dr. Wadden says.

Cravings for sweet, fatty foods like chocolate may be the body's way of responding to stress, Dr. Drewnowski says. These foods prompt the body to release mood-lifting brain chemicals called endorphins, he says.

This may be why women suffering the symptoms of premenstrual syndrome often crave chocolate. Some studies show these women produce unusually low levels of feel-good brain chemicals. The chocolate may temporarily correct the deficiency, Dr. Drewnowski says.

MEMORIES OF PAST DELIGHTS

Of course, we also crave certain foods simply because we've had them before and know they taste good, Dr. Wadden says. Most of us yearn for sweet and fatty or salty and fatty foods.

The sight of a chocolate brownie, a whiff of the sugar-perfumed air of an ice cream parlor or a bakery and the crackle of bacon frying are all external triggers that prompt us to eat certain foods even when we're not hungry. Certain colors also seem to stimulate the appetite. And music—depending on the tempo—can either stimulate or depress it.

In a world chock-full of stimulating sights, sounds and odors of food, the stress/eat/stress cycle is one many of us would like to escape. More than half of all American women consider themselves overweight, and many of us have trouble managing cravings. Tuning in internal eating cues—and tuning out external triggers—can help strike a balance between what you want and what you need.

REGULATING YOUR APPETITE NATURALLY

Occasionally a genetic glitch can throw the appetite's regulatory system off course and lead to obesity, says Dr. Drewnowksi. Nonetheless, Dr. Drewnowski estimates only 10 percent of us are overweight for genetic reasons. The other 90 percent can do something about our weight.

"If we listened to our internal cues only, overeating and overweight would be less of a problem," says Maria Simonson, Ph.D., Sc.D., professor emeritus and director of the Health, Weight and Stress Clinic at the Johns Hopkins Medical Institutions in Baltimore. It's the external eating cues that get us into trouble.

Here's some advice on how to zero in on your body's internal eating cues and work with your appetite and cravings instead of against them.

Eat carbs in the morning. In laboratory rats, levels of brain chemicals that stimulate an appetite for carbohydrates seemed to peak in the morning. A high-carb breakfast appeared to shut off the "eat carbohydrates" message, leaving the rats feeling sated.

So try whole-wheat pancakes, oatmeal and cold cereal in the morning, suggests Dr. Leibowitz. You may feel more satisfied than you would after a plate of eggs and bacon.

Don't overdo fat. High-fat meals at any time of the day seem to induce cravings for yet more fat, according to Dr. Leibowitz. She found that laboratory rats that ate meals that were more than 40 percent fat continued to produce high levels of a neurochemical that stimulates an appetite for fat.

"If you get a huge amount of calories in a small amount of food, it seems the basic regulatory system breaks down," Dr. Geary says.

A study by researchers at England's University of Leeds suggests this holds true for our regulatory systems. The study compared two groups of people: One was served a lunch that was 50 percent fat and the other received a lunch that had less than 25 percent fat. Though the members of the first group ate more calories at midday than the second group ate, they didn't compensate by eating fewer calories at dinner, when both groups were allowed to choose what they ate. A high-fat meal, it seems, simply isn't as satisfying as a high-carbohydrate meal, the researchers concluded.

Don't overdo simple carbohydrates (such as sugary foods and desserts) either. After you eat carbohydrates, your digestive system breaks them down into simple sugars that enter your bloodstream. When the sugars appear, your

SLIMMING INFLUENCES IN TABLE DECOR

Ever wonder why Howard Johnson's opted for that vivid orange color scheme?

Originally the restaurant chain was all decked out in light blue. It looked nice, but customers weren't biting. Sales were low. So the chain called in a food consultant, who suggested the brighter hue. Sales rocketed.

The consultant suspected what was later confirmed by research conducted by Maria Simonson, Ph.D., Sc.D., professor emeritus and director of the Health, Weight and Stress Clinic at the Johns Hopkins Medical Institutions in Baltimore: Bright colors like orange, red and yellow stimulate the appetite far more than dark ones like gray, black and brown.

If you have a problem controlling your appetite, color selection can make a difference: A dark tablecloth and napkins will tame the appetite tiger; bright colors will do the opposite.

pancreas secretes the hormone insulin, which regulates how quickly your cells dip into the sugar—or energy—supply.

If you eat too much sugar at one time, however, things don't go so smoothly. Your blood sugar levels shoot way up, and your pancreas reacts by dumping a lot of insulin into your bloodstream. That increases the rate at which cells tap the sugar supply, and suddenly your blood sugar levels plummet. The drop can leave you feeling tired and irritable and may bring on a craving, says Somer.

DEFENSE SHIELDS UP

If you're overstimulated by the sight, smell or suggestion of food—and your waistline shows it—these tips can help mitigate the effects of potent external eating cues.

Put fewer dishes on the table. The more entrées and side dishes are set before us on the table, the more calories we're likely to eat.

"It's clear that one of the major things that's difficult for people to deal with is the variety of good-tasting, calorically rich foods,'' Dr. Geary says. ''I'd try to avoid situations where there's a rich variety of very calorically rich foods.''

If you're serving pizza or steak or your mother's famous lasagna, then, be sure to balance the meal with a few leaner accompaniments, not a long lineup of other heavy hitters.

Stay out of the kitchen. Simply walking into the kitchen turns our thoughts to food and sets the scene for cravings, Dr. Wadden says. In an experiment, he and his colleagues asked people to go into different rooms in their homes and note how often they thought of or craved food. It rarely happened in the bathroom and basement, happened more often in the dining room and occurred almost continuously in the kitchen.

Think before you eat. If you find yourself raiding the refrigerator or making yourself a ham sandwich after dinner, ask yourself if you're really hungry or if the ham just looked too good to pass up. Eat only if you can honestly say you're famished, says Dr. Simonson.

Walk away from cravings. The kind of craving that kicks in at the sight of an ice cream sandwich may dissipate after 15 minutes or so if you get moving, says Dr. Simonson. So walk around the block a few times on the way to the vending machine. By the time you get there, the ice cream may have lost its appeal.

Fix a sweet craving with fruit. If you can't shake the craving for a sweet, Dr. Simonson suggests you try satisfying it with fresh fruit. The fruit will give you energy, but it won't cause your blood sugar levels to soar, then plummet—setting you up for another craving—the way candy will.

Trick your palate. Low-fat versions of the foods you crave may make you happy without making you fat. If a walk or a piece of fruit doesn't work, *one* serving of a low-fat goodie may be an acceptable compromise.

''The one thing you should avoid is the fat,'' Dr. Drewowski says. ''If you want sugar, indulge in LifeSavers and marshmallows. If you want potato chips, go for the new baked ones. If you want a dessert that's creamy and sweet, go for frozen yogurt and not premium ice cream.''

You might also try new versions of old favorites that are made with so-called fake fats or sugar substitutes or both, he says. It's not clear whether these will boost levels of much-

WHY WOMEN LOVE CHOCOLATE

If you seem to crave chocolate more than your husband, boyfriend or male coworker, you're not imagining things.

Women report cravings for chocolate even more often then men do, explains Harvey Weingarten, Ph.D., professor of psychology at McMaster University in Hamilton, Ontario, who has conducted one of the largest studies on gender differences and food cravings.

Women, in fact, crave chocolate more than any other food.

"We found that as a rule, men tend to crave things like meat and pizza," says Dr. Weingarten. "And some women report the same. But what stands out is how ubiquitous chocolate cravings are among women."

We're talking driving-in-a-blizzard-at-midnight-type cravings.

Why the incessant hankering for chocolate among the XX chromosome set? No one knows—but hypotheses abound. Research suggests we like chocolate primarily for its sweet, creamy, rich taste. In one experiment, scientists at the University of Pennsylvania in Philadelphia gave a group of cocoa-cravers a gelatin capsule that contained chocolate's active chemical compounds, like phenylethylamine, a substance that appears to improve mood—sort of a candy bar supplement. They gave a second group real chocolate. Only the group that got the real thing felt satisfied.

"It looks to us as though what people crave is the melt-in-the-mouth texture and flavor of chocolate," says Paul Rozin, Ph.D., professor of psychology at the university and a member of the research team. "But this doesn't mean hormones and other things don't play a role in initiating (chocolate) cravings."

ARE YOU A CHOCOHOLIC?

Some women who responded to our *Food and You* survey referred to themselves as chocolate addicts or chocoholics. Scientifically, experts aren't so sure anyone can actually be addicted to a particular food, Dr. Weingarten says. But self-described chocoholics do seem to have a few things in common with people who have bona fide addictions to alcohol or other chemical substances.

According to a study conducted in Scotland, most so-called chocolate addicts believe their consumption is excessive and causes problems—like preventing them from losing excess weight. Still, they don't (or can't) give it up. Like individuals who have chemical dependencies, they also report very frequent cravings for chocolate—an average of six a week. And they, too, feel better while indulging their cravings but guilty and depressed afterward.

How then to handle a yen for chocolate? Dr. Weingarten and others say there's no one "remedy" that's right for everyone.

Some studies suggest that trying to ignore a chocolate craving will only intensify it. So nutritionist Elizabeth Somer, R.D., author of *Food and Mood*, suggests eating a small piece when cravings overtake you.

That may be your best bet, since another study suggests that people who eat lots of chocolate get progressively more "desensitized" to the confection. "Thus, the consumer requires more and more of this food to obtain the same degree of pleasure and to produce an adequate degree of satiety," the authors of the study concluded.

NOT AS BAD AS YOU THINK

Though chocolate is high in saturated fat and calories, a small piece probably won't hurt you. Research suggests chocolate may not be as bad for your heart as you might expect. Scientists at Pennsylvania State University in University Park found that chocolate doesn't seem to raise blood levels of either total cholesterol or "bad" LDL cholesterol. The type of saturated fat in chocolate, stearic acid, appears to affect cholesterol levels differently than other types of saturated fatty acids do.

needed mood-lifting brain chemicals the way real sugar and fat do, he adds, but they may. In any event, sugar substitutes don't seem to stimulate the appetite the way early studies suggested.

Of course, don't go overboard on quantity, or you'll defeat the purpose.

Take a (small) bite out of chocolate cravings. Chocolate cravings are harder to resist than most, Somer acknowledges. If you can't resist, try getting by with a very small piece of something chocolatey. To make sure you only have a little, eat your treat with meals—you're less likely to overdo it than if you tackle a jumbo chocolate bar and nothing else.

Another strategy: If you must have chocolate, choose baked goods made with low-fat cocoa powder, she suggests.

Plan ahead. If you know you're susceptible to late-afternoon or late-night cravings, be prepared, Somer says. Be sure to have some nutritious snacks, such as cinnamon-raisin bagels, fruit, low-fat yogurt or graham crackers and peanut butter, on hand. Eat before the urge escalates into a craving or, worse yet, a binge.

Tune in some slow food/mood music. People chew faster and eat more to spirited tunes, such as marches, than to slow, restful strains, Dr. Simonson has found.

Eating in a crowd? Watch your plate! The worry isn't that someone else will gobble your meal but that you will. Researchers at Georgia State University in Atlanta have found that we all eat more when we dine with company. When dining in large groups, in fact, we tend to consume an average of 75 percent more than we eat when dining alone.

Get more exercise. "Good, healthy exercise can decrease the appetite," Dr. Simonson says.

A 20- to 60-minute workout—walking, swimming or tennis, for example—three to five times a week should do it. (If you're not in the habit of exercising, it's a good idea to get clearance from your doctor before you start. And go slowly at first.)

Remain vigilant. Our internal appetite regulators seem to do a better job when we're young. Researchers at the U.S. Department of Agriculture have found that young men do a better job adjusting food intake to meet changing energy needs than older men do. Researchers say it's not clear whether the same applies to women, but it's probably wise to keep closer tabs on what we eat as we age.

39

PREMENSTRUAL SYNDROME

A diet to relieve symptoms

Like tax season, the *Sports Illustrated* swimsuit issue, widowed socks and inexplicable fashion fads, premenstrual syndrome (PMS) shows up with unpleasant regularity.

With it come irritability, depression, insomnia, bloating, headaches, edginess, constipation, fatigue and breast tenderness—to name just a few pesky discomforts.

If that weren't enough, there's the out-of-control appetite and cravings for chocolate and chips that can accompany PMS—and seriously sabotage the best intentions to avoid fats, sugar, salt and other dietary bad guys. PMS can even exacerbate existing health problems like asthma or allergies.

QUIRKY MOODS, QUIRKY APPETITE

Unfortunately, no one's sure why some women get PMS and others don't, or why some of us have really distressing symptoms while others have mild ones. A lucky 15 percent of women actually report pleasant premenstrual side effects, like increased sex drive or creativity.

Levels of the sex hormones estrogen and progesterone fluctuate dramatically just before we menstruate. But that alone doesn't explain PMS. Studies show that women who don't have PMS go through the same hormonal fluctuations that everyone else does. If hormonal fluctuations were the culprit, every woman who menstruates would have PMS.

Research suggests a more complex explanation. Women who get PMS may actually have a slightly different (but still normal) brain chemistry from those who don't. In these women, say theorists, the brain chemicals known as neurotransmitters that transmit messages through the nervous system may behave differently.

"For some reason, their neurotransmitters respond differently to hormonal changes," says Andrea Rapkin, M.D., associate professor of obstetrics and gynecology at the University of California at Los Angeles.

Dr. Rapkin has found that women with PMS, for instance, produce lower levels of a feel-good neurotransmitter called serotonin than do women without PMS. A British study reports that deficiencies of other mood regulators, such as endorphins, could play a role in premenstrual distress.

Shortages of these chemicals or problems with the way the body uses them would explain some symptoms of PMS. Studies show that low levels of serotonin and other brain chemicals can cause depression and anxiety and trigger the kinds of cravings for combinations of fat, sugar and salt that many women report experiencing prior to their periods.

"There's a tendency for women to crave sweets and salty foods premenstrually," says Jean Endicott, Ph.D., professor of clinical psychology in the Department of Psychiatry at Columbia University College of Physicians and Surgeons and director of the Premenstrual Evaluation Unit at Columbia Presbyterian Medical Center, both in New York City. "It may not always be chocolate; it could be pretzels or peanuts."

Studies suggest these cravings could be the body's way of demanding a carbohydrate fix for a shortage of feel-good neurochemicals. When researchers at Massachusetts Institute of Technology in Cambridge fed women with PMS endorphin-boosting high-carbohydrate meals, the women reported feeling less depressed, fatigued and tense.

Research has also shown that drugs capable of boosting serotonin activity eliminate some symptoms of the syndrome—

suggesting that cravings could be an instinctive way of "self-medicating" with food.

A few studies suggest that calcium and magnesium, which play roles in the production of serotonin, may ease symptoms as well, notes James Penland, Ph.D., a research psychologist at the U.S. Department of Agriculture's Human Nutrition Research Center in Grand Forks, North Dakota.

IS IT REALLY PMS?

Chances are, if you have PMS, you know it. Usually the tell-tale symptoms arrive a week to ten days before your period, disappear one to three days after it's begun, then come back to haunt you two weeks later.

Evidence indicates that as many as 95 percent of us have at least a few symptoms of PMS. Some experience the same symptoms in the middle of the month but notice that they worsen premenstrually. About 5 percent of us have symptoms so severe that they interfere with work and relationships.

Just to be sure your symptoms are hormonally related and not due to stress, psychological or medical problems—thyroid disorders cause similar ones—you need to keep a daily symptom diary for at least two months, says Leslie Hartley Gise, M.D., associate clinical professor and director of the Premenstrual Syndromes Program at Mount Sinai School of Medicine in New York City. Each day, note where you are in your menstrual cycle, what your symptoms are and their severity.

Does a Klondike bar soothe your jangled nerves? Does insomnia send you to the fridge for a bowl of cold spaghetti? Do deadlines launch you on a chip binge? Given the choice, would you opt for chocolate over sex? Look for a pattern, for symptoms that appear before but not during or right after your period.

DIETARY FOES AND FRIENDS

If you experience PMS, a few changes in what you eat—and when—can help show symptoms the door.

Eat a little something before a craving strikes. Frequent small meals high in complex carbohydrates can help you shake the moodiness and cravings that go with PMS, says Dr. Endicott. "Anecdotal evidence suggests that you're more irritable about four hours after your last meal," she explains. "So we suggest women don't go more than three or four hours without eating something."

Your best bets: Make midmorning, midafternoon and after-dinner mini-meals of fresh fruit and vegetables, says Dr. Endicott. Get creative: Put half a grapefruit under the broiler to bring out its sweetness. Freeze bananas, puree them in the blender, then refreeze the mixture in ice cube trays to make banana "ice cream." Slice a pear and pair it with tiny slivers of low-fat cheese. Spread spicy apple or pear butter on a toasted whole-wheat English muffin.

Beware of sugar/fat combos. As mentioned, studies suggest that we yearn for chocolate and other sweets before our periods because sugar and fat mixtures raise levels of mood-lifting brain chemicals.

Unfortunately, sugary foods lift you up just to let you down, says Maria Simonson, Sc.D., Ph.D., professor emeritus and director of the Health, Weight and Stress Clinic at the Johns Hopkins Medical Institutions in Baltimore. Eat a lot of sweets and your blood sugar will soar, then plummet, she explains. You end up feeling more dragged-out than you did before the snack.

And if the sweets are both sugary and fatty, like chocolate cookies, you may also end up toting unwanted pounds.

Instead, reach for complex-carbohydrate snacks, like a toasted bagel or fresh vegetables dipped in hummus, suggests Joanne Curran-Celentano, R.D., Ph.D, associate professor of nutritional sciences at the University of New Hampshire in Durham. Or crunch some salt-free whole-wheat pretzels or sweet cherry tomatoes. They will keep your blood sugar and energy level on an even keel, says Dr. Curran-Celentano. You shouldn't eat your snack quickly but should savor and enjoy it, she says. You'll feel more relaxed and satisfied.

Drink your milk. Research shows that women who get roughly 1,500 milligrams of calcium daily have fewer pre-menstrual symptoms than those who get 500 to 600 milli-grams—the average day's intake for American women.

Shoot for at least 1,000 milligrams daily, advises Dr. Penland, preferably from calcium rich-foods (low-fat or nonfat

PMS
What Works

From pacifying cravings with pretzels to beating anxiety with frozen yogurt, women who responded to our *Food and You* survey shared their secrets for fighting PMS with food. Experts explain why these winning tactics work.

KELLY W., AGE 34

"I felt very depressed before every period. And I craved chocolate. Or I'd eat a whole bag of taco chips. I finally went to my gynecologist, and she recommended vitamin therapy. Now I take vitamin E, magnesium and B$_6$ when I feel the onset of symptoms. That eliminates the depression. I still have the food cravings. I try to eat unsalted pretzels—they're sugar-free and low in fat and sodium—or eat just a little of whatever food I crave."

Why it works: Both B$_6$ and magnesium seem to aid the production of a feel-good brain chemical known as serotonin, low levels of which are associated with depression, according to a report in the *British Medical Journal*. As for snacking on pretzels, women who eat carbohydrates tend to report fewer feelings of depression and other mood disturbances associated with PMS, according to research at the Massachusetts Institute of Technology in Cambridge. Salt contributes to water retention, says Andrea Rapkin, M.D., associate professor of obstetrics and gynecology at the University of California at Los Angeles Medical School, so unsalted pretzels are probably a good choice.

JANICE S., AGE 44

"I crave chocolate and sweets. So I suck on hard candy, because that takes care of the sweet craving. And I allow myself a small cup of frozen yogurt in the evenings. That helps me get over the chocolate craving. I also double up on B vitamins, which helps keep me from being uptight and cranky. I take them two weeks beforehand. And I really try to watch my caffeine."

Why it works: Hard candy usually contains no fat; an ounce of milk chocolate has almost nine grams. So Janice is satisfying her sweet tooth while saving on unwanted fat. As for yogurt, women who get a hefty supply of calcium from dairy products like yogurt experience fewer PMS symptoms, says James Penland, Ph.D., a research psychologist at the U.S. Department of Agriculture's Human Nutrition Research Center in Grand Forks, North Dakota. And as Dr. Rapkin notes, B_6 seems to aid production of serotonin. Evidence indicates that caffeine, a stimulant in coffee and chocolate, may magnify premenstrual anxiety, says Jean Endicott, Ph.D., professor of clinical psychology in the Department of Psychiatry at Columbia University College of Physicians and Surgeons and director of the Premenstrual Evaluation Unit at Columbia Presbyterian Medical Center, both in New York City. So staying away from caffeine helps ease jitters.

KATHY S., AGE 33

"I have chocolate cravings. What works is not taking the first bite of chocolate. If I do, forget it. If I'm overwhelmed by the craving, I satisfy it with a low-fat McDonald's chocolate shake. I sometimes feel bloated before my period, so I really watch the salt."

Why it works: Research done by behavioral neurobiologist Sarah Leibowitz, Ph.D., at Rockefeller University in New York City indicates that giving in to a craving for high-fat food tends to lead to cravings for more high-fat foods. So eating a low-fat version of whatever you crave helps keep PMS cravings under control. And as noted above, salt can worsen premenstrual water retention, says Dr. Rapkin.

milk, yogurt and cheese; collard and dandelion greens; or canned salmon with the bones). If you miss the mark, he says, consider a calcium supplement.

Look for B_6. Like magnesium and calcium, vitamin B_6 seems to aid in the production of serotonin, the feel-good brain chemical that may be in short supply in those with PMS, according to a report in the *British Medical Journal*. A 100-

HERBAL TEAS FOR PMS

"Thank God for tea!" effused English essayist Sydney Smith. And with good cause: Nothing soothes the nerves like a hot cup of tea. And depending on the brew, tea can help relieve bothersome symptoms of premenstrual syndrome, such as headaches or insomnia, says Melvyn Werbach, M.D., assistant clinical professor of anesthesiology and psychiatry at the University of California at Los Angeles, author of *Healing with Food* and co-author of *Botanical Influences on Illness*.

In one study, 89 percent of volunteers reported more restful sleep after drinking a cup of valerian tea. Substances in valerian root, from which the tea is made, appear to latch on to brain receptors that play a key role in sedation, Dr. Werbach explains.

Feverfew, another herb, has been winning praises as a headache remedy for 200 years. Twentieth-century scientific studies have upheld its reputation, Dr. Werbach says.

Both valerian and feverfew are considered generally safe, says Dr. Werbach, although as is sometimes the case with herbs, their safety in pregnancy is unproven. Feverfew is best used as needed, not continuously, because discontinuing its use after several years can, paradoxically, cause severe migraines. Also keep in mind that herbs are medicine and not always entirely free of side effects. If you feel worse instead of better, consider other options.

VALERIAN ROOT TEA FOR PREMENSTRUAL INSOMNIA

Valerian root powder is available at health food stores, either loose or in tea bags.

    1 teaspoon or 1 bag dried valerian root powder
    1 cup boiling water

Pour the water over the herbs. Cover the container to prevent volatile oils from evaporating and steep for 10 minutes. Strain, then drink.

FEVERFEW TEA FOR PREMENSTRUAL HEADACHE

Like valerian, feverfew is available at health food stores.
Drink one to two cups a day, in tablespoon-size doses, for
one week preceding menstruation.
    1 heaping teaspoon fresh or dried feverfew leaves
    1 cup boiling water
  Pour the water over the herbs. Cover to prevent volatile
oils from evaporating and steep for 10 minutes. Strain, then
drink.

milligram daily dose seems to help ease symptoms. Don't
exceed that amount, though—high levels of B_6 can cause nerve
damage. Try to get at least part of your daily quota from food.
Bananas, white-meat turkey, chicken breast, baked potatoes,
chick-peas, spinach, tomatoes, brown rice, rainbow trout and
fresh tuna are rich in B_6.

Toss the salt. Salty foods can make water retention worse.
If bloating is a problem, lose the salt shaker, says Dr. Rapkin.
Try flavoring your food with herbs or a salt substitute like
Mrs. Dash. And avoid salty prepared foods.

"Some women find they swell if they eat a lot of high-salt
foods like pizza," Dr. Rapkin says. "If they already have
swelling, it's reasonable not to eat those foods."

Quit caffeine. A mug of coffee may seem just the antidote
for premenstrual fatigue. But it can cause more problems than
it solves, says Dr. Endicott. There's some evidence that caffeine, a stimulant, will make you feel worse if you're anxious
and irritable, she says. It may also contribute to breast tenderness. So cut back on coffee, tea, cola and chocolate, she suggests. But do it gradually. "Don't stop abruptly, because you
are likely to get horrible headaches," she warns.

Start drinking a brew that's three-quarters regular and one-
quarter decaf. Move on to half regular and half decaf, then
graduate to all decaf.

Drink in moderation (if at all). Women who average ten
or more alcoholic drinks a week are more likely to have moderate to severe PMS than nondrinkers, according to a study

conducted at the Kaiser Permanente Medical Center in San Francisco.

Alcohol is also a depressant, so it'll make you feel worse if you're already blue, says Stephanie DeGraff Bender, clinical psychology director of the PMS Clinic in Boulder, Colorado. While dousing your spirits, alcohol will also lower your inhibitions, adds Dr. Endicott. And that's not necessarily beneficial.

"If you're angry, you're more apt to have an outburst if you've been drinking," Dr. Endicott says. "Angry outbursts, tearfulness and other impulsive actions may be facilitated by alcohol."

MORE DO'S FOR THE PMS BLUES

Dietary strategies against PMS are more likely to work if bolstered by other, nondietary strategies.

Exercise. Exercise can lift your mood, help you fight fatigue, relieve tension, make you more alert, help control your appetite and ease insomnia, according to the American College of Obstetricians and Gynecologists.

"It doesn't have to be aerobic dancing or in-line skating," Dr. Endicott says. "Twenty minutes of brisk walking helps. Do it throughout the month, but particularly when you're premenstrual. Studies on fatigue show that, as a pick-me-up, 20 minutes of rapid walking is as beneficial as a 20-minute nap."

As a bonus, extra exercise will also help keep your weight stable if you tend to eat more before your period, Dr. Rapkin says.

Quit smoking. The list of reasons to kick the habit keeps growing. Here's another: Nicotine has a simulating effect, but it wears off quickly, Dr. Gise warns, and you'll feel more fatigued than you did before you lit up.

Take time out to relax. Stress can magnify the symptoms of PMS, Dr. Gise says, but some form of relaxation can help. When researchers taught women to relax with the help of guided imagery, complaints of premenstrual symptoms decreased considerably. Other options include a few minutes of yoga or an exercise break, like a walk around the park, which may improve your outlook.

40

PREGNANCY AND POST-PREGNANCY

The best foods for baby and you

Never eat potatoes with spots, American midwives once warned pregnant women, or your baby will be deformed. Avoid chopped-up, mashed food, their Asian counterparts told expectant moms, or your baby will have a careless disposition.

Fill up on moose thyroid during pregnancy, suggested those in the know at the Arctic Circle. Dine on spider crabs, even if you have to go out of your way to get them, experts urged mothers-to-be in Fiji.

Any woman who's been pregnant knows that there's no shortage of advice on what to eat (and what not to eat) during pregnancy. In truth, though, a good prenatal (and preconception) diet isn't too exotic or complicated. The long and short of it is this: You need extra nutrients during pregnancy, but not as many extra calories as you might expect. The key is to choose what you eat more carefully, picking familiar nutrient-rich foods, say doctors. You're building a whole new person. The foods you eat are the raw (and the cooked) materials.

GETTING READY

These days, obstetricians are emphasizing the value of preconception health more and more. Ideally, you should build a solid nutritional foundation *before* you get pregnant, says Carl Keen, Ph.D., professor of nutrition and internal medicine at the University of California, Davis, although it's never too late to start. If possible, give yourself a few months to a year to get your body in nutritional balance before trying to conceive.

"Prepregnancy nutrition is as important as nutrition during pregnancy," says Dr. Keen. "Many times a woman doesn't know for several weeks that she's pregnant. And by that time, very critical developments have occurred in the growing fetus." Here's an eight-point prepregnancy plan.

Shoot for your ideal weight. According to the American College of Obstetricians and Gynecologists (ACOG), achieving an appropriate weight is paramount to a successful pregnancy. For some women, that means *gaining* weight. Women who are underweight when they conceive are more likely to deliver babies weighing less than 5.5 pounds, the minimum required for a strong, healthy child, according to the ACOG. Statistically, low-birthweight infants are more susceptible to infection or other serious problems and often need medical attention to survive.

At the same time, women who are overweight at conception are more likely to develop complications like gestational diabetes—a type that develops only in pregnant women.

If you need to lose weight, do it before you conceive, says Dorothy Barbo, M.D., professor of obstetrics and gynecology at the University of New Mexico in Albuquerque. Pregnancy is the worst possible time to diet, she says. "If you go on a reducing diet, the baby may not get adequate nutrition."

Re-educate your taste buds. Before you get pregnant, try to cultivate a taste for any nutritious foods you may be neglecting, advises Miami dietitian Sheah Rarback, R.D. Pregnancy is often accompanied by morning sickness, so if you've never cared for say, green vegetables, this isn't the best time to try to learn to love them.

Thrive on five. To construct a solid prepregnancy diet, says Kathleen Zelman, R.D., a nutritionist in Atlanta and spokesperson for the American Dietetic Association, start with a min-

SAY GOOD-BYE TO MORNING SICKNESS

The Wahungue Makioni tribe in Africa have a wonderful folk story concerning pregnancy: According to legend, the Morning Star gave birth to all the plants of the Earth after a pregnancy that lasted one blissfully short night.

Too bad all pregnancies aren't so brief—there'd be no morning sickness. A misnomer, morning sickness can rear its nauseating head at any time of day. It usually disappears after the first trimester, says Dorothy Barbo, M.D., professor of obstetrics and gynecology at the University of New Mexico in Albuquerque. But you can save yourself some of the misery. Here's how to reduce the nausea of real-life pregnancy, according to experts.

- Steer clear of strong odors, says Kathleen Zelman, R.D., a nutritionist in Atlanta and a spokesperson for the American Dietetic Association. Many expectant moms find that strong aromas, like coffee, bacon, cooking meat and strong perfume, make them queasy.
- To try to combat nausea, eat solid foods at one sitting and drink liquids at another, says Zelman. This seems to help.
- Eat crackers before you get out of bed in the morning. An empty stomach sets the scene for nausea, says Zelman.
- Ginger ale and other carbonated beverages may soothe your savage stomach, says Dr. Barbo.
- Shelve the spices. Some women find strong or savory seasonings hard to tolerate during pregnancy, says Wahida Karmally, R.D., director of nutrition at the Irving Center for Clinical Research at Columbia University in New York City.
- "For some women with extreme nausea and vomiting, vitamin B_6 may be worth taking," says Bonnie Worthington-Roberts, Ph.D., professor of nutritional sciences at the University of Washington in Seattle. Don't exceed ten milligrams of B_6 a day, though, as the vitamin may be dangerous in large doses. Also, get permission first from your obstetrician.

imum of five servings of fruits and vegetables a day. Include strawberries, green peppers or other choices rich in vitamin C, plus cantaloupe, spinach and other dark leafy greens and yellow or orange foods—all high in bete-carotene.

Get your fill of folate. If you're trying to get pregnant, says Dr. Keen, you need to include one more nutrient—folate, a B vitamin found in orange juice, leafy green vegetables, legumes, asparagus, broccoli and wheat germ. Folate can dramatically cut the odds of neural tube defects—serious spinal cord and brain abnormalities. The Recommended Dietary Allowance for pregnant women is 400 micrograms of folate a day. Unless you eat folate-rich foods daily, you may need a supplement, says Dr. Barbo.

Most obstetricians (and the ACOG) suggest you start taking 400 micrograms of folic acid (the supplemental form of folate) daily as soon as you start trying to conceive. A baby's neural tube forms within the first four weeks of pregnancy, and most mothers don't even know they're pregnant at that point, Dr. Barbo notes.

Go for calcium. Add two or three servings of calcium-rich dairy foods, like skim milk or low-fat yogurt, says Zelman. It's essential to the mother's bones and, during pregnancy, for the developing baby's skeleton.

Make good on grains. Shore up your prepregnancy diet with at least six servings of whole grains and other complex carbohydrates for energy, adds Zelman.

Add some protein. Top off your prepregnancy plan with two three-ounce servings of high-protein foods, like lean chicken or beef, fish or tofu for growth and development.

Jettison the alcohol and cigarettes. Booze can lead to brain damage and growth deficiency in the infant, so experts advise against alcohol if you think you're pregnant or are trying to conceive. And if you haven't quit smoking, do it now. Evidence indicates that smoking is a prime cause of underweight deliveries.

WHAT TO EAT WHEN YOU'RE PREGNANT

Once you're pregnant, it's time to shift to phase two of your make-a-baby nutrition plan.

Climb on the scale. Common practice dictates that if you're at your ideal weight when you conceive, you should eat enough over the next nine months to gain 30 to 37 pounds. Gaining too little will boost the odds that you'll deliver an underweight baby. Gaining too much, on the other hand, can raise the odds that you'll develop gestational diabetes or pregnancy-induced high blood pressure (also known as pre-eclampsia or toxemia), jeopardizing you and your developing child.

If you're overweight when you conceive—that is, you're 20 percent or more above your desirable weight—you can still gain 15 pounds or so and deliver a normal-weight baby, says the ACOG. If you're underweight, you may need to gain a bit more than average. Your obstetrician can help determine what's best for you.

During the first couple of months of pregnancy, some women have a hard time gaining any weight at all. Some *lose* weight at first—often due to morning sickness.

Shoot for an extra 300 calories per day. Continue to eat the same healthy diet you ate prior to conception, plus an additional 300 calories a day, says Zelman. Since you also need more protein, vitamins and minerals, the extra 300 calories needs to come from wholesome foods—a sandwich and a piece of fruit, for example—not candy, doughnuts or the like.

Customize your diet to your tastes. Be imaginative: Sandwiches aren't your thing? Have a skinless chicken breast and some crackers, a tofu burger or some whole-grain crackers with peanut butter or low-fat cheese instead. When fruit doesn't appeal to you, opt for a cold glass of fruit or vegetable juice instead, says Dr. Barbo. Or treat yourself to chopped vegetables with a yogurt dip.

Help yourself to milk. According to the National Institutes of Health, pregnant women need a minimum of 1,200 milligrams of calcium daily during pregnancy (200 milligrams above the minimum that you needed before pregnancy). And if you get even more from food sources like skim milk, that's all to the good. Studies suggest increased calcium intake may even reduce the risk of preeclampsia and premature delivery in high-risk women. Zelman recommends adding two cups of milk to your menu each day. That's a total of five eight-ounce glasses of skim milk (or the equivalent) a day.

If you can't bring yourself to drink that much milk, sneak extra calcium into your diet, says Wahida Karmally, R.D., director of nutrition at the Irving Center for Clinical Research at Columbia University in New York City. Add powdered milk to cream soups, casseroles, meat loaf and hamburger patties. Add low-fat cheese to your sandwiches and salads. Try yogurt, frozen yogurt, buttermilk and calcium-rich vegetables like broccoli. Sandwich sardines (with the bones, of course) between bread and enjoy 'em. Refresh yourself with calcium-fortified orange juice. Try some pudding made with milk.

Or make Karmally's favorite, a fruit-and-milk shake. Put low-fat milk, orange juice, vanilla and ice cubes into a blender, then blend. "It's delicious—like an Orange Julius," says Karmally.

Eat small meals often. Grazing accomplishes a number of things. It can help stave off nausea by putting something in your belly, and it helps you meet the increased need for nutrients that you have during pregnancy, says Zelman. Nibbling throughout the day also helps to keep your blood sugar and appetite under control, so you're less likely to grab junk food on impulse, says Warren Crosby, M.D., clinical professor of obstetrics and gynecology at the University of Oklahoma Health Sciences Center in Oklahoma City. Plus, small meals are easier to tolerate toward the end of pregnancy, when the baby is putting a lot of pressure on your digestive tract, says Zelman.

Don't skip breakfast. Some women complain of fatigue early in pregnancy, says Karmally. So be absolutely sure you eat first thing in the morning. "This will prevent you from feeling run-down in midafternoon," she says.

Curb caffeine. Some studies have found that consuming moderate amounts of caffeine during pregnancy—up to three cups of coffee a day or the equivalent—is safe for your baby. Other research suggests that two cups or less a day will raise risks of miscarriage. Err on the side of caution and avoid caffeine-containing colas, coffee, teas and chocolates, the ACOG advises.

Consider a supplement. Even the most diligent among us have a hard time getting all the extra nutrients we need without going overboard on calories, says Dr. Barbo, so most obstetricians prescribe a prenatal multivitamin. It's similar to general-purpose, over-the-counter multivitamins but includes higher doses of calcium, folate, iron and other key nutrients.

"By using a prenatal vitamin, pregnant women can be sure they're covered," Dr. Barbo says, adding, "though we still encourage them to eat plenty of fresh fruit and vegetables and so forth." If you want to take a supplement, do so only under supervision of your obstetrician.

Be wary of vitamin A. Consuming more than 25,000 international units of vitamin A during pregnancy can harm a baby's bones, urinary tract and central nervous system, says Bonnie Worthington-Roberts, Ph.D., professor of nutritional sciences at the University of Washington in Seattle. High doses could be particularly harmful in the first trimester—and some doctors recommend 15,000 international units as an upper limit. Just be sure not to exceed your doctor's recommendation—and don't self-prescribe.

Toast the new arrival later. Like drinking and driving, pregnancy and alcohol don't mix. Exposure to alcohol can cause brain damage and stunt the growth of your developing child. So at this time, abstaining is essential, says Avanelle Kirksey, Ph.D., professor of nutrition at Purdue University in West Lafayette, Indiana.

Befriend fiber. Throughout pregnancy, there's a tendency to become constipated. To combat this, consume more fiber-rich foods, such as legumes and grain products—and drink extra water, Zelman says. Bowel action is more irregular because of slower action due to hormones, says Dr. Barbo. Also, late in pregnancy the baby may compress the lower bowel, she adds.

Drink water. Counseling pregnant women in an arid clime like Albuquerque, Dr. Barbo tells them to drink 10 to 12 eight-ounce glasses of water a day. You may need less, but try to stay hydrated. A splash of lemon juice can make water more palatable; so can refrigerating your drinking water. And of course, drinking milk counts.

Add exercise. By eating nutritious, low-fat foods during pregnancy, you can both stack the deck in favor of a healthy baby and avoid excess weight gain. Exercise helps keep off excess pounds and is safe for most mothers-to-be, says Dr. Crosby. Walking and swimming are good choices, he says. So

FOR VEGETARIAN MOMS-TO-BE

If you're a vegetarian mother-to-be, you may need extra vitamin B_{12} and zinc, according to the American College of Obstetricians and Gynecologists, since meat is a prime source of both. If you don't eat dairy products, you may also need additional calcium, vitamin D or both. Ask your obstetrician if your prenatal supplement provides enough of these vitamins and minerals. Also increase your protein sources, such as milk, legumes (including soybean products such as tofu) and wheat products, says Dorothy Barbo, M.D., professor of obstetrics and gynecology at the University of New Mexico in Albuquerque.

are aerobics. But toward the end of your pregnancy, keep your heart rate down to 150, he advises.

"None of the things that even serious athletes do is going to hurt the baby," he says. "But pregnancy imposes an additional workload on the heart. So moderation is the bottom line. The higher the impact, the harder it's going to be for you. It's fine to maintain your workout level during pregnancy, but it's really not the time to intensify it."

You can expect to have a little extra weight left over after the baby's born, says Dr. Kirksey. "It's healthy. Ten pounds is about average. If the mother breast-feeds and exercises, in time, she'll lose the residual weight."

PUT CRAVINGS TO WORK FOR YOU

So much for what you *should* eat when pregnant. What should you avoid? When queried, experts single out foods such as candy, pastries, chips, fried chickens, cream and sour cream—they're low in nutrients and high in fat—and, of course, alcohol.

Unfortunately, the list of foods women crave most during pregnancy looks suspiciously like the list of worst foods. An estimated 66 to 85 percent of all pregnant women report either cravings for or aversions to foods (or both). According to researchers at the University of Tennessee in Knoxville, pregnant teens crave sweets, chocolate, fruit and fruit juices, pickles, ice cream, pizza, beef and chips more than any other foods. (They turn up their noses at coffee, alcohol, Italian food, meat and eggs.)

When it comes to pregnancy, almost no craving is too weird. Researchers aren't exactly sure why expectant moms have food cravings. Some cravings seem to stem from cultural expectations—you have heard that pregnant women get yens for things like pickles and ice cream, so you do, too. Some cravings may be signals that something is missing from your diet. (Ice cream does supply calcium, after all.) Here are some suggested ways to turn pregnancy cravings from a liability to an asset.

Analyze your cravings. Talk to your obstetrician about your cravings, suggests Karmally. In some cases, they may provide a clue to a possible nutritional deficiency.

Substitute, substitute, substitute. If you're dreaming of biting into rich, dark chocolate truffles, satisfy the longing while satisfying some nutritional needs. Treat yourself to a calcium-rich serving of low-fat chocolate frozen yogurt, Karmally suggests.

If you crave a bag of crunchy chips, try a handful of carrot sticks dunked in yogurt-and-chive dip instead, says Karmally. Next time you cook, cut up some extra vegetables and store them in a plastic bag in the refrigerator so they're readily available when you get the munchies, says Zelman.

Eat just a little. If these surrogate snacks don't work, it's okay to indulge in the real thing (like chips), provided you eat a small amount and combine them with something more nutritious (like a turkey sandwich and vegetables), says Karmally. That way, you don't make a whole meal out of snack food.

ADVICE FOR NURSING MOMS

After your baby's born, your nutritional needs change once more. If you don't breast-feed, you can return to your healthy prepregnancy diet, according to the ACOG. Bear in mind, though, that breast-feeding has certain advantages. The first few weeks, nursing moms pass important immunity to their babies through their breast milk. And studies suggest that breast-fed babies have fewer developmental problems than bottle-fed ones. So if you do breast-feed, you need about 500 calories more each day than you needed before pregnancy, or 200 more than you needed while pregnant.

Make up the difference with a calcium-rich snack such as yogurt, ice milk, low-fat cheese and other choices mentioned previously, says Dr. Barbo. Your obstetrician will probably suggest you also continue to take prenatal vitamins while breast-feeding, she adds.

41

MENOPAUSE

Natural dietary sources of protective estrogen

A few years back, researchers studying menopausal symptoms began to notice something very peculiar going on. Or rather, not going on.

They noticed that women in Japan rarely mentioned experiencing hot flashes during menopause. In the United States, on the other hand, women complained of hot flashes more often than any other menopausal symptom.

Intrigued by the relative coolness in the Land of the Rising Sun, scientists decided to take a closer look—one that paid off in a big way.

Did something in the Japanese diet prevent certain symptoms of menopause? they wondered. Possibly.

One hunch was that tofu, miso soup and other soy foods that figure prominently in Japanese diets—and play a minor role in American cuisine—might explain the mystery of the missing hot flashes.

The hunch was a good one. As it turns out, soy foods contain phytoestrogens, plant compounds that, during digestion, are converted into hormonelike compounds that behave surprisingly like the female sex hormone estrogen. Japanese women get many times more phytoestrogens from their diets than American women do.

But phytoestrogens are only part of the reason that Asian women have fewer symptoms during menopause.

"Oriental women also tend to eat a low-fat diet, and that too could account for the difference," says Margo Woods, Ph.D., associate professor at Tufts University School of Medicine in Boston, who researches phytoestrogens.

EXPLORING THE MISSING LINK

Phytoestrogens occur in two general forms: isoflavones and lignans. Isoflavones are found primarily in soy foods; lignans are present in grains, fruits and vegetables. The theory that a diet rich in these estrogen-like substances could alleviate menopausal symptoms makes sense, researchers believe. Menopause occurs when your ovaries produce less estrogen. The hot flashes, headaches, insomnia and other side effects associated with menopause are, in effect, your body's response to an estrogen "work stoppage." So, say researchers, a continued supply of estrogen-like chemicals, such as phytoestrogens, could tame symptoms of decreased production.

Officially, menopause begins when you have your final menstrual period (average age, 51) and lasts until your body adjusts to the new hormonal order and symptoms end. But menopause isn't an overnight phenomenon: Your body starts producing less estrogen a decade or so before your periods end. By your late forties, estrogen production drops significantly, and you enter what's known as "perimenopause." At this point, many women first start to experience "mini-symptoms" of bigger changes to come.

Hot flashes are the most common sign of menopause, but not the only one. At the height of menopause, women may experience any or all of a variety of other symptoms, including (but not limited to) insomnia, fatigue, headaches, vaginal dryness, urinary tract problems, joint pain and constipation.

For some, menopause is like premenstrual syndrome. We may feel unusually blue during menopause—or extra-jittery. Many of us put on weight, possibly due to cravings for chocolate and other sweets.

Over time, our bodies eventually adjust to the hormonal changes and symptoms disappear. But the loss of estrogen has a dramatic impact on our bodies. It makes us more vulnerable to heart disease and osteoporosis. After menopause, when estrogen levels nose-dive, risks of both jump considerably.

MORE THAN JUST HOT FLASHES

The symptoms of menopause are wide-ranging because so many parts of your body are sensitive to estrogen, explains Brian Walsh, M.D., assistant professor of obstetrics, gynecology and reproductive biology at Harvard Medical School and director of the Menopause Clinic at Brigham and Women's Hospital in Boston. Cells in your brain, your heart, your skin, your bladder and your genitals all have receptors for estrogen—tiny switching stations that pick up and relay instructions that tell your body to behave a certain way. When estrogen latches onto and starts relaying messages via these receptors, it affects all sorts of reactions in your body. When estrogen production starts tapering off at menopause, everything has to readjust to the hormone's absence. And the transition can be shaky.

Doctors caution that research on phytoestrogens in food is preliminary. They're not yet ready to write prescriptions for, say, tofu. But the connection between phytoestrogens and menopause relief is scientifically sound: Phytoestrogens, says Dr. Woods, seem to latch on to your body's estrogen receptors, just like the estrogen your body generates on its own. (Before menopause, it seems that phytoestrogens even compete with estrogen for receptors, hogging as many as they can get.)

Once phytoestrogens link up with receptors, they may relay partial instructions in some of the same ways your own estrogen does, though not as powerfully or accurately. So their effect is somewhat unclear. They are still being investigated. After menopause, when real estrogen is in short supply, phytoestrogens continue to latch on to receptors and act in some ways like estrogen. The presence of phytoestrogens has a buffering effect on the drastic decrease of estrogen that usually takes place during menopause, explains Dr. Woods.

"Our hypothesis is that in Oriental women, the net change in estrogen levels may not be as great as in American women," Dr. Woods says.

TRYING TO CONCEIVE?
Skip Soy

While phytoestrogens in soy foods may be the right stuff for women in menopause, they may be the wrong thing for would-be moms.

Because plant estrogens behave like circulating estrogens, the plant chemicals could have the same effect as a weak birth control pill, says Charles Hughes Jr., M.D., Ph.D., associate professor of comparative medicine and obstetrics and gynecology at the Bowman Gray School of Medicine at Wake Forest University in Winston-Salem, North Carolina. In fact, Dr. Hughes speculates that some vegetarians may have trouble conceiving because their diets are too rich in phytoestrogens. A vegetarian who is trying to conceive, says Dr. Hughes, might do well to steer clear of phytoestrogen-rich foods like soy, whole rye flour and alfalfa sprouts.

Phytoestrogens may stave off more than hot flashes: One study found that fewer Asian women than American women complained of other menopausal symptoms. Other studies suggest that phytoestrogens may help protect postmenopausal women from osteoporosis the way estrogen does. In separate studies in Hungary and Italy, women going through menopause who were treated with phytoestrogens showed a significant increase in bone density.

GIVE SOY A CHANCE

Charles Hughes, Jr., M.D., Ph.D., associate professor of comparative medicine and obstetrics and gynecology at the Bowman Gray School of Medicine at Wake Forest University in Winston-Salem, North Carolina, speculates that at some point, phytoestrogens might prove to be an alternative to synthetic hormone replacement therapy (HRT), which alleviates menopausal symptoms and cuts risks of heart disease and osteoporosis but appears to raise the risk of breast cancer.

Phytoestrogens may actually help defend against breast cancer, says Dr. Hughes, who's doing research with phytoestrogens at Wake Forest. Compared with American women, Japanese women have a lower incidence of breast cancer, he says. Why? Exposure to high levels of estrogen seems to set the stage for breast cancer. But a diet rich in phytoestrogens may ensure that the body is exposed to only moderate levels of the hormone. That's because phytoestrogens compete with estrogen for receptors. When phytoestrogens latch onto receptors—thereby keeping estrogens at bay—their effect on the body is similar to, though weaker than, the effect of the hormone. With a lot of phytoestrogens around, says Dr. Hughes, the body in effect gets a diluted dose of estrogen.

Because research on phytoestrogens is fairly new, doctors aren't yet sure what the optimal intake for women might be. Wulf Utian, M.D., Ph.D., director of the Department of Reproductive Biology at Case Western Reserve University in Cleveland, suggests that women take the lead from Asian women and include a serving or two of soy food in their daily diets.

Dr. Hughes agrees. "It's reasonable to include more soy protein in the diet for general health, and more use of soy foods might provide enough plant estrogens to impact on menopausal symptoms." he says.

If you're not wild about tofu (it takes some getting used to), try one of the new tofu burgers on the market, suggests Dr. Hughes. They're surprisingly good. Or maybe miso soup or soy milk is more to your liking. (For a list of reliable food sources of phytoestrogens, see "A Shopping List of Estrogen-Like Foods" on page 286.)

MORE DIETARY STRATEGIES AGAINST MENOPAUSE

Along with soy, health professionals offer these other nutritional guidelines for easing through menopause. (For more information on nutrition through the years, see chapter 42.)

Beat blahs, build bones with milk. Calcium's effectiveness against osteoporosis is well-documented and is discussed in chapter 27. Research suggests that calcium may also alleviate premenstrual mood swings, and by the same token, a dose may bring you down to earth again if you're riding an emotional roller coaster during menopause, says Chicago nutritionist Alicia Moag-Stahlberg, R.D.

Doctors agree that you need more calcium after menopause than you do before. The National Institutes of Health (NIH) recommend 1,500 milligrams a day (as much as you'd get from four eight-ounce glasses of skim milk) for postmenopausal women who aren't receiving HRT. Women on HRT need slightly less—1,000 milligrams daily, according to the NIH.

Don't like milk? Disguise it. Add dry milk powder to puddings and soups, suggests Moag-Stahlberg. Or try low-fat or nonfat yogurt and cheese. Pick up calcium-fortified breakfast cereals and orange juice. If you still can't get enough, a supplement can make up the difference. She recommends no more than 500 milligrams, taken as calcium carbonate or calcium citrate; if you take more, less calcium is actually absorbed.

Remember *D*, for *dense* (bones, that is). "Vitamin D is essential for absorbing calcium," says Colleen Pierre, R.D., a nutritionist in Baltimore. Sunshine is a good catalyst for the manufacture of vitamin D in your skin. Pasteurized milk is fortified with D, but other dairy products like cheese and yogurt aren't. So if you're not a milk-drinker and you don't go outside much, you may need a D supplement or multivitamin, says Tammy Baker, R.D., of Scottsdale, Arizona, a spokesperson for the American Dietetic Association. Two hundred international units of vitamin D a day should do it.

Pierre says that most people make all the vitamin D they need. All people need is 15 minutes of sunshine a day with their hands and face exposed. We could actually store enough from summer to get us through the winter, but some elderly people and those who live north of Boston may need greater exposure or a supplement. The elderly need more time outdoors or a supplement because their skin can't convert sunlight to vitamin D as well as younger skin can.

Ease up on animal protein. Too much protein makes your body lose calcium, say nutritionists. Two three-ounce servings of high-protein foods like chicken, veal and fish per day should suffice for everyone, says Pierre. On some days, opt for soy or other plant proteins instead of meat dishes. In countries where the intake of animal protein is low, the incidence of hip fractures is lower than in Western countries, according to Mark Messina, Ph.D., author of *The Simple Soybean and Your*

A SHOPPING LIST OF ESTROGEN-LIKE FOODS

Looking to take advantage of natural, estrogen-like compounds in food? Here's where to find them, says Charles Hughes Jr., M.D., Ph.D., associate professor of comparative medicine and obstetrics and gynecology at the Bowman Gray School of Medicine at Wake Forest University in Winston-Salem, North Carolina.

BEST SOURCES

- Soybeans and soy flour

NEXT BEST (IN DESCENDING ORDER)

- Alfalfa and clover sprouts
- Tofu, miso soup and other processed soy products
- Whole-grain rye
- Split peas, pinto beans and lima beans

Health. One reason may be that soy protein causes less calcium to be lost through urine than animal protein does.

Follow the "three-quarters rule." Need a simple self-check to see if your diet is meeting these nutritional rules of thumb? It's simple: Before you dig in to a meal, take a look at what's on your plate. "At least three-quarters should be fruit, vegetables and grains," Baker says. "No more than a quarter of your meal should be animal protein."

Opt for olive oil over butter and cream sauces. Estrogen seems to protect your heart by keeping cholesterol levels in line. A number of studies have found that women have higher levels of LDL (bad, artery-clogging cholesterol) and lower levels of HDL (good, artery-cleaning cholesterol) in their bloodstreams after menopause.

A raft of research shows that a low-fat diet will reduce your risk of heart disease after menopause. Limiting fat to from 25 to 30 percent of your daily calories will help keep the bad stuff under control. So will eating the right kind of fat. (For more details, see chapter 20.)

Saturated fats like lard, animal fats (cream, bacon, fatty

meats and so forth) and tropical oils (such as coconut oil) seem to raise levels of LDL cholesterol. So avoid them. Monounsaturated fats like olive oil and polyunsaturated ones like corn oil won't boost LDL levels and are your best bet, Dr. Walsh says.

Say, "A skinny decaf latte, please." Like excess animal protein, excess caffeine leads to calcium loss. Researchers at Harvard Medical School have found that women who drank more than three cups of coffee a day had thinner bones than light coffee drinkers. So limit coffee, cola, tea and chocolate. That'll also help take an edge off the insomnia that keeps some menopausal women up at night.

42

NUTRITION

The perfect eating plan for women

A hot fudge sundae is an essential part of a nutritious diet.

Well, okay—it's not true. Chances are it got your attention, though.

The truth is, nutrition is a lot more interesting than those lectures on the four basic food groups you heard in high school health class. Then again, your health teacher made *sex* sound boring, too.

Actually, sex is what makes nutrition interesting. As a woman, you have some distinct nutritional needs, many of which are influenced by uniquely female milestones like motherhood and menopause.

All told, you need about two dozen nutrients every single day, says Cheryl Rock, Ph.D., professor of nutrition at the University of Michigan at Ann Arbor. But don't worry—you don't have to memorize food groups in order to eat right. What follows is a detailed, meal-by-meal guide to what every woman needs—and how to get it—without blowing your calorie budget.

The calorie count for the ideas suggested here is around 1,500 calories a day, and the plan is designed to give you all the major nutrients you need for good health, says Dr. Rock.

If you're getting even a minimum amount of exercise—such as a 20-minute walk three times a week—you can follow this plan without gaining weight, she says. The more you exercise, the more you can eat. A more active woman can easily consume anywhere from 1,800 to 2,000 calories a day, says Dr. Rock. But remember, if you eat sensibly, reduce the fat in your diet and exercise regularly, calorie-counting needn't be a concern.

Here are the foods that are best for you.

BREAKFAST—YOU'VE GOTTA HAVE IT

You can't wait until noon to lay in provisions for the day. And not just any breakfast will do.

Figure on fruit. Dr. Rock's number one rule is, "Every meal should include a fruit or vegetable."

That includes breakfast. Since few people can face broccoli first thing in the morning, Dr. Rock says fruit is the logical choice. Concentrate on deep yellow fruits like cantaloupe, which provide beta-carotene and other carotenoids, along with vitamin C. Together, these antioxidant compounds help protect against cancer, heart disease and stroke.

Or, suggests Pittsburgh dietitian Pat Harper, R.D., a spokesperson for the American Dietetic Association, try a peach, a mango or a half-cup of berries. Other options include half a banana or half a grapefruit, a quarter-cup of raisins, or if you like, a half-cup of stewed prunes.

Drink some juice. Six ounces of orange, cranberry or strawberry-kiwi juice will also do the trick, says Dr. Rock. They supply vitamin C. When researchers in Spain compared women who'd developed breast cancer with others who were cancer-free, they found that the latter ate far more fruits and vegetables than the former. What's more, the women with breast cancer included less vitamin C in their overall diets.

Juice is also a rich source of beta-carotene, which is similarly protective. Consider the Harvard University Nurses' Health Study (an ongoing study of 115,000 women considered a landmark source of evidence regarding women's health). Researchers found that, among more than 87,000 women, those who were eating 15 to 21 milligrams of beta-carotene (found in fruits and vegetables) had a 22 percent lower risk of heart attack than those who consumed less than 6 milligrams. They also had 40 percent less risk of stroke.

Pour yourself some milk. You should also get some protein at breakfast, says Dr. Rock. Calcium-rich dairy products like milk are good choices, because calcium is one of the nutrients that women rarely get enough of, says Dr. Rock. Since our bones are often more fragile than men's, we're at greater risk for osteoporosis than they are. The best defense against this bone-thinning disease is, of course, to build strong bones while you can. Unfortunately, your body gets out of the bone-building business after you turn 35. From then on, the best you can do is preserve what you've got, says Gail Frank, R.D., Dr.P.H., professor of nutrition at California State University in Long Beach.

Or think yogurt. Low-fat and nonfat yogurt are other good choices because they also offer both protein and calcium, Dr. Rock explains. According to the National Institutes of Health, women between the ages of 25 and 55 need at least 1,000 milligrams of calcium a day—what you'd find in four eight-ounce glasses of skim milk or three cups of low-fat yogurt. If you're pregnant or nursing, you'll need a significantly higher amount—in the range of 1,200 milligrams. If you don't opt for hormone replacement therapy after menopause, you'll need even more calcium—at least 1,500 milligrams a day.

Low-fat yogurt tends to be higher in calcium than regular or nonfat (since low-fat yogurt is often fortified with powdered skim milk), so it's the best choice, says Dr. Rock.

Consider lactase. To use calcium, your body also needs vitamin D. Milk is a terrific source of both. It's such a good deal for your bones that you should include it in your diet even if you have lactose intolerance and can't digest milk sugar, says Mary Frances Picciano, Ph.D., professor of nutrition at Pennsylvania State University in University Park. If you have trouble tolerating lactose, simply add a few liquid lactase drops (Lactaid Drops) to the carton of milk about an hour before you have a glass. The drops, available at most pharmacies, will digest the milk sugar for you.

REAL FOOD VERSUS INSTANT BREAKFASTS AND ENERGY BARS

It's one of those mornings: You slept through the alarm, your kids missed the bus and you tore a hole in your last pair of stockings.

If you're going to have breakfast, it's gotta be fast.

In emergencies, there's nothing wrong with relying on fortified instant breakfast mixes, says Cheryl Rock, Ph.D., professor of nutrition at the University of Michigan in Ann Arbor. All you have to do is add milk. But there's a caveat.

"With instant breakfasts, you get certain vitamins but none of the fiber or protective nutrients (called phytochemicals) offered by real food," says Dr. Rock. Adding a piece of fresh fruit to your instant breakfast makes for a more nutritious meal, she says. You add fiber, vitamins (especially beta-carotene and vitamin C if you choose yellow fruit like cantaloupe or citrus fruit like oranges). Adding fruit also assures that you're getting protective phytochemicals, hundreds of which scientists are just beginning to study but which don't necessarily show up in factory-formulated foods.

What about lunch on the run? Will an energy bar do?

"If you're really strapped for time, they're okay," says Dr. Rock. But add an apple, peach or other nutritious fruit that's easily consumed out of hand, she says, to get the phytochemicals, vitamins and minerals that energy bars don't provide.

Take a tab or two. You can also find relief with lactase tablets (Lactaid Caplets) taken with milk or dairy products (or immediately afterward).

Buy lactose-friendly dairy products. Try yogurt, frozen yogurt and sweet acidophilus milk. They contain no lactose. But keep in mind that yogurts and cheeses don't contain vitamin D.

Chill that milk. If you don't much like the taste of milk, make your relationship even chillier. Drinking milk from a thick, frosty glass mug improves its flavor.

Remember cereal and milk—they're not just for kids.
With your fruit, protein and calcium you need a serving or
two of grains. That makes cereal and milk the perfect centerpiece for breakfast, says Dr. Rock.

Most breakfast cereals are fortified, so they're good sources
of many vitamins and minerals, Dr. Rock says. If you're trou-
bled by constipation (more common during pregnancy and after age 50), a high-fiber bran cereal is probably a good idea
every day, she says. Sprinkle on some plump raisins (more
fruit) or a sliced peach.

Or you can add a quarter-cup of chopped dried fruit or a
half-cup of fresh fruit (like apricots or strawberries) to your
cereal, suggests Chris Rosenbloom, R.D., Ph.D., a Georgia nutritionist and spokesperson for the American Dietetic Association.

Whole grains are also reputable sources of zinc, a mineral
with many functions, one of which is to maintain your immune
system. Your body needs 12 milligrams of this mineral per
day to stay up to snuff, Dr. Picciano says. If the stresses of
academics, work and family leave you vulnerable to frequent
bouts with colds or other infections, your immune system may
need a boost.

Grill a cheesy English muffin. Another quick way to combine dairy and grains, says Dr. Rock, is to melt two ounces of
low-fat cheese over a hot, crusty English muffin.

Or toast up a peanut butter bagel. For variety, spread
two tablespoons of peanut butter on toast or a bagel, says Dr.
Rock. Serve with milk.

Peanut butter is a fairly good source of vitamin E, another
antioxidant. Yes, peanut butter is high in fat, but it's unsaturated fat, which is less likely to raise the level of cholesterol
in your blood.

When it comes to breads, muffins and bagels, Dr. Rock
suggests you alternate between white and whole-grain choices.
Like fortified cereals, refined breads are enriched with iron.
But whole-grain breads offer more fiber. Studies suggest a diet
high in fiber will spare you from constipation and lower both
your blood cholesterol and your risk of heart disease and colon
cancer, two of the top four causes of death in women. We all
need at least 20 to 30 grams of fiber daily.

MAXI-NUTRIENTS, MINI-CALORIES

Nutritionally, some foods are far superior to others, offering lots of nutrients without a lot of high-calorie baggage. According to Janis Jibrin, R.D., a nutrition consultant in Washington D.C., a diet based primarily on fruits, vegetables, nonfat dairy foods and whole-grain complex carbohydrates like pasta and brown rice is a balanced approach to healthy eating. Since most Americans are getting too much protein in their diets, limit your meat to three-ounce portions, or better yet, says Jibrin, substitute beans for meat whenever you can. To make sure you're getting maximum nutrition for your caloric intake, Jibrin recommends you focus on these nutrition-packed standouts.

FOR THIS NUTRIENT	LOOK FOR
Antioxidants, other vitamins	Broccoli, carrots, collards, swiss chard, citrus fruits, papaya, cantaloupe
Folate	Oranges, orange juice, dark green leafy vegetables
Calcium	Nonfat yogurt, most dark leafy greens, calcium-fortified orange juice, (calcium and folate) skim milk, sardines
Iron	Fortified cereal; beans, especially chick-peas, pinto and white beans; most dark green leafy vegetables
Magnesium	Dark green leafy vegetables, whole grains, nuts and beans such as black beans and chick-peas

FOR THIS PROTEIN SOURCE	LOOK FOR
Meat	Select (extra-lean) cuts, particularly flank steak and top round
Fish	White fish, flounder, red snapper and most other fish

Poultry	Chicken (skinless), turkey (skinless), ground turkey (ground without the skin)
FOR THIS PROTEIN SOURCE	**LOOK FOR**
Legumes (beans)	Dried beans such as chick-peas, kidney and black beans, soybeans and soy-based foods such as tofu, tempeh and soy milk

"If you're eating a minimum of five fruits and vegetables and choosing some whole grains every day, you really don't need to count fiber grams," Dr. Rock says. "Chances are, you'll hit your quota."

Select apple butter and fat-free cream cheese. "A lot of women still think grains are fattening, but the truth is, it's what you put on top of them, like butter, that's fattening," Rosenbloom adds. Try nonfat or low-fat cream cheese on your bagel. Spread fruit butter on your toast, suggests Dr. Rock.

THE ART OF THE MIDMORNING SNACK

Snacking is an opportunity to bolster your nutritional intake, provided you go about it methodically.

Borrow from breakfast. If you're not especially hungry when you first wake up, eat your raisins or drink your juice as a midmorning snack, says Dr. Rock.

Crackers and fruit beat a Danish. The ideal midmorning snack, says Dr. Rock, might consist of fruit and whole-wheat crackers. You get carbohydrates (for quick energy), fiber and—as a bonus—folate, an essential B vitamin.

MAKE THE MOST OF LUNCH

Your stomach empties out and trips the hunger alarm every four hours or so. So by lunchtime, you'll be ready for more food.

Think beyond cold cuts. A tuna or chicken salad sandwich gives you protein and grain, says Dr. Rock. Use lots of celery and carrots for added fiber and beta-carotene.

Adding a couple of tablespoons of low-fat mayonnaise to your chicken salad or roast beef sandwich will make it tastier and help you absorb the vitamins in your diet, Dr. Rock explains. Fat carries vitamins A, D, E and K through your body and performs other essential tasks, explains Rosenbloom. And because fat is a natural component of body tissues, you need some fat in your diet, she says. And it makes food taste better all around. The trick is to keep the amount of fat you eat to a minimum.

Otherwise, there's nothing wrong with a lean roast beef sandwich—a couple of ounces of meat between slices of whole-grain or even white bread, says Dr. Rock. In moderation, red meat is a perfectly fine addition to your menu. In fact, three ounces of lean red meat three times a week will give you a significant percentage of the iron you need to keep going, Dr. Picciano explains.

Red meat is a particularly good dining companion if you're premenopausal. When you have your period, you lose iron via menstrual flow. To make up for the loss, you need 18 milligrams of iron in your diet daily, one and a half times as much as you need after menopause.

Nutritionists suggest just three ounces of meat a day. Men and women alike eat more protein than they need, says Philadelphia nutritionist Mona Sutnick, R.D., Ed.D., a spokesperson for the American Dietetic Association. When you eat excess protein, your body excretes calcium, so women who eat too much meat risk doing their bones harm. Get only the amount of protein you actually need. A three-ounce serving is about the size of a deck of cards.

Fortified breads also add needed iron, adds Dr. Rock, as do dark green leafy vegetables, chick-peas (garbanzo beans), tomato juice and raisins. If you're a vegetarian, though, you should know that the iron you get from vegetable sources isn't as easily utilized by the body. If you don't eat meat, ask your doctor whether you should be taking a multivitamin that includes iron, suggests Jodie Shield, R.D., adjunct instructor of nutrition communication at Rush University in Chicago and a nutritionist in Kildeer, Illinois.

Rendezvous with fruits and vegetables. Dr. Rock recommends including a vegetable or two with lunch. Carrot sticks are tops—they're rich in beta-carotene and other cancer-fighting carotenoids. Tomatoes, cantaloupe and other deep yellow and orange fruits and vegetables are also rich in these key nutrients. Or have a frosty glass of tomato juice or some tomato soup, both loaded with vitamin C.

Diversify your vegetable portfolio. The more varied your vegetable repertoire, the better, say dietitians. No single food will give you all the nutrients your body needs, notes Harper. Some carotenoids (there are about 400 different kinds), for instance, occur in certain fruits and vegetables but not others. Yet these nutrients, close cousins of beta-carotene, may help to ward off illness.

Broaden your lunchtime palate. Pasta (like shells stuffed with ricotta or other low-fat cheese) gives you two servings of grain, two or three ounces of protein and little fat, says Dr. Rock. Chicken breast strips and vegetables stir-fried in a few drops of vegetable oil and served over rice are fine, too, Dr. Rock says.

MIDAFTERNOON DELIGHT

Even on a waist-watching plan, you can afford a midafternoon snack, says Dr. Rock. Here are your options.

Carry over from lunch. Save the vegetable juice or banana or a piece of bread from lunch and eat it at midafternoon, suggests Dr. Rock.

Fruit and crackers make a fine pick-me-up. If you like, have an orange or some whole-grain crackers with a dab of jelly at midafternoon, Dr. Rock says.

JUST-RIGHT DINNERS

Call it dinner, supper, whatever you prefer, the evening meal is your last chance to pack in essential nutrients and have some gustatory fun before toddling off to bed for the night. Dr. Rock's second rule about a nutritious menu is, "Enjoy what you eat." Her suggestions, which follow, reflect that advice.

Your dinner plans should include two servings of grains, a bit of fat and a modest amount of high-protein food.

Beef? Make it lean. If you didn't have roast beef for lunch, consider a couple of ounces of red meat, like an extra-lean hamburger patty, beef kabobs or thinly sliced flank steak, says Dr. Rock.

Serve soup as an entrée. Lots of vegetables and delicious broth make a little meat go a long way, says Diane Woznicki, R.D., a nutritionist at Albright College in Reading, Pennsylvania.

Make a pasta or rice dish. And garnish it with thinly sliced beef or chicken, says Woznicki. That way, you can stretch two or three ounces of meat into a meal.

Veg-e-size your fajitas. Use lots of peppers and onions but only three strips or so of meat.

Catch some fish. Tuna, mackerel, herring, oysters, clams and halibut are good sources of B vitamins, making fish a valuable option. Birth control pills can deplete your body's B vitamin stores, including folate, says Rosenbloom. So if you take the Pill, watch your B vitamin intake. For most people over 65, the body is less efficient at absorbing vitamins B_6 and B_{12} and folate, says Jeffrey Blumberg, associate director of the Jean Mayer USDA Human Nutrition Research Center on Aging at Tufts University in Boston. That's another time to eat more B-rich foods.

Seafood is also a good source of zinc, needed for immunity.

Befriend beans. Beans are a good protein choice, since they're low in fat and cholesterol. A cup of black beans will give you as much protein as two ounces of lean ground beef. If you're past menopause, you need less iron and should eat fewer calories and less fat and cholesterol. For you, beans are ideal.

The fiber in beans can help lower your risk of colon cancer, as well. Comparing people who got roughly 30 grams of fiber in their diets with those who consumed around 12 grams daily, researchers at the Harvard School of Public Health found that the first group had a 50 percent lower risk of developing colon tumors.

Finally, beans—like so many other plant foods—contain various protective substances collectively known as phyto-chemicals. Studies have found that women who eat diets rich in these plant chemicals have a lower risk of breast cancer than those who don't.

QUICK TAKE
What to Eat, When and Why

This one-day menu, compiled by Cheryl Rock, Ph.D., professor of nutrition at the University of Michigan in Ann Arbor, exemplifies the perfect eating plan. Post it on your fridge for easy reference.

EAT THIS	FOR THESE NUTRIENTS
Breakfast	
6 ounces mango, papaya or tangerine juice mixtures	Beta-carotene, vitamin C, folate
Whole-wheat bagel with 2 ounces melted low-fat cheese	Fiber, folate, calcium, protein
Midmorning Snack	
Handful of whole-grain crackers	Folate, carbohydrate
Lunch	
Spinach salad with 2 tablespoons Italian dressing made with olive oil	Beta-carotene, iron, magnesium, monounsaturated oils
6 ounces tomato juice	Vitamin C
3 ounces roast beef between 2 slices of rye bread	Iron, zinc, protein, carbohydrate
Midafternoon Snack	
Small bran muffin	Fiber, carbohydrates
Dinner	
Kale sautéed in olive oil and garlic	Magnesium, beta-carotene, monounsaturated oils
3 ounces tuna steak, broiled with lemon	B vitamins, protein
½ cup brown rice	Fiber, carbohydrate
Small roll	Fiber, carbohydrate

EAT THIS	FOR THESE NUTRIENTS
Dessert	
½ cup frozen yogurt with fresh strawberries	Calcium, vitamin C

You can cook red beans in vegetarian chili and serve it with mashed potatoes, roll black beans in tortillas, dip pita shells in mashed chick-peas or simmer beans into a beautiful dinnertime soup served with crusty French bread.

Cheese and pasta, the perfect mates. If you haven't had two servings of milk, yogurt or cheese yet, serve yourself a dinner of pasta primavera sprinkled with two ounces of shredded nonfat mozzarella, says Dr. Rock.

If it's Friday, this must be pizza. Homemade pizza—a low-fat crust topped with low-fat cheese and steamed vegetables—can go a long way toward meeting your remaining nutritional requirements for the day, says Dr. Rock.

Calling all vegetables. Speaking of vegetables, you should invite at least one vegetable over to your dinner plate, two if you didn't have two at lunch. At least one should be dark green or deep yellow. Small and round but intriguing—truly the Danny DeVito of vegetables—brussels sprouts are a good choice. They're a respectable source of both calcium and iron. Kale, swiss chard, beet greens and broccoli are top picks, too. You can add broccoli to your stir-fry, toss greens in a salad with dressing or sauté them in a couple of tablespoons of olive oil and some garlic. That way, you'll get the fat you need to absorb all those good vitamins, plus a lot of great taste.

Garnish your dinner entrées with a couple of slices of apple. It's half a serving, says Rosenbloom, but it counts.

Put dessert to work for you, not against you. Few things taste as refreshing as fresh seasonal fruit. Have some. If you're lagging in the calcium category, a frosty dish of frozen yogurt topped with fruit (and maybe a dab of chocolate syrup) would be ideal.

Make fruit sorbet. Puree fresh fruits like strawberries, then pour the mixture into ice cube trays and freeze, says Rosenbloom.

Shake it up. Make an exquisitely delicious fruit shake by mixing sliced banana, skim milk, cinnamon and vanilla in the blender, says Rosenbloom.

As you can see, with those pointers, good nutrition doesn't have to be a chore. You can choose and prepare deprivation-free, good-for-you meals—without a fuss.

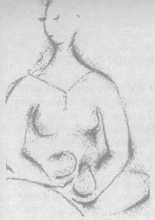

43

SUPPLEMENTS

Not a substitute for food

There's great literature, and then there are Cliffs Notes. There's romance, and there are romance novels. There's Europe, and there's Epcot Center. There's food, and there are dietary supplements.

With food, as with so many other good things in life, much is lost in imitation.

Food offers an enticing aroma, sensuous textures, an intoxicating array of flavors and, if you make the right choices, all the nutrients you need for good health. Dietary supplements offer whatever is listed on the label—no more, no less.

A supplement is just that, an addition to a diet, not the sole source of nutrients. If your food choices lean heavily in the direction of buffalo wings and ice cream, you can't expect a pill to provide the wherewithal to keep you going, say nutrition experts.

So think food first, then supplements—maybe.

WHERE WOMEN'S DIETS FALL SHORT

Women need more than 20 different vitamins and minerals each day. (Daily requirements established by the government are expressed as Daily Values, or DV.) For some nutrients, women's needs vary from those of men. Since women are generally smaller-boned, you're at higher risk for osteoporosis and need more calcium. If you're menstruating, you need extra iron. If you're trying to conceive, you need extra folate. And if you're pregnant or nursing, you need higher amounts of almost everything.

Food is the best source of the nutrients we need. While most multivitamin/mineral supplements contain essentials like folic acid (the supplement form of folate), calcium and iron, they offer no protein, fiber or carbohydrates, which are major building blocks of nutrition. What's more, most supplements can't possibly offer the hundreds of other protective substances (collectively known as phytochemicals) that are found in fruits, vegetables and grains and are now believed to be just as vital to a woman's health as vitamins and minerals, notes Martha L. Rew, R.D., assistant clinical professor of nutrition at Texas Woman's University in Denton. Some studies suggest phytochemicals can help protect us against bone loss, heart disease and even cancer.

That said, surveys indicate that a gap exists between what women eat and what they need. According to one study conducted by the U.S. Department of Agriculture, only about one out of ten women eats even one nutrient-dense dark green or deep yellow vegetable daily, let alone three to five, as authorities recommend. And most eat only a quarter of the calcium-rich foods they should.

If women have a hard time getting the nutrients they need from food, it's not entirely for lack of trying. Since women tend to be smaller, they don't have as many calories to work with as men do. Women who cut back on calories intentionally to lose weight or avoid gaining weight cut back on good and bad foods alike, and they lose out on nutrients in the bargain.

When dietitians at Utah State University in Logan tried to design menus that supplied the Recommended Dietary Allowances of the vitamins and minerals women need, they were hard-pressed to keep the calorie count below 2,200. That's as many as 700 calories more than some of us can enjoy without gaining weight.

FILL THE FRIDGE, FILL THE GAP

Many nutrition experts recommend dietary supplements for some women to help fill the gaps that can occur when we don't eat as we should.

"When women have difficulty meeting some of these requirements, resorting to nutrient supplements is perfectly reasonable," says Jeffrey Blumberg, Ph.D., associate director of the Jean Mayer USDA Human Nutrition Research Center on Aging at Tufts University in Boston. "I want to emphasize that I don't think nutrient supplements should be used as nutrient substitutes. They don't really replace good food. But they can help ensure the intakes necessary for maintaining health and preventing disease." Other experts agree.

"There are certainly individuals who do not eat a balanced diet," explains John Pinto, Ph.D., associate professor of biochemistry in medicine at Cornell University Medical College and director of the Nutrition Research Laboratory at Memorial Sloan-Kettering Cancer Center, both in New York City. "For them, taking supplements would be a form of insurance."

VITAMINS: A LA CARTE OR A MULTI?

You can go about getting your nutritional insurance in one of two ways, say experts. One is to take a supplement or supplements of only the individual nutrient or nutrients you need. The other approach is to take a multivitamin/mineral.

Both approaches have merit, say researchers. If you're trying to eat better but aren't there yet, your best bet is to analyze your diet, see where you've got a deficiency and choose the supplements that are necessary to take up the slack, says Mark Levine, M.D., senior investigator at the Cell Biology and Genetics Laboratory at the National Institutes of Health (NIH) and director of the Nutrition Program of the National Institute for Diabetes and Digestive and Kidney Diseases of the NIH in Bethesda, Maryland.

If you don't or can't drink much milk, for instance, it's likely you could use a calcium supplement, says Dr. Levine. If you eat fewer than three to five servings of fruits and vegetables a day, your folate, beta-carotene and vitamin C intake could be flagging. If you limit meat intake to avoid the fat and calories, your iron stores might be low—and so on.

If, on the other hand, your dietary stock-taking shows you're missing the boat on several vitamins and minerals, you should consider a multivitamin/mineral supplement, says Dr. Levine.

Some women are better off with a "multi" in the first place. For one thing, multis usually pack the right combination of vitamins and minerals, says Dr. Pinto. Most multis that offer calcium, for instance, also include vitamin D, which is needed to absorb calcium, he says.

"Nutrients work in a coordinated fashion," says Dr. Pinto. "They depend on one another for their activities." And, he adds, most multivitamins won't give you megadoses of isolated nutrients—more than three times the DV. For some nutrients, like vitamins A and D, excessive doses can be dangerous, say experts.

The balanced nutritional insurance that multivitamins provide can pay off. A study conducted in Hungary, for example, found that women who took multis prior to conception and early in pregnancy were less likely to deliver babies with neurological defects than those who took a supplement containing only copper, manganese, zinc and a low dose of vitamin C. Studying people over 65, scientists in Canada found that those who took a multi were sick only half as many days per year as those who took a placebo (an inactive look-alike pill). The supplemented group had only 23 days of infection-related illnesses, compared with 48 days for the placebo group.

THE CASE FOR ADDED CALCIUM

The best multis, say researchers, are those that provide 100 percent of the DVs for women. But don't expect to find all the calcium you need in any multivitamin formula. According to the NIH, women should get at least 1,000 milligrams of calcium daily, and those who are pregnant or nursing or have opted not to have hormone replacement therapy after menopause should get at least 1,500 milligrams. A multi supplying all that calcium would be impractical to swallow; most multis contain 200 milligrams or less. But you can get the balance by adding individual calcium supplements.

If you're not including milk products in your daily diet, says Neva Cochran, R.D., a nutritionist in Dallas and spokesperson for the American Dietetic Association, you may well need to take supplementary calcium, in doses divided over the course of a day, in addition to a multivitamin.

EXTRA ANTIOXIDANTS, EXTRA PROTECTION

Getting 100 percent of the DVs may spare you from deficiency-related disorders like osteoporosis. But getting *more* than 100 percent of certain nutrients—like the antioxidant vitamins C and E and beta-carotene—may give you an edge against a whole range of other diseases, according to research. One of the most exciting discoveries in nutritional science was evidence that certain vitamins block the process of oxidation, a natural process that generates harmful substances known as free radicals. Free radicals in turn damage cells and, it's believed, contribute to a variety of health conditions from heart disease to premature aging.

Studies suggest that an intake of antioxidants at higher-than-DV levels, for example, may lower your risks of cataracts, high blood pressure, heart disease and cancers of the breast, mouth, stomach, esophagus and cervix.

Unfortunately, it's not entirely clear whether you can get all of this additional protection from antioxidants in supplement form or whether it's necessary to get these vitamins from food, says Thomas Wolever, Ph.D., associate professor of nutritional sciences at the University of Toronto.

Some research indicates that supplements may do the trick. When scientists in China gave men and women a supplement that supplied more than the DV for vitamin E (along with beta-carotene and selenium), fewer people than average died of cancer.

Other studies suggest that you need to get antioxidants from food, where they're accompanied by other known phytochemicals and possibly by other potentially beneficial and as yet undiscovered nutrients, says Dr. Wolever. Research indicates the combination of antioxidants, phytochemicals and other nutrients, rather than the antioxidants alone, may provide the best protection, he says.

"The studies showing antioxidants are beneficial are the ones that look at people who eat more fruits and vegetables than average," says Dr. Wolever, shoring up the argument that as a general rule supplements are no substitute for nutrient-rich foods.

Nonetheless, other experts contend that there's enough evidence suggesting that antioxidant supplements have enough value to warrant taking them if your diet doesn't provide plenty of these important nutrients. "So if this description fits you, safeguard your health with supplements," says Tom Watkins, Ph.D., laboratory director at the Jordan Heart Research Foundation in Montclair, New Jersey. "It makes sense to take several supplements, not just a multiple and not just extra antioxidants," says Dr. Watkins.

"It's quite clear to me and many others, though it's certainly very controversial, that current DVs for antioxidants are really inadequate for optimal health," Dr. Blumberg agrees. "They provide enough to prevent scurvy or vitamin E deficiency, but they're not the levels that are associated with reduced risk of heart disease or cataracts. Those intakes are much higher."

SUPPLEMENTS: TAILOR-MADE FOR YOU

To get on a supplement program that's most beneficial to your health, you should consult your doctor or a qualified nutrition expert. Be prepared to answer the following questions.

Do you regularly eat carrots and other rich sources of beta-carotene? If you're not averaging two to three servings of fruits and vegetables rich in beta-carotene (like carrots, apricots, papaya, tomatoes, pumpkin and mangoes) a day, take ten milligrams of beta-carotene in supplement form, Dr. Blumberg suggests. If your multi doesn't supply that much or if you're not taking one, pick up a separate beta-carotene supplement. If your eating habits are erratic—you eat two servings each of tomatoes and carrots one day but no trace of beta-carotene the next—it's still perfectly safe to take that supplement every day, says Dr. Blumberg.

Do you regularly drink vitamin C–rich juice or eat citrus fruits, peppers and other good sources of vitamin C? Unless you're averaging two large glasses of orange juice or two large servings of cantaloupe or other foods high in C each day, you'll need some extra C, says Dr. Blumberg. He recommends a daily intake of 250 to 1,000 milligrams—more than four times the DV.

Research suggests that higher-than-DV doses of vitamin C reduce the risks of cancer, heart disease and cataracts. One study of 50,000 American women found a 45 percent lower risk of cataracts among those who took 250- to 500-milligram supplements of vitamin C daily for ten or more years.

Again, if you're not taking a multi or yours doesn't supply 250 milligrams of C, add an individual vitamin C supplement. And yes, it's safe to take it even on those days when you're getting C from your diet, Dr. Blumberg says.

Do you smoke cigarettes (or have you quit recently)? Smokers in particular should make a point of getting more than the DV of vitamin C, says Howerde Sauberlich, Ph.D., professor in the nutrition department of the University of Alabama in Birmingham. Smoking appears to deplete the body's antioxidant stores, Dr. Sauberlich explains.

Are you at high risk for heart disease? Like C, vitamin E may help protect you from heart disease.

The Harvard University Nurses' Health Study (an ongoing study of 115,000 women considered a landmark source of evidence regarding women's health) found that, among more than 87,000 women, those taking 100 international units of vitamin E each day were 34 percent less likely to have heart attacks than those who weren't taking E. This suggests the vitamin could be particularly important for older women who face a higher risk of heart disease.

Researchers like Dr. Blumberg suggest 100 to 400 international units of vitamin E daily. Unfortunately, most foods rich in E—like oils and nuts—are also rich in fat. "You'd have to have lots of fat to get protective amounts of E in your diet," notes Dr. Blumberg. To get 100 international units of E, for instance, you'd need to eat 1½ cups of peanut butter. So Dr. Blumberg recommends supplements. If your multi doesn't give you 100 international units or you're not taking one, make up the difference with individual E capsules, he says.

Do you drink milk and eat yogurt, cheese, ice milk, frozen yogurt, broccoli, spinach or canned salmon with the bones? Your bones need a minimum of 1,000 milligrams of calcium every day to ward off osteoporosis. They need at least 1,500 if you're pregnant or nursing or if you're past menopause but aren't taking hormone replacement therapy.

Good sources of calcium include skim milk (300 milligrams per serving) nonfat yogurt (450 milligrams) and part-skim ricotta cheese (335 milligrams). But even if you ate a serving of each of these foods each and every day, you'd still have a calcium shortfall. And let's face it, most of us don't eat that well every day.

"In my mind, there's no doubt—you've got to take a calcium supplement every day," Dr. Blumberg says.

If you drink a glass of milk every morning at breakfast (and get the accompanying 300 milligrams of calcium), take another 700 to 1,200 milligrams in supplement form, advises Dr. Blumberg. If you never eat dairy foods or your milk-drinking habits are erratic, he recommends upping the dose to 1,000 to 1,500 milligrams. It's safe to take that much even on those days when you do remember to drink your milk and eat your broccoli, Dr. Blumberg says.

Since most multis give you only 200 milligrams of calcium, you'll need individual supplements to reach your goal. Choose a brand that gives you the mineral as calcium citrate or calcium carbonate, the most easily absorbed forms, advises Cochran.

Do you get vitamin D in your diet? Your body needs D to use calcium effectively. Good dietary sources include milk, herring, sardines and salmon. And your skin will produce the vitamin when exposed to sunlight; just five to ten minutes in the morning or late-afternoon sun three times a week will do it.

If you're running a deficit of D from either food or sunlight, make a habit of taking a multi that provides 100 percent of the DV, says Walter Willett, M.D., Dr.Ph., professor of epidemiology and nutrition and chairman of the Department of Nutrition at the Harvard University School of Public Health. It's safe, even when you get your sun and drink your milk. But vitamin D tablets are not recommended. They come in doses much higher than those in a multiple, and vitamin D can be toxic in large amounts.

Is meat on your menu? The DV for iron is 18 milligrams. Red meat is a particularly good source. Soybeans, lentils and enriched cereal grains, including cream of wheat, also contain a fair amount of iron. But your body can make better use of the type of iron found in meat than of the form found in plant foods, says Mary Frances Picciano, Ph.D., professor of nutrition at Pennsylvania State University in University Park. If you don't eat three servings of red meat a week (averaging three ounces per serving), you may need an iron supplement, she says. To be sure, ask your doctor.

If necessary, an iron-fortified multi supplying 18 milligrams is your best bet, Dr. Willett says. And yes, it's also safe to take it even on those days when you're eating iron-rich food, he says.

Do you plan to get pregnant? Orange juice is probably the best source of folate around, Dr. Willett says. Even then, you'd have to drink three or four eight-ounce glasses to get the folate you need if you're trying to conceive or are expecting a baby. Numerous studies suggest that an adequate supply of folate during the first month of pregnancy can help prevent birth defects like spina bifida.

Since it's so hard to get enough folate in your diet, Dr. Willett suggests taking a multi that provides 400 micrograms of folic acid (the supplemental form of folate), even on days when you've downed a few glasses of OJ.

Are you past menopause? After menopause, you still need folate. Folate may help lower the risk of cardiovascular disease, cancer of the cervix and cancer of the colon, says Joel B. Mason, M.D., assistant professor of medicine and nutrition at Tufts University.

Are you age 70 or over? Women over 70 should get slightly higher doses of certain B vitamins, calcium and vitamin D, Dr. Blumberg says.

As we age, we absorb calcium and the B vitamins less efficiently, he explains. Our skin, which produces vitamin D when exposed to sunlight, also starts doing its job less efficiently.

Dr. Blumberg suggests one of the newer special-formula multivitamin supplements that are geared toward older people, one that provides two to three times the DV for vitamins B_6, B_{12} and folate.

MAKE THE MOST OF SUPPLEMENTS

If you find supplements are warranted, nutrition experts offer the following tips for optimal safety and effectiveness.

Maximize your multi. When shopping for a multi, choose one that supplies 100 percent of the DVs of most vitamins and minerals, suggests Joanne Curran-Celentano, R.D., Ph.D., associate professor of nutrition and food sciences at the University of New Hampshire in Durham. Remember, though, no multi will include all the calcium you need.

Look for selenium and chromium. There are no official DVs for these nutrients, but it's a good idea to include them in your supplement program, says Dr. Blumberg. Deaths from heart disease rose dramatically among residents of an Italian village after their public water supply was switched from wells that supplied water high in selenium to those whose water was low in the mineral. And preliminary studies suggest chromium may lower cholesterol levels.

Dr. Blumberg suggests a multi with 25 to 70 micrograms of selenium and 50 to 200 micrograms of chromium.

Compare products formulated for women. Women's formulas may be more likely to include the 400 micrograms of folic acid you'll need daily if you're trying to conceive or are pregnant, says Dr. Curran-Celentano. But multis specially formulated for women aren't necessarily more complete than general, all-purpose multis meant for everyone, says Stephanie Sturiale, R.D., a nutritionist in New York City. Compare labels, suggests Dr. Curran-Celentano.

Be cautious. There's a big difference between the supplement levels used in medical studies and what doctors recommend for general good health. No matter how old you are, you want to avoid taking potentially harmful megadoses of vitamins and minerals. Consult "Vitamins and Minerals: What Women Need" on page 311 for the optimal amounts recommended by experts. For most nutrients, two or three times the DV should be the limit, according to Dr. Blumberg.

Separate calcium and iron. Your body can't absorb certain nutrients in the presence of others. Calcium and iron are a case in point, says Dr. Pinto, so try to take calcium supplements and multivitamin-with-iron preparations at different times of the day.

Pair your iron with orange juice. Your body does a better job of absorbing iron when vitamin C is around, says Dr. Pinto. So consider taking your multivitamin with iron with your orange juice or other vitamin C-rich juice, he says.

Swallow with food. "Vitamins are more efficiently absorbed in the presence of food," Dr. Pinto explains. "There's increased blood flow through the intestines, and the absorption mechanism is more effective."

Cork the bottle. If you have wine or cocktails with dinner, wait a couple of hours after your last drink before taking your vitamins, Cochran says. Alcohol can interfere with absorption. By the same token, you shouldn't wash down your supplements with any form of alcohol.

VITAMINS AND MINERALS
What Women Need

Does your diet provide all the nutrients you need? Do you need to take supplements? If so, which ones? To find out what vitamins and minerals you should be getting—and how much you need for optimal health—consult the following chart, which is designed for today's active women. If you feel the condition of your health or your lifestyle might cause nutritional deficiencies, talk with your doctor about tailoring a personal supplement program.

VITAMINS

Vitamin A
Action in body: Helps maintain normal vision in dim light; forms and maintains normal structure and functions of mucous membranes to assure healthy eyes, skin, hair, gums and various glands; helps build bones and teeth; maintains strong immunity.
Daily Value (DV): 5,000 international units.
Optimal amount: 5,000 international units.
Especially important if you: Are a smoker, have diabetes, eat lots of junk food, are fighting an infection, are

VITAMINS AND MINERALS—*CONTINUED*

recovering from surgery or are exposed to high levels of pollutants.

Recommended food sources: Carrots, fortified skim milk, pumpkin, sweet potatoes, dark green leafy vegetables (like spinach and kale), winter squash, tuna, halibut, cantaloupe, mangoes, apricots, broccoli and watermelon.

Thiamin

Action in body: Critical for energy; important for carbohydrate metabolism; maintains nerve function, muscle tone, normal appetite and a healthy mental attitude.

Daily Value (DV): 1.5 milligrams.

Optimal amount: Not established.

Especially important if you: Drink alcohol heavily, are on a weight-loss diet or drink lots of coffee or tea. Women over age 70 who eat poor diets or are recovering from surgery may be at risk for a thiamin deficiency.

Recommended food sources: Lean pork, sunflower seeds, wheat germ, pasta, peanuts, legumes, watermelon, oranges, brown rice and oatmeal.

Riboflavin

Action in body: Essential for growth and tissue repair; important for carbohydrate, fat and protein metabolism; aids in the formation of red blood cells in bone marrow and in the functioning of the adrenal gland.

Daily Value (DV): 1.7 milligrams.

Optimal amount: Not established.

Especially important if you: Exercise daily or exercise strenuously (or both), fail to eat a variety of nutritious foods, are pregnant or nursing or drink alcohol heavily. Women over age 70 with poor diets may be at risk for riboflavin deficiency.

Recommended food sources: Skim milk, fat-free or low-fat cottage cheese, enriched cereals, avocados, tangerines, prunes, asparagus, broccoli, mushrooms, lean beef, salmon and chicken.

Niacin

Action in body: Important for carbohydrate, fat and protein metabolism; needed for oxygen use by cells.

Daily Value (DV): 20 milligrams.

Optimal amount: Not established.

Especially important if you: Have high cholesterol or a history of cardiovascular disease (or both).

Recommended food sources: Lean meat, poultry, fish, peanut butter, legumes, soybeans, whole-grain cereals and breads, broccoli, asparagus, baked potatoes. (Also, skim milk is high in tryptophan, which converts to niacin in the body.)

Vitamin B_6

Action in body: Important for carbohydrate, fat and protein metabolism; aids in production of red blood cells; maintains integrity of the central nervous system. Of all the B vitamins, vitamin B_6 is the most important for maintaining a healthy immune system.

Daily Value (DV): Two milligrams.

Optimal amount: Three to five milligrams.

Especially important if you: Are on the Pill, are pregnant, have symptoms of premenstrual tension or are over age 70.

Recommended food sources: Fish, soybeans, avocados, lima beans, poultry, bananas, cauliflower, green peppers, potatoes, spinach and raisins.

Folic Acid

Action in body: Important for synthesis of DNA and RNA, which make up the genetic code vital to all cells in the body; aids in red blood cell development.

Daily Value (DV): 400 micrograms.

Optimal amount: 400 micrograms.

Especially important if you: Drink alcohol heavily, are pregnant, are on a low-calorie diet, have sickle cell disease, are trying to conceive a child, are past menopause or are over age 70.

Recommended food sources: Legumes, poultry, tuna, wheat germ, mushrooms, oranges, asparagus, broccoli, spinach, bananas, strawberries and cantaloupe.

Vitamin B_{12}

Action in body: Important for red blood cell formation; maintains nerve tissue; aids in carbohydrate, fat and protein metabolism.

Daily Value (DV): 6 micrograms.

Optimal amount: 10 to 20 micrograms.

VITAMINS AND MINERALS—*CONTINUED*

Especially important if you: Smoke, are on a vegetarian or macrobiotic diet or are over age 70.

Recommended food sources: Salmon, low-fat cottage cheese, swordfish, tuna, clams, crab, mussels, oysters and lean beef or pork.

Biotin

Action in body: Important for carbohydrate, fat and protein metabolism.

Daily Value (DV): 300 micrograms.

Optimal amount: Not established.

Especially important if you: Are on long-term oral antibiotics, eat poorly or are on a very low calorie weight-loss diet.

Recommended food sources: Peanut butter, oatmeal, wheat germ, poultry, cauliflower, nuts, legumes, fat-free or low-fat cheese and mushrooms.

Pantothenic Acid

Action in body: Important for carbohydrate, fat and protein metabolism; aids in formation of red blood cells, hormones and nerve transmission substances; helps maintain normal blood sugar levels.

Daily Value (DV): Ten milligrams.

Optimal amount: Not established.

Especially important if you: Have rheumatoid arthritis.

Recommended food sources: Fish, whole-grain cereals, mushrooms, avocados, broccoli, peanuts, cashews, lentils and soybeans.

Vitamin C

Action in body: Antioxidant—protects cells from damage by seeking out and neutralizing free radicals that cause oxidation in the body; builds and maintains collagen, the substance that binds body cells together; promotes healing of wounds and burns; maintains healthy gums, teeth, bones and blood vessels; increases absorption of iron.

Daily Value (DV): 60 milligrams.

Optimal amount: 500 to 1,000 milligrams.

Especially important if you: Smoke or are exposed to tobacco smoke, have diabetes, are recovering from surgery, drink alcohol heavily or are pregnant.

Recommended food sources: Oranges, grapefruit, bell peppers, strawberries, tomatoes, spinach, cabbage, melons, broccoli, kiwifruit, raspberries and brussels sprouts.

Vitamin D

Action in body: Increases calcium absorption; helps build bones and teeth.

Daily Value (DV): 400 international units.

Optimal amount: 400 international units.

Especially important if you: Drink alcohol heavily, do not drink milk, do not receive adequate exposure to sunlight or are over age 70.

Recommended sources: Sunlight, fortified skim milk, tuna, salmon, sardines and fortified cereals.

Vitamin E

Action in body: Antioxidant—protects cells from damage by seeking out and neutralizing free radicals that cause oxidation in the body; important for stabilizing cell membranes; protects lung tissue from air pollution.

Daily Value (DV): 30 international units.

Optimal amount: 100 to 400 international units.

Especially important if you: Are exposed to pollution.

Recommended food sources: Nut and vegetable oils, wheat germ, mangoes, blackberries, apples, broccoli, peanuts, spinach and whole-wheat breads.

Vitamin K

Action in body: Controls clotting of blood; helps maintain normal bone and aids in the healing of fractures.

Daily Value (DV): Not established.

Optimal amount: 70 micrograms.

Especially important if you: Are on a very low calorie diet or are on a long-term oral antibiotic therapy.

Recommended food sources: Green tea, spinach, broccoli, brussels sprouts, cabbage, asparagus, parsley, chick-peas, cauliflower, lentils, carrots, avocados and tomatoes.

MINERALS

Calcium

Action in body: Builds bones and teeth; maintains bones; aids in nerve transmission, muscle function and blood clotting; maintains strong immunity.

VITAMINS AND MINERALS—*CONTINUED*

Daily Value (DV): 1,000 milligrams.

Optimal amount: 1,200 to 1,500 milligrams.

Especially important if you: Are a postmenopausal woman not on hormone replacement therapy, drink alcohol, are inactive, are on a low-calorie, high-protein or high-fiber diet, are lactose intolerant or are pregnant or nursing. Postmenopausal women not on hormone replacement therapy and all women over age 65 should get 1,500 milligrams.

Recommended food sources: Skim milk, fat-free or low-fat cheese, fat-free yogurt, salmon and sardines with bones, broccoli, green beans, almonds, turnip greens and fortified orange juice.

Chromium

Action in body: Aids carbohydrate, fat and protein metabolism; contributes to the effectiveness of insulin.

Daily Value (DV): Not established.

Optimal amount: 125 to 200 micrograms.

Especially important if you: Are pregnant, engage in regular strenuous exercise (like running) or are over age 70.

Recommended food sources: Blackstrap molasses, whole grains, broccoli, grape juice, orange juice, lean meat, black pepper, brewer's yeast and fat-free or low-fat cheese.

Copper

Action in body: Facilitates absorption of iron; helps form red blood cells; develops and maintains blood vessels, tendons and bones; aids in the functioning of the central nervous system; required for normal hair color; important for fertility.

Daily Value (DV): Two milligrams.

Optimal amount: Not established.

Especially important if you: Are taking zinc supplements (zinc and copper should be balanced at a 10:1 ratio) or are over age 70.

Recommended food sources: Oysters and other shell-fish, nuts, cherries, cocoa, mushrooms, gelatin, whole-grain cereals, fish and legumes.

Fluoride

Action in body: Maintains bones and teeth; helps prevent tooth decay.

Daily Value (DV): Not established.

Optimal amount: Usually obtained from fluoridated drinking water.

Especially important if you: Live where the water is not fluoridated.

Recommended dietary sources: Fluoridated water, fish and tea.

Iodine

Action in body: Makes up thyroid hormones, which are involved in energy production, growth, nerve and muscle function and circulation.

Daily Value (DV): 150 micrograms.

Optimal amount: Not established.

Especially important if you: Have fibrocystic breasts.

Recommended food sources: Spinach, lobster, shrimp, oysters, skim milk and iodized salt.

Iron

Action in body: Carries oxygen in blood; contributes to energy metabolism.

Daily Value (DV): 18 milligrams.

Optimal amount: 10 to 18 milligrams.

Especially important if you: Are premenopausal, are on a low-calorie diet, are pregnant or nursing, are vegetarian or are over age 70 with poor long-term dietary habits.

Recommended food sources: Clams, asparagus, lean meat, chicken, prunes, raisins, spinach, pumpkin seeds, soybeans and tofu.

Magnesium

Action in body: Essential for every major body process, including glucose metabolism, cellular energy, muscle contraction and nerve function; helps build bones and teeth.

Daily Value (DV): 400 milligrams.

VITAMINS AND MINERALS—*CONTINUED*

Optimal amount: 400 to 800 milligrams.

Especially important if you: Are on a low-calorie diet, have diabetes, drink alcohol, are pregnant, take diuretics, exercise regularly and strenuously or are over age 70.

Recommended food sources: Molasses, nuts, spinach, wheat germ, pumpkin seeds, sesame seeds, seafood, fat-free or low-fat cheese, baked potatoes, broccoli and bananas.

Manganese

Action in body: Helps form bone; aids growth of connective tissue; contributes to blood clotting; aids in carbohydrate, fat and protein metabolism.

Daily Value (DV): Not established.

Optimal amount: Not established.

Especially important if you: Are taking large doses of calcium or iron supplements, are on a low-calorie diet or are being fed intravenously.

Recommended food sources: Nuts, whole-grain cereals, legumes, tea, dried fruits and spinach and other green leafy vegetables.

Molybdenum

Action in body: Aids in carbohydrate, fat and protein metabolism; a component of tooth enamel.

Daily Value (DV): Not established.

Optimal amount: 75 to 250 micrograms.

Especially important if you: Are on a low-calorie diet or are being fed intravenously.

Recommended food sources: Legumes, lean meats, whole-grain cereals, breads and skim milk.

Phosphorus

Action in body: Helps build bones and teeth; maintains bone; builds muscle tissue; aids in carbohydrate, fat and protein metabolism; is a component of DNA and RNA, which make up the genetic code vital to all cells in the body.

Daily Value (DV): 1,000 milligrams.

Optimal amount: Not established.

Especially important if you: Drink alcohol heavily or use magnesium-containing or aluminum-containing antacids regularly.

Recommended food sources: Lean meats, fish, poultry, fat-free or low-fat dairy products and cereals.

Potassium

Action in body: Maintains acid/base balance in the body; involved in muscle function, energy production and protein synthesis; required for the release of insulin by the pancreas; maintains normal blood pressure; works with sodium to maintain fluid balance.

Daily Value (DV): 3,500 milligrams.

Optimal amount: Not established.

Especially important if you: Have high blood pressure or take prescription diuretics.

Recommended food sources: Baked potatoes, avocados, dried fruits, fat-free or low-fat yogurt, cantaloupe, spinach, bananas, mushrooms, skim milk and tomatoes.

Selenium

Action in body: Contributes to certain antioxidant functions; maintains strong immunity.

Daily Value (DV): Not established.

Optimal amount: 100 micrograms in supplement form.

Especially important if you: No special considerations.

Recommended food sources: Lean meats, whole-grain cereals, fat-free or low-fat dairy products, fish, shellfish, mushrooms and Brazil nuts.

Sodium

Action in body: Maintains water and acid/base balance in the body; helps make up bile, sweat and tears; involved in muscle contraction; contributes to nervous system function.

Daily Value (DV): 2,400 milligrams.

Optimal amount: Not established.

Special considerations: Sodium is prevalent in many commonly eaten foods, especially processed foods, so there is no need to pay special attention to intake.

VITAMINS AND MINERALS—*CONTINUED*

<u>Zinc</u>
Action in body: Maintains strong immunity; helps fight disease; maintains normal skin, bones and hair; aids in digestion and respiration; important for the development and functioning of reproductive organs; involved in wound healing; maintains normal sense of taste.
Daily Value (DV): 15 milligrams.
Optimal amount: 15 milligrams.
Especially important if you: Are a vegetarian, are on a low-calorie diet, are taking diuretics, have diabetes, drink alcohol heavily, sweat excessively or are over age 70.
Recommended food sources: Oysters, lean beef, wheat germ, seafood, lima beans, legumes, nuts, poultry, skim milk and low-fat Cheddar cheese.

NOTE: The Daily Value is based on the levels of intake established by the National Research Council that are judged to provide adequate nutrition for a healthy person. The optimal amount gives you added benefit, based on available scientific research as interpreted by Jeffrey Blumberg, Ph.D., professor of nutrition at Tufts University in Boston. Food sources were reviewed by Joanne Curran-Celentano, R.D., Ph.D., associate professor of nutrition and food sciences at the University of New Hampshire in Durham.

PART 4

FOOD AND YOUR WEIGHT

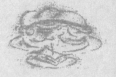

44

YOUR IDEAL WEIGHT

How much should *you* weigh?

Of the 200 women who responded to our *Food and You* survey, half said they needed to lose weight. Some said they needed to lose as much as 100 pounds, others as little as 3 to 5 pounds.

The survey respondents included women who are striving to achieve prepregnancy weights. Or they just want to fit into their jeans again after an annual bout of "winter weight gain." Others had achieved their ideal weight and said they're struggling to maintain it.

It's no surprise that the results of our small informal survey correspond to statistics from major studies. According to one nationwide survey, nearly one out of every two adults queried said they considered themselves overweight. Women were more likely to consider themselves overweight than men: About 40 percent of the women surveyed were trying to lose weight.

A similar study conducted by the Calorie Control Council, an Atlanta-based association of manufacturers of low-calorie and reduced-fat foods and beverages, revealed that 69 percent of adult women in this country say they need to lose weight, and 30 percent are currently on a diet.

Yet just what constitutes the ideal weight? That question

has perplexed women for years. It's a rare woman who's satisfied with the number she sees on her bathroom scale.

So what's going on? Do all of these women truly need to lose weight, or are they needlessly obsessing? Here's what the experts have to say.

EVERYBODY (AND EVERY BODY) IS DIFFERENT

For years, women (and men) have relied on height/weight charts issued by the Metropolitan Life Insurance Company or other authorities, such as the U.S. Department of Agriculture and the Department of Health and Human Services.

But some equally well-respected authorities argue that the MetLife tables, revised in 1983 to allow for more weight, are too lenient. In fact, the American Heart Association has urged people to ignore those guidelines. According to current MetLife tables, for example, 155 pounds is within the desirable weight range for a large-framed woman who is five feet five inches tall. A weight of 145 would be better.

Here's the problem: The MetLife tables are based on death rates and vital statistics from millions of insurance holders in the United States. But as William P. Castelli, M.D., medical director of the Framingham Heart Study, points out, the MetLife tables don't account for the fact that many thin people who die are cigarette smokers or are otherwise ill. If sick people and smokers had been eliminated from the current calculations, he says, desirable weights would be lower.

In other words, if you really want to know what constitutes a healthy weight, look at healthy people, not sick people and smokers, says F. Xavier Pi-Sunyer, M.D., director of endocrinology, diabetes and nutrition at St. Luke's—Roosevelt Hospital Center in New York City.

Instead of the height/weight tables, weight-loss experts are advocating use of two alternative criteria for optimum weight: body mass index (BMI) and waist/hip ratio (WHR).

A BETTER WAY TO MEASURE WEIGHT

Body mass index is a simple formula that compares your height to your weight.

HOW TO CALCULATE YOUR BODY MASS INDEX (BMI)

The body mass index (BMI) is a simple formula for determining weight-related health risks. To find your BMI, locate your height in the left column of this chart. (If you've lost inches over the years, use your peak adult height.) Move across the chart to the right until you find your approximate weight. Then follow that column down to the corresponding BMI number at the bottom of the chart.

HEIGHT WEIGHT (lb.)

HEIGHT														
4'10"	91	96	100	105	110	115	119	124	129	134	138	143	148	153
4'11"	94	99	104	109	114	119	124	128	133	138	143	148	153	158
5'0"	97	102	107	112	118	123	128	133	138	143	148	153	158	163
5'1"	100	106	111	116	122	127	132	137	143	148	153	158	164	169
5'2"	104	109	115	120	126	131	136	142	147	153	158	164	169	174
5'3"	107	113	118	124	130	135	141	146	152	158	163	169	175	180
5'4"	110	116	122	128	134	140	145	151	157	163	169	174	180	186
5'5"	114	120	126	132	138	144	150	156	162	168	174	180	186	192
5'6"	118	124	130	136	142	148	155	161	167	173	179	186	192	198
5'7"	121	127	134	140	146	153	159	166	172	178	185	191	197	204
5'8"	125	131	138	144	151	158	164	171	177	184	190	197	203	210
5'9"	128	135	142	149	155	162	169	176	182	189	196	203	209	216
5'10"	132	139	146	153	160	167	174	181	188	195	202	207	215	222
5'11"	136	143	150	157	165	172	179	186	193	200	208	215	222	229
6'0"	140	147	154	162	169	177	184	191	199	206	213	221	228	235
BMI	**19**	**20**	**21**	**22**	**23**	**24**	**25**	**26**	**27**	**28**	**29**	**30**	**31**	**32**

"Compared to the MetLife tables, the BMI is more precise, making it the better of the two methods," says James O. Hill, Ph.D., associate director of the Center for Human Nutrition at the University of Colorado Health Sciences Center in Denver.

"The BMI is also easier to use," says Dr. Pi-Sunyer. "So most of us have gone over to using the BMI." How do you calculate your BMI?

1. Divide your weight (in pounds) by your height (in inches) squared. If you're 130 pounds and five feet three inches tall, that's 130 divided by 3969 (63 × 63), which is 0.032.
2. Multiply the number you get by 705 (0.032 × 705 = 23). The number you get is your BMI.

Or you can use the table on the previous page, which does all the arithmetic for you.

Most likely, your BMI will fall somewhere between 19 and 32. Within that range, the experts generally agree that a BMI between 20 and 25 is desirable. "We say that 25 to 27 is the upper limit of a healthy BMI," says Dr. Hill, a member of the Dietary Guidelines Advisory Committee that advises the U.S. Public Health Service on establishing healthy weight goals.

In other words, as with cholesterol, there's no one BMI that's "right." The ideal BMI for you depends on your particular risk for certain weight-related health concerns. To help determine your ideal BMI, ask yourself these questions.

Are you at risk for heart disease? One large-scale study, the Harvard University Nurses' Health Study, points to a BMI of below 22 as ideal for preventing heart disease. Researchers based at Harvard and Brigham and Women's Hospital in Boston followed 115,886 initially healthy American women ages 30 to 55 for eight years. During that time, 605 of the women experienced coronary artery disease. There was no elevated risk of heart disease among women whose BMIs were under 21. The risk rose gradually for women with BMIs from 21 to 25, compared with women whose BMI was less than 21. For BMIs higher than that, the health risks rise more rapidly: They were 80 percent higher for a BMI of 25 to 29 and 230 percent higher for a BMI greater than 29.

Do you have or are you at risk for diabetes? According to the American Diabetes Association, women with a BMI of 28 or higher are at increased risk for this condition. Dr. Pi-Sunyer says 27 or lower is better.

Do you have other chronic conditions? "Your risk for diseases such as gout, arthritis and high cholesterol or high triglycerides is higher when your BMI is over 27," says Dr. Pi-Sunyer. "Data shows that the higher the number, the greater the risk. At a BMI of 27, the risks increase sharply, so we consider 27 the cutoff point."

Are you at risk for breast cancer? "For people with a family history of breast cancer, a BMI below 27 is better," says Susan Zelitch Yanovski, M.D., obesity expert with the National Institute of Diabetes and Digestive and Kidney Diseases at the National Institutes of Health in Bethesda, Maryland.

How old are you? "If you're under 35 years old, try to maintain a BMI of below 25," says Dr. Yanovski. The reasoning is twofold, she says: You may gain weight as you age, and a BMI of below 25 may be more protective of health than 26 or 27.

Regardless of your age or individual risk factors, most scientists agree that a BMI over 27 is potentially hazardous to your health.

"I'd rather see a woman with a BMI of 21 than 27—she'd have fewer health problems," says Dr. Pi-Sunyer. "Besides, it's easier to not gain it than to lose it once you've gained it," he says.

Are you underweight? What if your BMI is off the low end of the chart? "A lot of people have a BMI under 18, and they are fine and doing everything right," says Dr. Hill. "But there's a chance you may be too underweight. We recommend that women whose BMI is under 18 see their physicians. It may be worth checking into."

YOUR WAIST/HIP RATIO

Calculating body mass is one gauge of ideal weight, but it's not the only parameter: *Where* you carry that weight also factors in, says Dr. Pi-Sunyer. Carrying too much in your midsection puts you at greatest health risk, he says.

Researchers have determined that the fat most associated with health risks is on the upper body—the abdomen and

HOW TO DETERMINE YOUR WAIST/HIP RATIO (WHR)

Experts in weight control say that for women, measuring your waist and hips is a better way to assess your health risks than stepping on a bathroom scale. The ratio of these two measurements, called the Waist/hip ratio, tells you *where* your fat is distributed, says F. Xaviėr Pi-Sunyer, M.D., director of endocrinology, diabetes and nutrition at St. Luke's–Roosevelt Hospital Center in New York City.

To find your WHR:

1. Feel for the top of your hip and the bottom of your ribcage on one side.
2. Place the tape measure halfway between those points and measure your waist.
3. Measure your hips at the widest point.
4. Divide your waist measurement by your hip measurement (___inches ÷ ___inches = ___waist/hip ratio).

For women, if the ratio is greater than 0.8 you may be at high risk for heart disease, stroke, diabetes, high blood pressure and perhaps even breast cancer.

above (known as central obesity or an apple shape)—rather than on the thighs and hips (a pear shape).

"Increasingly, experts find that body fat—especially body fat distribution—may be more important than body weight in determining risk," says Kelly D. Brownell, Ph.D., director of the Center for Eating and Weight Disorders at Yale University. "So any measure that tells us about body fat distribution is more informative than just knowing weight."

That's where the waist/hip ratio comes in.

"If someone had a BMI of 26 with a lot of central fat versus someone with a higher BMI with all her fat below the waist, I'd be much more aggressive about getting the first woman to lose weight because of the location of her fat," says Dr. Pi-Sunyer.

For most people, and especially women, say researchers, the WHR seems to be a fairly good gauge of an individual's risk of cardiovascular disease. That's because upper-body fat is strongly correlated with visceral fat—fat that's packed around our internal organs, according to Dr. Castelli.

PUT THE BRAKES ON MIDDLE-AGE WEIGHT GAIN

The bathroom scale still has a place as a gauge of what you should weigh, says Dr. Pi-Sunyer. You need to know how much you weigh to determine your BMI. The lower your body weight, the lower your BMI. If you gain weight, your BMI increases.

Weigh yourself no more than once a week. Some daily or weekly weight fluctuation, primarily water weight, is extremely common—and normal, says C. Wayne Callaway, an obesity specialist at George Washington University in Washington, D.C. "Bathroom scales are not very accurate for measuring short-term changes. You may be gaining weight through fluid accumulation associated with the menstrual cycle, not increases in body fat or muscle."

That's good news for people who are overly obsessed with what their bathroom scale tells them from day to day and week to week. "I was obsessed with the scale," confesses Deb H., one of our *Food and You* survey respondents. "I would weigh myself, exercise for two hours and weigh myself again—and when the needle didn't move down, I would become depressed."

"People can become too obsessed with the scale," Dr. Hill acknowledges. "But if you look at weighing yourself as a part of a behavior-monitoring program, that's helpful."

Chart your weight over the long haul. Stick a sheet of graph paper to your bathroom mirror. Each vertical square represents 2-pound increments over 100; each horizontal square represents a week. Pencil in a dot for your current weight and repeat weekly. That will help you keep track of your weight without giving undue importance to minor fluctuations.

"Often we're in love with a particular number on the scale, and we feel like failures if we can't reach and maintain that number," says Stephen P. Gullo, Ph.D., president of the Institute for Health and Weight Sciences and former chair of the National Obesity and Weight Control Education Institute of the American Institute for Life-Threatening Illness at Columbia Medical Center, both in New York City. "But what's important for your health is not just how low your weight is but how long you stay at a healthy weight."

"What you want to prevent is slow, creeping weight gain," says Dr. Pi-Sunyer. Data from one component of the Harvard University Nurses' Health Study headed by Walter C. Willett, M.D., professor of epidemiology and nutrition at Harvard School of Public Health, gives clear-cut evidence that midlife weight gain increases women's health risks significantly. Researchers found that for every 2.2 pounds gained after age 18, women's risk of heart attack rose by 3.1 percent. "Even modest weight gains can increase the risk of high blood pressure and diabetes and have a negative effect on blood cholesterol," says Dr. Willett.

"If you're 35 or 40 and put on 10 pounds, it's important to make a permanent adjustment in your lifestyle immediately and not wait until you've gained 30 or 40 pounds and your risks for heart attack have taken hold," says Dr. Willett.

YO-YO DIETING: NOT A PROBLEM AFTER ALL

If you've been riding the weight-loss roller coaster for much of your life, you may have been reluctant to launch yet another diet after hearing reports that yo-yo dieting—repeatedly losing and gaining weight—is actually *worse* for your health than remaining overweight. As it turns out, though, yo-yo dieting (also called weight cycling) may do more psychological harm than physical harm. Seeing the number on the scale go up and down hurts self-esteem, says Dr. Brownell. But according to a report by the National Institutes of Health in Bethesda, Maryland, losing the same 10 or 20 pounds time and again doesn't wreck your metabolism, raise your cholesterol or wreak havoc with your blood pressure, as early reports suggested. Nor does repeatedly losing and gaining weight make subsequent efforts to lose weight more difficult.

Lose excess weight and keep it off. "There is no evidence in humans, or in animals, for that matter, that weight cycling is a real problem,'' says Dr. Pi-Sunyer. And while no one is recommending weight cycling, ''if you're overweight, you should try to lose weight, even if you've had a history of weight cycling,'' he says.

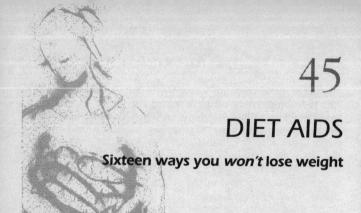

45

DIET AIDS

Sixteen ways you *won't* lose weight

We all know women who don't play the lottery, who hang up on sales calls for real estate in Sinkhole, Florida and who are leery of questionable-sounding deals of any kind but who nonetheless have lost lots of money and little weight on quick weight-loss schemes.

So powerful is the allure of instant thinness, even the most savvy consumers can get sucked in.

According to the Food and Drug Administration (FDA) and the Federal Trade Commission, Americans fork over an estimated $30 billion each year for a nearly endless array of diet plans and aids: high-protein diets; no-protein diets; grapefruit pills; liquid shakes; thigh wraps; thigh creams; weight-loss teas. The list goes on.

"The idea of a quick fix is very appealing," says Susan Zelitch Yanovski, M.D., director of the Obesity and Eating Disorders Program at the National Institute of Diabetes and Digestive and Kidney Diseases of the National Institutes of Health in Bethesda, Maryland. "It's rare that any woman who's significantly overweight hasn't tried at least one fad diet or weight-loss gimmick sometime in her life."

If the diet gimmicks worked, $30 billion would be money well spent. But they don't, says John Renner, M.D., who heads the resource center for the National Council against Health Fraud in Independence, Missouri.

Some diet aids and programs can help you lose weight in the short run. In the long run, though, you gain it back.

"If it doesn't work in the long term—and that's what matters—it's not effective," says Frances Berg, licensed nutritionist, adjunct professor of family wellness at the University of North Dakota School of Medicine in Grand Forks and author of *Health Risks of Weight Loss.*

"If there were a magic diet or weight-loss pill, everyone would be on it and no one would be overweight," says Dr. Yanovski. "It's just not out there."

Not only are many of these gimmicks useless and ineffective, some are dangerous. Here's what weight-loss experts have to say about what's on the market these days.

HIGH-CARBOHYDRATE DIETS: DON'T GO OVERBOARD

High-carbohydrate foods like grains, fruit and vegetables fill you up without filling you out, and these diets capitalize on that ability. The Life Choice Program, directed by Dean Ornish, M.D., president and director of the Institute for Preventive Medicine in Sausalito, California, and the Pritikin Program are good examples. The regimens put heavy emphasis on fresh fruits, vegetables and whole grains, deriving roughly 80 percent of calories from these high-carbohydrate foods, 10 percent from protein sources and 10 percent from fat. The Ornish plan is essentially a low-fat vegetarian diet. The Pritikin plan allows you roughly four ounces of lean meat a day. As the names suggest, these regimens are billed not as diets but as healthy lifetime food plans.

Do they work? They do for some people, says Judy E. Marshel, R.D., director of Health Resources in Great Neck, New York and former senior nutritionist for Weight Watchers International.

Because carbohydrates are both filling and relatively low in calories, people do lose weight on plans like Pritikin's and Ornish's, Marshel says. And because they don't feel deprived, people find it easier to stick with the plans for the long haul and keep the weight off.

"You just have to watch quantities—that's the one way people can go wrong with these plans," she adds. Although carbohydrates have fewer than half the calories of fats (four calories per gram versus nine calories per gram), they're not *calorie-free*, Marshel notes. So you can't wolf down bags of fat-free cookies and expect to lose (or even maintain) weight.

Are they safe? High-carbohydrate diets are generally safe, as long as they include sufficient protein, says Sachiko St. Jeor, R.D., Ph.D., professor of nutrition and director of the Nutrition Education and Research Program at the University of Nevada School of Medicine in Reno. At least 10 percent of daily calories (or at least 50 grams) should be protein, Dr. St. Jeor says.

Protein is essential. If you don't get enough from the food you eat, your body will break down your own muscle tissue—including heart tissue—to get the protein it needs, Marshel explains.

"To avoid excess calories, you can always eat vegetable protein sources like beans," she says. "You don't have to go with animal protein."

It's safe to follow a high-carbohydrate, low-fat eating plan of your own devising as long as it gives you enough protein, vitamins and minerals, Marshel adds. Make sure you eat at least two servings of fruit, three servings of vegetables, four ounces of protein such as chicken or the equivalent and two servings of calcium-rich foods such as low-fat or nonfat milk or cheese daily.

One caveat with high-carbohydrate diets: They're a bad idea for people with insulin resistance, Dr. Renner says. If you have this problem—key symptoms are fatigue and difficulty losing weight—your cells don't make efficient use of carbohydrates once they're broken down and absorbed into your bloodstream. If you suspect you are insulin-resistant, Dr. Renner suggests you see your doctor for a glucose tolerance test.

OVER-THE-COUNTER APPETITE SUPPRESSANTS: NOT WITHOUT RISKS

Inexpensive, brightly packaged and often touted by svelte celebrities, appetite suppressants such as Dexatrim and Acutrim contain phenylpropanolamine (PPA) as an active ingredient. These pills pass muster with the FDA.

Do they work? Over-the-counter appetite suppressants help curb hunger pangs temporarily, says Paul Lachance, Ph.D., professor of nutrition and food science at Rutgers University in New Brunswick, New Jersey. At first they'll help you feel a bit more satisfied with fewer mouthfuls, so you may lose weight over the short haul. But long-term success is another story, say experts.

"Once people stop taking the pills, the weight comes back," says John Foreyt, Ph.D., director of the Nutrition Research Clinic at Baylor College of Medicine in Houston.

Why? Because appetite comes back. Rely on pills to help muffle your appetite's insistent voice, say experts, and you'll never learn to manage your appetite and eat so that you're neither hungry nor overfed.

Women who try appetite suppressants soon learn the limits of these weight-loss aids.

"I didn't learn how to eat properly when I was using appetite suppressant pills," says Maria L., who responded to our *Food and You* survey. "I was afraid that if I stopped taking the pills, even for one day, I wouldn't be able to control my eating."

Can you just pop the pills the rest of your life? No. As Dr. Lachance explains, you can develop a tolerance to over-the-counter diet drugs. After several weeks they stop working, so with or without the pills, your appetite returns and, unless you've modified your eating habits, so does the weight.

Are they safe? Even though you can buy appetite suppressants off the drugstore shelf, they're not risk-free, says Dr. Lachance. The active ingredient, PPA, can raise blood pressure. In fact, the warning label on a typical package makes for pretty scary reading. Warnings caution that these pills have been associated with "stroke, seizure, heart attack, arrhythmia, psychosis" and, last but not least, "death." You're advised to steer clear, except under a doctor's supervision, "if you are being treated for depression or an eating disorder or have heart disease, diabetes, thyroid or any other disease."

That said, we should mention some non-life-threatening but bothersome side effects we heard about from women like Maria.

FDA APPROVAL
What It Means

Don't assume that every weight-loss product on the market has been reviewed and approved by the Food and Drug Administration (FDA), says Denise Bruner, M.D., an obesity and bariatric medicine specialist in Arlington, Virginia.

Many haven't.

"The FDA doesn't look at everything," says Dr. Bruner.

The FDA spot-checks products to determine if low-calorie foods and diet drinks like Slim-Fast actually contain the ingredients that are listed on the labels. The FDA also requires manufacturers of weight-loss drugs like Dexatrim (an over-the-counter product) and fenfluramine (Pondimin, a prescription drug for obesity), to submit studies showing that their products are safe and effective. But that still leaves a lot of untested diet aids on the shelves.

"The problem is, many products don't explicitly claim to promote weight loss but suggest they do, with names like Dieter's Tea," says FDA spokesman Brad Stone. Unless the claim is specific, the agency can't require the manufacturer to submit supporting scientific evidence before going to market.

If the FDA hears enough complaints about a product causing harm or failing to produce results, the agency can investigate and order the product off the market if necessary. Meanwhile, consumers are on their own.

Even if a product earns FDA approval, it doesn't mean it's *always* effective or free of harmful effects for everyone, says Steven Jonas, M.D., professor of preventive medicine at the School of Medicine of the State University of New York at Stony Brook. Rather, it means that the health benefits of the weight loss that the product helps achieve outweigh any side effects.

Read the fine print. The take-home lesson for consumers, says Dr. Jonas, is to read package labels carefully.

Proceed with caution, if at all. Side effects such as stroke can be pretty alarming, but for certain diet aids, they do sometimes occur.

"If a label indicates that there have been serious side ef-

fects, you've got to be cautious about using it, and you
may want to consult your physician before doing so," says
Dr. Jonas. "There's a big difference between FDA approval
of a product and medical recommendation of that product," he adds. No aid is safe and effective for everyone.

Be a skeptic. If a label is vague or confusing, skip the
product.

"The pills made me nervous and irritable, and I snapped at
everyone," she told us. "I'd never take them again."

The bottom line: If you take appetite suppressants, you'll
most likely regain any weight you lose, risk serious health
consequences *and* probably feel jumpy in the meantime. So
while these pills are legal, they're not advisable, say experts.

DIET SHAKES: TEMPORARY RESULTS—AT BEST

Ads for these flavored, fortified drinks and drink mixes promise to give you the nutrients you need without excess calories
you don't want. Also known as liquid protein diets, these
shakes pack an average of 200 calories a serving—about the
same as a cup of low-fat fruit-flavored yogurt.

You add water or skim milk to the mixes or simply pop
open cans of the already prepared stuff. Popular brands like
Slim-Fast and Nestlé Sweet Success come in chocolate, straw-
berry and other dessert-type flavors.

Most manufacturers suggest you chug one of their shakes
for breakfast and another for lunch, then eat a normal meal at
dinnertime.

Do they work? Assuming you substitute the drinks for meals
that would pack more calories than the shakes do, you can lose
a moderate amount of weight on these regimens, says Dr.
Lachance. This, of course, is simple weight-loss arithmetic.
Fewer calories equal fewer pounds. The regimen, says Dr.
Lachance, will also help you maintain weight loss—as long as
you stick with it.

And there's the rub. Women who've tried these shakes told
us the regimen is boring and not particularly satisfying.

"I tried to lose weight with a popular diet shake two or

three times, but I never lasted more than a week," says Pam M., another woman who responded to our survey. She found the taste insipidly sweet, and she was always hungry. "After one shake in the morning and another in the afternoon, you're supposed to eat a 'sensible dinner,' " says Pam. "But by dinnertime, I'd be starving, so I'd eat a *huge* dinner."

What's more, some experts say the products encourage bad eating habits.

"What these products do, unfortunately, is distort people's normal eating patterns," says Berg, who is also editor of *Healthy Weight Journal.* "Drinking instead of eating—or not eating when you're hungry—aren't healthy eating patterns. So in my view, these cause more harm than good," she says.

Instead of relying on premixed shakes, you need to learn to choose a variety of filling yet nutritious foods, to eat them when you're hungry and to stop when you're full, says psychologist Ronna Kabatznick, Ph.D., a consultant to *Weight Watchers Magazine.* Premixed shakes are a no-think solution. Ultimately, it's important that you learn the skills to choose from a wide variety of nutritious foods on your own, says Dr. Kabatznick.

"These products are unlikely to lead to long-term, sustained weight loss," concludes Dr. Yanovski.

Are they safe? Early versions of diet shakes and mixes that hit the shelves in the 1970s were linked with a number of deaths. Investigators found the products nutritionally lacking (lack of potassium and/or poor-quality protein triggered fatal heart irregularities), and the products were taken off the market.

Experts tend to agree that today's drinks are vastly improved, but some nutritionists still have concerns.

"I think these products are unhealthy," says Faye Berger Mitchell, R.D., spokesperson for the District of Columbia Dietetic Association in Washington, D.C. "The average woman needs 1,600 to 2,000 calories a day. If you use these products for breakfast and lunch, they may provide a total of only 500 calories. By midday, you should have eaten 800 to 1,000 calories. This calorie deficit puts the body into a starvation state. And you may not get all the nutrients you need from your third meal. Furthermore, people can only stick with this routine for a few days because they just get too hungry."

Women who are under 18, pregnant or nursing have higher-than-average nutritional needs and should not be using these liquid diet plans, Berg warns. Others would be wise to limit themselves to one diet shake or so a week, says Dr. Renner.

"If someone's trying to lose weight and they take a can of Slim-Fast to work instead of running out and getting a deli sandwich with a lot of fat, then it may be helpful," says Dr. Renner.

If you opt for an occasional diet shake, check the nutrient analysis on the label. Dr. Lachance suggests you select one that supplies 25 to 35 percent or more of the Daily Values for calcium, iron, vitamin A and other essential nutrients.

VERY LOW CALORIE DIETS: BY PRESCRIPTION ONLY

Also known as liquid fasts, these very low calorie cousins of over-the-counter liquid diet plans supply fewer than 800 calories a day and are available by prescription only. You consume little or nothing but prepared fortified drinks for weeks or months while you're following very low calorie regimens. Popular brands include Optifast and Medifast.

Do they work? "They *can* work," Dr. Lachance says. "The problem is, if your diet is this low in calories, you may get a quick weight loss initially, then hit a plateau and get frustrated."

How come? Because your metabolism slows. The human body is genetically programmed to interpret a very low calorie diet as a sign of impending famine, explains Linn Goldberg, M.D., professor of medicine and head of the health promotion and sports medicine section at Oregon Health Sciences University in Portland. In an effort to save you from perceived starvation, your brain turns down the idle on your metabolism. You burn fewer calories, and the pounds get harder to drop. Unfortunately, after you start eating real food again, it takes your metabolic rate a while to get back up to speed. A few months after you've switched to a higher-calorie diet, your metabolism is still plodding along at its slower rate. When that happens, you *gain* weight.

"All the published data suggest that most people regain

weight once they discontinue use of these products," Dr. For-eyt says.

Like their over-the-counter counterparts, prescription liquid diets don't let you practice the healthy eating habits needed to keep weight off long-term, says Berg.

Very low calorie diets are appropriate for the severely obese only—women who are 40 percent above their ideal weight— whose lives are threatened by weight-related health problems like heart disease, says Louis Aronne, M.D., who heads the Comprehensive Weight Control Center at the New York Hos-pital—Cornell Medical Center in New York City. Prescribed for limited periods of time, the diets can help the extremely obese lose weight and improve their health faster than other regimens can, say experts.

Are they safe? While extreme overweight poses health risks, this extreme weight-loss strategy poses risks of its own. The rapid weight loss associated with the diets can cause very se-rious problems (gallbladder disease, anemia, heart rhythm dis-turbances, abdominal pain, muscle cramps and diarrhea) or less threatening but bothersome problems (moodiness, irritability, poor concentration and other emotional problems). Never try a very low calorie diet except under a doctor's supervision, experts warn.

FASTING: A BAD IDEA

As diet gimmicks go, fasting couldn't get any simpler: You eat nothing and drink water—maybe juice. That's all.

Does it work? Say *fast*, and people think: fast weight loss. But fasting is no quick fix, says Dr. Renner.

"You can only fast for so long," says Susan Olson, Ph.D., a clinical psychologist and consultant to the Southwest Bari-atric Nutrition Center in Scottsdale, Arizona. "Afterward, you usually end up bingeing because you're just so hungry and deprived."

Like most other quick weight-loss schemes, fasting gives you no practice at eating sensibly, says Steven Jonas, M.D., professor of preventive medicine at the School of Medicine of the State University of New York at Stony Brook. You end the fast no better equipped to eat sensibly than you were when you began. So naturally, you regain weight.

Is it safe? It's a good thing most people can't put up with a fast for long, since fasting can be risky, says Berg. Also, common side effects include moodiness, light-headedness and inability to concentrate, according to Berg.

A 24-hour fast probably won't hurt you, as long as you drink enough water, says Dr. Lachance. If you have diabetes, however, even a day-long fast *can* be harmful, he warns. Diabetics should never consider fasting for any length of time without talking to their doctors, says Dr. Renner. The rest of us should avoid regular or prolonged fasting (going without food for more than a day). It can lead to serious nutritional deficiencies and health problems, says Dr. Renner.

So while fasting is tempting, it sets you up to fail *and* jeopardizes your health.

FOOD COMBINING: NOT MAGIC

In the 1980s, a couple of popular diet gurus resurrected the notion that eating foods from just one food group at a time (say, fruit for breakfast) hastens weight loss, while eating foods from different food groups in combination (eating both fruit and chicken at the same meal, for instance) adds pounds.

Does it work? Weight-loss experts find this theory hard to swallow.

"From a biochemical standpoint, your body is able to digest whatever foods you consume at whatever time and in whatever combinations you consume them," says Mitchell. "To say otherwise may sound intriguing, but it's a lot of baloney."

Is it safe? As long as you eat all the food components you need—protein, carbohydrate and fat—within a 24-hour period, a food-combining diet isn't necessarily unhealthy, says Dr. Jonas. And it's not dangerous. But don't expect to see dramatic weight loss.

HIGH-PROTEIN DIETS: OUT-AND-OUT DANGEROUS

Heavy on the meat, chicken, fish, eggs, milk and cheese, high-protein diets are essentially high-fat, low-carbohydrate diets—

stingy with the grains, fruits and vegetables. A typical menu on a high-protein diet: an omelet, three ounces of tomato juice, a sliver of bran crispbread and coffee or tea for breakfast; a chef's salad with ham, cheese, chicken and egg and iced tea for lunch; seafood salad, poached salmon, two-thirds cup of vegetables and a half-cup of strawberries in cream for dinner. High-protein diets hark back to the early 1970s and resurface every few years, with new names.

Do they work? Despite their inordinately high fat content, people do lose weight on these diets—partly because the portions and your choices of food are so limited, says Dr. Lachance.

A good share of the "weight" you lose, however, is water weight, he says. A high protein intake prompts your body to excrete higher-than-normal amounts of water, Dr. Lachance explains.

Water loss is not real weight loss, though. As soon as you start eating normally, you regain the water weight and then some, says Dr. Lachance. Again, on regimens like these you don't learn how to eat the low-fat, low-calorie meals featuring fruits, vegetables and grains that are the real secret to staying slim the rest of your life.

The author of *The Scarsdale Diet*, the late Herman Tarnower, M.D., suggested that adherents follow the regimen for just a couple of weeks at a time. You could probably stay on it longer, according to Dr. Tarnower's book, but switching off for two weeks before resuming the diet allows you to choose from a wider variety of foods in the interim. Many women, however, find that even a couple of weeks on high-protein diets are rough going.

"I was on a high-protein diet where you could eat all the steak, other red meat and chicken you wanted, but no bread or dairy," recalls Kathy S., who responded to our *Food and You* survey. "I had ungodly cravings, mostly for salt—I'd eat deli pickles like crazy. It worked—I lost pounds. But when I started to eat regularly again, I quickly regained the weight."

Are they safe? In a word, no. Diets of this ilk are nutritional disasters, according to Dr. Lachance.

For starters, he says, high-protein diets shortchange you on a range of nutrients found in vegetables, fruits and grains.

"Nutrient analyses we've done show these diets are not nutritionally balanced," he says.

The diets also give you more protein than your body needs. Consuming all that extra protein creates a surplus of waste products that puts a strain on your kidneys, he adds.

To top it off, the diets' high fat and cholesterol content can contribute to heart disease, says Dr. Lachance.

Finally, there's the problem of ketosis. Without carbohydrates, your body can't burn fat completely, so it produces substances called ketones, by-products of incomplete fat metabolism. Ketones can cause nausea and increase blood levels of uric acid, a waste product that contributes to gout and kidney failure.

High-protein diets are bad for everyone, and they're particularly bad for women with high blood pressure, high blood cholesterol and triglyceride levels and diabetes, says Dr. Renner. He cautions teenagers and pregnant and nursing women in particular against these diet plans.

ALL-FRUIT DIETS: NUTRITIONALLY LACKING

Evoking the cachet of one of America's most fashionable addresses, the Beverly Hills Diet is among the better-known fruit diets.

Typically, your diet is made up primarily of fruit. The premise behind these diets is that fruit contains enzymes that can magically "burn" fat.

Do they work? Fruit diets can help you lose weight for some of the same reasons that high-protein diets can help you lose weight. They limit your choices so you're hard-pressed to eat more than a few hundred calories over the course of a day, Berg says. And they're so low in protein that they can also cause flulike symptoms, including nausea, after a few days. You're so nauseated that you can't eat, so you lose weight, says Dr. Lachance. But the fruit doesn't "burn" fat.

"No food burns fat," Dr. Renner says. "Exercise burns fat by burning calories."

Furthermore, staying on regimens like the Beverly Hills Diet is tough. Most people regain once they go off the diet, says Dr. Lachance.

"I once went on an all-fruit diet," Pam M. told us. "The first day you'd only eat one type of fruit all day, then the next day you'd eat another type of fruit. I ended up with mouth sores from all the citric acid! I felt terrible—and hungry."

Are they safe? No. In general, any diet that focuses on one food group to the exclusion of others is a bad deal. "You run the risk of deficiencies of certain nutrients," warns Mitchell.

GRAPEFRUIT PILLS: A FRUITY IDEA

Available at health food stores, grapefruit pills supposedly contain special enzymes found only in grapefruit that miraculously melt fat.

Do they work? No. Fruit doesn't "melt" fat, and pills made from fruit don't melt fat either, says Dr. Renner. There's no scientific basis for this diet aid at all, he says.

"There is no evidence that grapefruit or products made from grapefruit contain enzymes—or anything else—that will burn fat," says Dr. Renner. "It's ridiculous! Eat grapefruit pills to lose weight and you're wasting your money."

Are they safe? They're probably harmless but "entirely worthless," says Peter D. Vash, M.D., assistant clinical professor of medicine at the University of California at Los Angeles.

CHROMIUM PICOLINATE: A BOGUS TACTIC

An essential trace mineral, chromium has emerged from obscurity thanks to some heavy promotional efforts by supplement manufacturers. Some ads for chromium supplements claim the pills can help burn fat and build muscle.

Does it work? Since you probably don't need to take supplements to begin with, they're not likely to help you lose weight, says Forrest H. Nielsen, Ph.D., director of the U.S. Department of Agriculture Human Nutrition Research Center in Grand Forks, North Dakota.

"You need only a tiny amount of chromium—as little as between 25 and 50 micrograms—each day," Dr. Nielsen says. "And most people get that in the average American diet. Once you satisfy your requirement for chromium, you don't need more. Taking an excess won't melt away fat.''

Is it safe? The amount of chromium found in standard chromium supplements—up to 200 micrograms—is safe, says Dr. Lachance. But if you take them with the hope of burning fat, you're wasting your money.

HERBAL DIET AIDS: STEER CLEAR

Teas and capsules promoted as weight-loss aids usually contain one of two herbs, ma huang or senna. Ma huang is a potent (and dangerous) appetite suppressant. Senna is a powerful laxative.

Do they work? Ma huang dampens your appetite, and senna induces diarrhea because it has irritating compounds. So technically, you lose weight—at great cost to your health.

Are they safe? To the contrary, says Dr. Vash. The active ingredient in ma huang is ephedrine, a powerful stimulant, which can cause insomnia and dry mouth or leave you feeling like you're on amphetamines. Ma huang can cause high blood pressure and rapid heart rate and boost your risk of stroke and heart attack. It's dangerous. ''No one should take ma huang,'' says Dr. Lachance.

According to FDA spokesman Brad Stone, a number of complaints about ma huang have led the agency to investigate the herb.

As for senna, it's a potent purgative that can cause dehydration and wreak havoc with levels of electrolytes—sodium, potassium and other minerals that regulate your heartbeat—triggering dangerous heart rhythm irregularities. Used for more than two weeks, it causes lazy bowel syndrome—you can't move your bowels without a stimulant. Best advice: Steer clear.

NEW WAVE DIET PILLS: MUCH PROMISE, LITTLE WEIGHT LOSS

A variety of prescription diet pills (notably fenfluramine, phentermine, diethylpropion and phendimetrazine) act on serotonin and other brain chemicals that regulate appetite. The drugs are supposed to help reduce appetite, so you eat less.

Do they work? Researchers claim that regimens combining more than one drug (phentermine and fenfluramine, for example) seem to offer the best results. Not that the weight comes off all that fast—less than a pound a week, according to some studies. That's a fraction of a pound more than what the same people lost when taking an inactive, look-alike pill. In one study, overweight men and women who took fenfluramine and phentermine off and on for two years lost weight much more slowly—about a pound a month—for a total of 24 pounds.

Even the researchers who are most optimistic about the new drugs don't suggest that the pills alone will do the trick. You still have to watch what you eat and you still have to exercise, they say.

"These drugs are most effective when used with modest caloric restriction and a planned consistent exercise program," says Arthur Jacknowitz, Pharm.D., professor of clinical pharmacy and chairman of the clinical pharmacy department at West Virginia University in Morgantown. Yet one long-term study showed that after three years of diet, exercise and drug therapy, one group of severely overweight men and women lost an average of 20 pounds—not much better than people treated with drugs alone. (Other factors, such as cardiovascular fitness and improved blood fat levels, are favorably influenced by proper diet and exercise, adds Dr. Jacknowitz.)

Part of the reason total weight loss isn't greater is that people seem to stop losing weight and hit a plateau after about six months, according to a study at Indiana University School of Medicine in Indianapolis. Some researchers speculate that weight loss plateaus after several months because people develop a tolerance to the drugs, so the hunger-reducing effects wear off.

Moreover, most of those who have lost weight with these new drugs have regained it after they've stopped taking the pills.

"The problem is, if they come off the drugs, most people regain the weight," says Dr. Jonas.

Are they safe? The pills may be most effective if prescribed continuously, like high blood pressure drugs, Dr. Jonas says. Yet experts are cautious about who should take these drugs—they're not for everyone, and they're certainly not for the mildly overweight. Each type of pill has its own set of potential side effects, but the more common adverse effects are rashes, insomnia, allergies and dry mouth. Some of the drugs may also cause neurological damage or increase the risk of heart failure, Dr. Jonas says, although the research is not conclusive.

One thing is clear: If you need to lose 20 pounds or more, it's going to take time and effort, whether you diet and exercise or take drugs when they are appropriate. Because of the known side effects and potential risks, experts recommend obesity drugs only for those who are so severely overweight that their health is in immediate jeopardy and only when monitored closely by a physician.

CELLULITE CREAMS: FAT-DISSOLVERS THAT DON'T

Massaged into bumpy thighs, these creams are supposed to smooth away cellulite. The so-called active ingredient in the creams is a small amount of aminophylline, a prescription drug used to treat asthma and bronchial conditions.

Do they work? Despite the hype that accompanied their debut, the creams have yet to prove themselves in scientific studies, according to Stone. "We've never seen data substantiating the claims," he says. If these creams penetrated the skin and worked, they'd be considered a drug and, like the asthma medicine, they would be available by prescription only. But no prescriptions are necessary.

Are they safe? People with sensitive skin have complained of rashes after using cellulite creams, says Stone. So while cellulite creams don't appear to be dangerous, they certainly seem pointless.

THIGH WRAPS: SHEER NONSENSE

Kind of kinky, thigh wraps are sheets of thin plastic or fabric that you bind around your thighs, mummy-style. Some are impregnated with herbs. The theory is, if you wrap yourself tightly, your thighs will shrink, and they'll stay trimmer even after you unwrap the sheeting.

Do they work? Will a leg of lamb shrink if you wrap it in

plastic wrap? No. And neither will your thighs.

"Thigh wraps don't do anything except constrict circulation and probably irritate the skin," says Dr. Renner. "They're like a girdle for your thighs, nothing more. People are conned into thinking they're thinner, but there's no scientific evidence that they work."

Are they safe? No. If you pull the wrapping too tight, these products can cause dangerous circulation problems, Dr. Renner says. People who already have circulatory problems—due to phlebitis or diabetes—should definitely avoid these wraps, he adds.

DIET PATCHES: A COVERUP

Slap a special patch on your wrist and it'll apply pressure to an acupressure point that curbs appetite, claim the manufacturers of so-called diet patches.

Do they work? There's no evidence that these diet patches do anything at all. "You might as well just wear an ordinary Band-Aid," Dr. Renner says.

Are they safe? Diet patches appear to be as harmless as they are ineffective, Dr. Renner says.

EXERCISE TABLES: ON SHAKY GROUND

Don't want to exercise? Let a machine exercise for you.

That's the message from the manufacturers of these devices. One variety, known as continuous passive motion exercise tables, shake various parts of your body. Another type, called electrical muscle stimulators, transmit tiny electrical impulses that move your limbs.

Do they work? No. "You can't lose weight by letting a machine move your arms and legs for you," says Dr. Renner. If you're going to burn calories and lose weight, *you* have to move your muscles, he says.

Are they safe? Not for your wallet. "As far as I know, the only danger is that people are being scammed," says Dr. Renner.

As for electrical muscle stimulators, they have a legitimate use in physical therapy but not weight loss, according to the

FDA. Regardless, if used incorrectly, the machines can cause electrical shocks and burns.

When all is said and done, says Dr. Yanovski, the guaranteed safe and effective way to lose weight is to eat a low-fat diet—which will fill you up and meet your nutritional needs without busting your calorie budget—and to exercise so you have a bigger calorie budget.

46

LOW-FAT LIVING

Why eating less fat is a woman's number one priority

Salad dressing "on the side." Lean cuts of meat trimmed of all visible fat. Sorbet, not ice cream, for dessert. If you've adopted low-fat eating habits like these—or would like to— you're in good company.

In a nationwide survey done for the American Dietetic Association (ADA), women dieters said that cutting dietary fat is one of their major weight-loss strategies. With up to two-thirds of American women between the ages of 18 and 64 trying to shed excess pounds, that means a lot of us are choosing skim milk over whole milk, eating chicken without the skin and avoiding the butter dish.

Why a leaner cuisine? Women say their motivation goes beyond looking svelte in a swimsuit. While 23 percent of dieters told the ADA they simply wanted a more attractive appearance, nearly twice as many—42 percent—hoped to improve their health. And another 34 percent aimed to accomplish both.

Trimming the fat and calories, experts say, is one of the most effective dietary routes to both goals.

"There are certainly a lot of benefits to a low-fat diet, including weight loss and decreased health risks for heart disease, cancer and diabetes," says Susan Zelitch Yanovski,

M.D., an obesity expert with the National Institute of Diabetes and Digestive and Kidney Diseases at the National Institutes of Health in Bethesda, Maryland.

"Maintaining a healthful, low-fat diet does take some vigilance, because we're bombarded with advertisements for pizza, super-premium ice cream and fast food," Dr. Yanovski notes. "But in another sense, it's easier than ever. There are more fat-free foods available these days. The key is moderation—if you've had a fat-free breakfast of skim milk, cereal and fruit, you *can* enjoy a little ice cream later on."

Lowering fat is probably the most important thing you can do with your diet to achieve and maintain lower body weight, says JoAnn E. Manson, M.D., associate professor of medicine at Harvard Medical School, co-director of women's health at Brigham and Women's Hospital in Boston and co-principal investigator of the cardiovascular component of the Harvard University Nurses' Health Study (an ongoing study of 115,000 women considered a landmark source of evidence regarding women's health).

"In terms of health, 50 percent of all chronic diseases in the United States are related to obesity," Dr. Manson says. "Cutting fat and exercising are the best ways to prevent obesity."

As a bonus, you'll feel more energetic. And when your diet shifts from french fries, cheeseburgers and other high-fat fare to fruits, vegetables and whole grains, you're giving yourself more of the nutrients your body needs, too.

"And you can eat more!" says Dr. Yanovski. "You could have a big bowl of fruit salad for the same calories as a few bites of cheesecake!"

EAT LEAN, STAY LEAN

What makes a woman fat? Well, *eating* fat, for one thing!

Many of us eat too much. The average American gets 38 percent of calories from fat, according to researchers at the National Cancer Institute. That's a far cry from the 25 to 30 percent doctors recommend.

"Gram for gram, fat contains more than twice the calories found in carbohydrates or protein," says Steven Jonas, M.D.,

THE TEN "MOST UNWANTED" FAT FOODS

Here's a hit list of the foods that, according to the U.S. Department of Agriculture, are responsible for most of the fat calories consumed nationwide, along with fat-free or reduced-fat substitutes recommended by experts.

1. Salad dressing. (Buy and use low-fat and fat-free versions.)
2. Margarine. (Use fat-free cream cheese or all-fruit spread instead.)
3. Cheese. (Use low-fat and fat-free cheese.)
4. Ground beef. (Use extra-lean ground beef or ground turkey breast without skin for burgers, meat loaf and meatballs.)
5. Luncheon meats and sausages. (Use turkey breast without skin for sandwiches.)
6. Beef cuts. (Use beef not marbled with fat, with the fat on the outside so it can be cut off easily.)
7. Whole milk and whole-milk beverages. (Drink 1 percent milk, skim milk or skim milk with added milk solids.)
8. French fries, potato chips and other fried potatoes. (Try to avoid these completely.)
9. Poultry. (Remove the skin and use only white meat.)
10. Vegetable shortening. (Oil pans with nonfat cooking spray.)

Ph.D., professor of preventive medicine at the School of Medicine of the State University of New York at Stony Brook.

With nine calories per gram, a little fat packs a big caloric wallop. (In contrast, there are about five calories in a gram of protein and four in a gram of carbohydrate.) Excess fat calories can easily become excess pounds: Spreading your dinner roll with two teaspoons of butter, for example, would add 68 calories to your daily total. Do it for two months, and you'll put on an extra pound.

But the trouble with excess fat goes beyond mere calories.

When researchers at Indiana University in Bloomington looked closely at the diets of 32 women, what they found came as a surprise: Obese women took in only slightly more calories than lean women, but they got significantly more of those daily calories from fat. Do fat calories make us fatter than, say, calories from an apple? It's possible.

"Your body converts dietary fat into body fat very easily," explains Dean Ornish, M.D., president and director of the Institute for Preventive Medicine in Sausalito, California. "It's much more difficult to convert protein and carbohydrates into body fat—in fact, your body actually *burns* calories metabolizing protein and carbohydrates. Consequently, the more closely you can adhere to a very low fat diet, the less fat will remain on you."

Women who eat a lot of fat also tend to eat fewer fruits, vegetables and high-fiber bread and cereal. In a study of 11,758 women, researchers from the National Cancer Institute found that women who consumed the least fat ate nearly 20 servings of fruit and vegetables weekly, while high-fat eaters ate less than 13. This "produce gap" probably explains why the fat-lovers had lower intakes of vitamin C, folate, fiber and beta-carotene, the researchers noted.

"Fruits and vegetables are your best natural sources of antioxidant vitamins and a whole host of micronutrients and phytochemicals that are important for health but can't be found in vitamin pills," says Dr. Manson. "You get them on a low-fat, high-fiber diet."

Just what foods do high-fat aficionados favor? Red meat. Butter. Whole milk and cheese. Salty snacks and rich desserts. In short, a diet rich in animal fat—a primary source of saturated fats that medical researchers say are linked to a greater risk of heart disease, diabetes and cancer.

LESS FAT MEANS BETTER HEALTH

Medical research has good news for women: Eating lean can have a powerful and positive impact on your health, reducing the threat of major diseases now and in the future. Here's what a low-fat diet can do.

- Clear your arteries. A report published by the U.S. Department of Health and Human Services states that reducing saturated fat can lessen the risk of coronary heart disease.

"For every 1 percent drop in cholesterol levels in your blood, you get a 2 to 3 percent reduction in the risk of coronary heart disease," says Dr. Manson. "And a low-fat diet can lower cholesterol levels."

- Defend against diabetes. Your risk of developing Type II (non-insulin-dependent) diabetes doubles if you're mildly overweight (20 percent above ideal weight), goes up fivefold if you're moderately overweight (20 to 30 percent above ideal weight) and is ten times higher for severely overweight women (30 percent or more above the ideal).
- Give you a possible edge against breast cancer. Most medical studies have not found a strong link between dietary fat and breast cancer. But rates of breast cancer in countries such as Japan and China, whose residents have a low fat intake, are about one-fifth those of the United States. Although these differences could be due to other factors, some nutrition experts advise women to reduce fat—particularly animal fat—to less than 30 percent of total daily calories.

But other elements of a low-fat diet do seem to confer protection. A University of Toronto study that followed 56,837 Canadian women compared the 519 women who developed breast cancer with 1,182 cancer-free women and found that those consuming the most fiber and whole-grain cereals had about a 30 percent lower breast cancer risk. The reduction of risk was not as strong for those who ate fruits and vegetables.

- Promote healthier ovaries, and more. In a three-year study of 631 women, Yale University School of Medicine researchers found a definite link between saturated fat in the diet and the development of ovarian cancer. How can you lower your risk? Reduce saturated fat and eat more vegetables.

In a study conducted by Louise Brinton, Ph.D., chief of environmental studies at the National Cancer Institute, women who ate a diet low in fat enjoyed a 34 percent lower risk of endometrial cancer than women who ate a diet high in fat. Diets high in animal fats like hamburgers or whole milk and fried foods, in particular, were related to increased risk. On the other hand, women who consumed diets high in breads and cereals had a 40 percent lower risk of this cancer.

- Guard against colon cancer. Studies of individuals with colon polyps seem to bear out the dietary link. A study of 236 men and women conducted by researchers at the University of North Carolina at Chapel Hill concluded that a diet low in fat and high in complex carbohydrates and fruit and vegetable fiber cuts the risk of colon polyps, which could develop into colon cancer.

- Put a stopper on lung cancer. At the National Cancer Institute, researchers studied the diets of 429 women with lung cancer and 1,021 women who were free of lung cancer. Their findings? While cigarette smoking is the primary cause of lung cancer, diet may play a role: Women who consumed the highest levels of saturated fat (15 percent of daily calories) had six times the lung cancer risk of women who got 10 percent of their calories from saturated fat.

- Sidestep skin cancer. When 38 men and women with a precancerous skin condition caused by sun damage were put on a 20 percent fat diet for two years, the number of new premalignant lesions was lower than in the group that ate their normal diet and did not restrict their fat intake, according to researchers at the Veterans Affairs Medical Center and Baylor College of Medicine, both in Houston.

NO MORE "FAT HANGOVER"

A number of women responding to our *Food and You* survey mentioned that once they cut fried foods, rich desserts and other fatty items from their diet, a surprising thing happened: Not only didn't they feel deprived, they had more energy than ever.

Experts confirm the effect.

"To me, the most important benefit of going low-fat is that you feel better," says Dr. Jonas. "Very often, people who eat too much fat wake up the next day feeling sluggish and bloated. I know from experience that if I eat a lot of chocolate or cheese late at night, I'll feel uncomfortable the next morning," he says. "In general, I feel much more comfortable if I eat less fat, more carbs and a moderate amount of protein."

Dr. Ornish concurs. "I grew up in Texas, eating a lot of meat—I liked the taste. But I found I felt so much better when I didn't eat meat that it seemed like a worthwhile choice," he says. "Once you really pay attention to how your body is reacting after you've eaten a steak or a cheeseburger, you might find that you're feeling sleepy and sluggish and your thinking is fuzzy. But if you substantially cut the fat from your diet, you'll probably feel so much better right away that the wise food choices will seem obvious to you."

DIETARY FAT: HOW LOW SHOULD YOU GO?

So the consensus seems to be that women are better off curbing their taste for fat. Just how little fat should you aim for? As with calculating your ideal weight, the ideal percentage of calories from fat is not absolute. Rather, the ideal is a range that depends on individual health concerns.

"The need to limit dietary fat depends on a number of factors," says James J. Kenney, R.D., Ph.D., nutrition research specialist at the Pritikin Longevity Center in Santa Monica, California. "Your family and your own health history will help determine the relative dangers of the amount and type of fat you're eating."

Is your cholesterol high or borderline high? Are your HDL (high-density lipoprotein) levels low? "The higher your cholesterol, the more likely you are to develop blocked arteries," says Dr. Kenney. So if blood tests show your cholesterol is high, says Dr. Ornish, you should talk to your doctor about trying a very low-fat diet (10 to 15 percent of calories from fat) such as that used in either Dr. Ornish's program at the Institute for Preventive Medicine or Dr. Kenney's at the Pritikin Longevity Center. Both doctors report tremendous success in reversing heart disease in people they've treated. The same applies if you have high blood triglyceride levels, high blood pressure, diabetes or heart disease (or a family history of heart disease) or if you've had a heart attack, say Dr. Ornish and Dr. Kenney. Those conditions increase your risk for heart disease.

"If, for example, your cholesterol is high and you're overweight, 30 percent of calories from fat might be too much, and you may need to lower yours to as low as 15 percent,'' says Georgia G. Kostas, R.D., director of nutrition at the Cooper Clinic in Dallas and author of *The Balancing Act Nutrition and Weight Guide*. Start by reducing your fat calories to 30 percent; if you are already eating 30 percent, try 20 percent, then 15 percent if needed to lower cholesterol, she suggests.

Are you at risk for other fat-related conditions, like cancer? Then 25 to 30 percent of calories from fat is prudent.

''It's clear that the healthiest diet is a Pritikin/Dean Ornish sort of diet, with about 10 to 15 percent of calories from fat,'' says James W. Anderson, M.D., professor of medicine and clinical nutrition at the University of Kentucky College of Medicine in Lexington. ''But it's also true that a diet only works if people follow it, and nine out of ten people (or more) can't follow such a low-fat diet. Every woman, however, can lower her fat intake to 25 to 30 percent—it's easy to achieve and a good recommendation for everyone.''

Are you overweight? A diet in the 25 to 30 percent range is compatible with weight loss, as long as you include five servings a day of high-fiber fruits and vegetables and couple your diet with regular exercise, says Dr. Anderson.

Are you in good health? If you're one of the lucky few with no pressing health concerns—slim and trim, favorable cholesterol, easy-going blood pressure, a healthy insulin level—then up to 30 percent of calories from fat would be fine, say some experts.

''A woman who's slender, fairly active and doesn't have a family history of diabetes or fat-related cancers, like breast or colon cancer, can probably take in more dietary fat than someone who's overweight and has a family history of breast cancer and diabetes,'' says Dr. Kenney. ''If you've got good genes, you can probably get away with a little more fat, particularly if it comes from fish, nuts (except coconuts), tofu, avocado and seeds such as pumpkin or sunflower.''

''Generally, it's healthy and reasonable if a woman or a man sticks to the 20 to 30 percent range,'' says Kostas.

A LITTLE GOES A LONG WAY

A very small amount of dietary fat is essential for good health, says Dr. Kenney. The key is to make sure that when you do eat fat, it's the right kind, say experts.

"Small amounts of omega-3 (found in cold-water fatty fish such as mackerel and sardines) and omega-6 fatty acids (found in whole grains and most other plant foods) are essential," says Dr. Kenney. "In fact, a little omega-3 fat seems to reduce the risk of breast cancer. Eskimo women who eat large amounts of fish containing omega-3's have relatively little breast cancer."

Furthermore, certain kinds of vegetable oils—namely mono-unsaturated oils (like canola and olive oil) and polyunsaturated oils (like corn and soybean oil)—have been found to lower total blood cholesterol when substituted for saturated fat (animal fat). They also are carriers of fat-soluble vitamins, which are essential for optimal health. Be careful, though, all fats are concentrated sources of calories, says Alice H. Lichtenstein, D.Sc., associate professor of nutrition and a research scientist at the Jean Mayer USDA Human Nutrition Research Center on Aging at Tufts University in Boston.

On the other hand, saturated fat and cholesterol (found primarily in red meats, full-fat dairy products and fatty cream and sauces) are totally expendable, says Dr. Kenney. Limit calories from saturated fat to no more than 7 percent of calories from fat if you have high cholesterol or heart disease and 10 percent if you don't, says Margo A. Denke, M.D., associate professor of internal medicine at the Center for Human Nutrition at the University of Texas Southwestern Medical Center in Dallas and a member of the American Heart Association's Nutrition Committee. On a 2,000-calorie-a-day diet, that 7 percent adds up to 140 calories from fat—about 15 grams a day (the amount in one hot dog).

"There is no nutritional need for saturated fat, and you should keep it as low as possible in your diet, particularly if you're at risk for heart disease," says Dr. Kenney.

FAT MATH: THE RULE OF THIRDS

Figuring out your daily allotment of fat is simple: Say you're eating 2,000 calories a day—the standard allotment from nutrition experts. Say, too, that you're shooting for 25 percent of calories from fat. The idea, then, would be to limit your intake of calories from fat to 500 a day, or about 55 grams total. If you're on a very low-fat diet—say 10 percent of calories from fat—your daily limit is 20 grams of fat total.

Follow the rule of thirds. As for the type of fat that makes up those 55 grams or so, Kostas offers a handy rule of thumb.

"At the Cooper Clinic, we use the 'rule of thirds' recommended by the American Heart Association," says Kostas. "That is, one-third of the fat grams should come from monounsaturates, up to one-third from polyunsaturates and one-third (at the most) from saturates.

"The easiest way to hit those proportions," says Kostas, "is first, use olive oil and limited amounts of vegetable margarine; second, limit meals featuring red meat to three times a week (and stick to lean cuts and three-ounce servings) and third, have fish, chicken, beans and low-fat dairy products the rest of the week. Let the rest of your diet consist of nonfat plant foods like fruits, vegetables, beans and whole grains.

"Do that," says Kostas, "and you'll automatically get about one-third of each of the three types of fat without having to burden yourself with counting types of fat grams."

OTHER HANDY WAYS TO SUBTRACT FAT

Here are inside ways to trim the fat without sacrificing flavor.

Think "substitutions." Low-fat living begins with smart shopping choices—especially when you're most vulnerable, such as when you're ravenous or your only ready source of food is a convenience store. Here are five "emergency tactics" from Rodman Starke, M.D., senior vice-president in the Office of Scientific Affairs of the American Heart Association.

- Instead of a candy bar, have a banana or an apple.
- Instead of a package of nuts, have ready-to-eat cereal.
- Instead of cookies, have graham crackers.
- Instead of chocolate, have licorice.

▪ Instead of a hot dog with chili, have a microwaved bean burrito.

Buy low-fat treats. When the Girl Scouts of the U.S.A. (or their moms and dads) peddle their cookies in your neighborhood or office, you don't have to be a Scrooge just because you're trying to cut fat, says Judy E. Marshel, R.D., director of Health Resources in Great Neck, New York, and former senior nutritionist for Weight Watchers International. Ask for their low-fat or nonfat cookies, she advises. Then help yourself to just one or two and leave the rest in the lunchroom for others to share.

Never eat standing up. Follow this rule and you automatically eliminate many places that high-fat foods are dispensed: pizzerias, hot dog stands and ice cream wagons, to name just three, says Steven Gullo, Ph.D., president of the Institute for Health and Weight Sciences and former chair of the National Obesity and Weight Control Education Institute of the American Institute for Life-Threatening Illness at Columbia Medical Center, both in New York City.

Lean toward loin. If you must eat meat at least occasionally, select loin cuts—sirloin, tenderloin and, if you like pork occasionally, center-cut loin chops, advises Dr. Jonas. They're lower in fat. According to Jayne Hurley, R.D., senior nutritionist with the Center for Science in the Public Interest in Washington, D.C., round steak, either bottom or top round, is the leanest cut of beef available, leaner than loin cuts.

Substitute ground turkey for ground beef. But don't assume that ground turkey is low-fat, warns Hurley. Most of the ground turkey sold contains turkey skin which, like any poultry skin, has fat. So look for products labeled 'ground turkey breast,' " says Hurley. "You'll get breast meat only, no skin."

Grilling? Try fat-free or low-fat hot dogs. Chicken or turkey franks may not necessarily be the best option for frankfurter fans, says Hurley. Some brands are indeed quite low in fat; others contain as much as 12 grams of fat apiece (compared to 15 or 16 for oversize or jumbo franks). Scrutinize labels and consider one of the fat-free varieties. With a little mustard and ketchup, you'll hardly know the difference.

Sample before you spread. If you tend to go on auto-pilot when adding butter to your bread or dressing to your salad,

LOW-FAT EQUALS LOW-CALORIE?
Not Always

Doctors are noticing that a lot of people are scrupulous about buying only fat-free products yet still can't lose weight. Some even *gain* weight.

What's going on?

Reading nutrition labels provides one important clue. Take that luscious-looking chocolate frozen yogurt, for example, that boasts a mere four grams of fat per half-cup serving. Before you fill 'er up, take a second look at the label. As it turns out, one serving of this treat also contains 140 calories—about as much as in the same amount of regular ice cream.

Further detective work reveals that other fat-free or low-fat products may also be quite high in calories. Sure, they may not have much fat. But *something* makes them taste good, and in some cases, that "something" adds calories. According to James J. Kenney, R.D., Ph.D., nutrition research specialist at the Pritikin Longevity Center in Santa Monica, California, fat-free products don't automatically cut calories or lead to weight loss, because the fat in the products has been replaced with sugar and white flour, actually increasing the calorie density.

"Products are formulated to achieve a fatlike taste, appearance and texture, and each manufacturer blends a variety of ingredients to do that," explains Angela Miraglio, R.D., head of AMM Nutrition Services in Chicago. "Some products end up with fewer calories, and some do not. It depends on the particular mix of ingredients."

Here's the math: If you have a cookie that contains four grams of fat, at 9 calories per gram (the number of calories in one gram of fat), the total calories from fat are 36, says Miraglio. If the manufacturer makes a fat-free version of the cookie, you "save" four grams of fat and 36 calories. But to maintain a flavorful cookie, the cookie-makers might put in, say, a bit of emulsifier, an additive that might contain nine calories per gram (the same as fat). Or they may add extra sugar (which contains no fat), accounting for a fair number of calories. Add it all up, and a fat-free cookie *might* have fewer calories than a regular cookie. But don't count on it.

In fact, some fat-free products have more calories than the original, notes G. Ken Goodrick, Ph.D., assistant professor of medicine at Baylor College of Medicine in Houston. "It's possible to have a very low-fat diet and eat so many calories that you gain weight."

"Yes, sugar is fat-free," says Dr. Kenney. "That doesn't mean it's good for you and will help you to lose weight. Sugar has 45 calories per tablespoon."

Contributing to the problem is the fact that many people buy a fat-free product, then eat the whole box or bag, not one portion, says Miraglio. "People often fool themselves," she says. "If you eat a pint of fat-free frozen dessert, you might still be eating 300 to 400 calories."

The solution to the low-fat-food dilemma? Stick to single-size portions, says Miraglio. And don't expect to lose much weight simply by substituting fat-free products for your regular treats, says Dr. Kenney. "You'll just end up eating a lot of sugar and refined carbohydrates instead of fat."

---

forgo added fat as an experiment. "Plain, unadorned rolls and bread taste great without butter," says Dr. Jonas. "Make a pact with yourself to never put oil or butter on any dish before you've sampled it first," he advises.

Spear and dip. Don't smother your salads in oil or dressing. Spear a piece of salad with your fork, then dip it into the dressing for a lighter, lower-fat lunch or starter, says Dr. Jonas.

Drizzle, don't drench. "If you must use butter or sour cream on your potatoes, for example, use only a fraction of what you'd normally add," says Marshel. "Also, if you're making home fries or french fries, don't fry them in a pan of oil. Instead bake them on a lightly greased cookie sheet. They'll soak up far less fat."

Nix the fat—or nix the mix. "Pilaf and rice mixes are always asking you to add butter, oil or margarine," says Elizabeth Ward, R.D., a nutritionist for the Harvard Community Health Plan, an HMO in Boston, and a spokesperson for the ADA. "Skip the fat—you don't need it. The rice still tastes great.'' The other alternative, of course, is to make your own from scratch, sans fat.

In many recipes, you can delete the fat or cut it considerably, says Linda Van Horn, Ph.D., professor of preventive medicine at Northwestern University Medical School in Chicago. "Recipes often call for twice as much fat as they really need, especially desserts. I can easily take any recipe for anything and immediately reduce it. For example, I often use applesauce, pureed prunes or other highly concentrated sweet food that can take the place of fat. If you're creative with flavors and textures, your mouth doesn't miss the fat."

MENTAL TACTICS FOR EATING LEAN

With low-fat eating, half the battle is learning to enjoy what you do eat. Here are some tips from weight-loss experts on how to "think low-fat."

Try aversion therapy. Tempted by fatty foods? Use your imagination to lessen their appeal, suggests Susan Olson, Ph.D., a clinical psychologist and consultant for the Southwest Bariatric Nutrition Center in Scottsdale, Arizona. "If you're tempted by a display of cheesecakes at the local deli or bakery, for example, visualize the confections for what they are—an amalgam of grease and sugar. In fact, picture auto grease seeping directly into your arteries. The image could dampen the appeal and help you pass up dessert."

Sample, don't splurge. "Give yourself permission to eat a little bit of what you want, including candy," says Dr. Olson. "If you know you can have it, it loses a lot of its power. Plan to go to the store once a week to buy one or two pieces." When you make deliberate choices, you'll probably reduce the amount of fat you want because you won't feel deprived, she says.

Meditate a moment. To enable himself to eat (and enjoy) tiny amounts of high-fat foods, Dr. Ornish has developed what he calls his Häagen-Dazs meditation.

"I eat one teaspoon of ice cream, close my eyes and meditate on the rich flavor, the cold rush and the wonderful sensations as the ice cream melts on my tongue," says Dr. Ornish. "It's exquisitely satisfying. I much prefer a small teaspoonful of chocolate Häagen Dazs to an entire pint of a fake-fat frozen dessert.''

Give up your worst fat nemesis for 40 days. Choose one of your high-fat favorites and, like giving up meat for Lent, give it up for 40 days, says Marshel. At the end of that period, you may lose your taste for it altogether.

Wait out the food flashes. Beware of those I-want-it-now sensations that draw you toward high-fat foods with the force of a high-powered refrigerator magnet, warns Dr. Gullo. ''A food flash hits quickly, but it passes quickly, too. The trick is to move *away* from the desired food.''

Forget the all-or-nothing attitude toward fat. Certain food beliefs can inadvertently prompt you to OD on high-fat food despite good intentions, says Dr. Olson. ''Just because you allow yourself one cookie doesn't mean you have to eat the whole box. Know that you can choose to have it at another time.''

Eat rich, not fat. What do broiled lobster, a baked potato with zingy salsa and mango sorbet have in common? They're all low in fat. Treating yourself to a fancy but low-fat meal reinforces the idea that low-fat eating is fun, not a hardship, says Marshel.

47

SUGAR AND SUGAR SUBSTITUTES

Moderation, not deprivation

Not so long ago, Debbie Q. had a series of lusty love affairs with some luscious hunks. Monday, it was a hunk of cheesecake. Tuesday, a hunk of pumpkin pie. Wednesday, carrot cake slathered with thick cream cheese frosting.

When this 37-year-old ended the affairs and switched to diet soda, she lost 20 pounds. "But I still miss the sugar," says Debbie, who responded to our *Food and You* survey.

Sugar. We love it, we hate it, we crave it—and for good reason. Experts say human beings are born with a hankering for its sweet taste. It's a prehistoric survival instinct. A preference for sweet tastes probably kept our ancestors alive thousands of years ago.

"That sweet tooth is wired in," says Adam Drewnowski, Ph.D., professor and director of the Human Nutrition Program at the University of Michigan School of Public Health in Ann Arbor. "We evolved to like fruits and other plant products because their sweet taste denoted calories and the presence of fat. Think of mother's milk. Or the biblical reference to the land of milk and honey—fat and sugar."

Yet what evolved as a survival tool has become a sticky trap, particularly for women. Studies show we crave modern sweets packed with added sugars—from Oreos to cinnamon buns to Snickers bars—more often than men do. And today's sweets are often loaded with fat and devoid of the nutrients women need for good health—calcium for strong bones, carotenoids for cancer protection or iron for mental and physical energy, for example.

"Our taste buds are programmed prehistorically to seek out sweets," says Michael Steelman, M.D., president of the American Society of Bariatric Physicians and founder of the Steelman Clinic in Oklahoma City.

The difference is that thousands of years ago sweets meant fruit, and even grains and some vegetables. Today it's Twinkies, Devil Dogs and ice cream sundaes. "Prehistoric sweet foods had high nutrient and fiber value and not all that much fat," says Dr. Steelman. "These days, it's different. We have sweet foods that are high in fat, high in calories and low in nutrition."

Contributing to sugar's bad reputation is its knack for promoting tooth decay by nourishing enamel-melting bacteria. (All carbohydrates do that.) If you have diabetes, too much sugar or any other carbohydrate could make the control of blood sugar levels difficult. And if you eat sweets packed with concentrated sugar—like a candy bar—the rapid rise and fall in your blood sugar levels could leave you feeling irritable and fatigued.

LIMIT SWEETS

These days, a typical American woman consumes approximately a quarter-cup of added sugar between breakfast and bedtime.

We're not talking about the natural sugars found in fruits and even in vegetables, grains and dairy products. The problems come from the extra stuff—spooned into your coffee, sprinkled on your cornflakes or included in soft drinks and desserts.

The trouble with added sugar? Strike number one: It's empty calories—and not much else.

Read the ingredient list of a food label, and the forms of added sugar you're apt to encounter include sucrose, dextrose, lactose, maltose, honey, corn syrup, molasses, sorbitol, mannitol and xylitol. Whew! Whether it's extracted from sugar cane, corn, sugar beets or other sources, at about 16 calories per teaspoon, added-sugar calories can add up quickly. "A typical soda contains 150 calories, at least 100 of which are from sugar," says Dr. Steelman. "So if a woman drinks one extra soda a day, she could gain a pound in a month and ten pounds in ten months."

Strike number two: Sugar is often paired with fat.

"We call desserts sweets, but what they really are is fat—the sugar is coupled with butter, margarine, oil, milk fat or even cheese," says Maggie Powers, R.D., a nutrition consultant in St. Paul, Minnesota. "That's where calories and health problems come into play."

If pies and cakes take the place of fruits, vegetables, grains and dairy products on your plate, you may be skimping on nutrition while loading up on fat and excess calories, says Chicago nutritionist Alicia Moag-Stahlberg, R.D., a spokesperson for American Dietetic Association (ADA). "If you skip lunch and have a mega-size candy bar, you've exchanged all the nutrients you could have gotten at lunch for calories coming from sugar and fat," she says.

Here's proof: When researchers at the National Institutes of Health compared the diets of 15,368 women and girls, they found that those who consumed the most sugar took in 11 percent less calcium than those who consumed the least sugar. As a group, the sugar-lovers got an average of 13 percent less of 11 important nutrients, including vitamins A and B_6. Why? Researchers think the sugar-lovers ate less fruit, vegetables and dairy products.

How do you strike a balance? The ADA and other authorities suggest limiting calories from added sugars to no more than 10 to 15 percent of your total daily calories. For a woman whose optimal calorie intake is 2,000 calories a day, that's between 200 and 300 calories—about as much as you'd get from consuming, say, two teaspoons of sugar in your morning coffee, a 12-ounce can of cola and a large fig bar from the office snack machine.

Or you could experiment with calorie-free artificial sweeteners that mimic the sweet taste of sugar.

MEN CRAVE MEAT, WOMEN CRAVE SWEETS

You might call psychologist Marcia Pelchat, Ph.D., the Sherlock Holmes of food cravings. Tell her what you crave (chocolate? double cheeseburgers?) and chances are, she can identify you by sex and age.

When 145 women and men confessed their deepest food desires to Dr. Pelchat and other researchers at the Monell Chemical Senses Center in Philadelphia, a surprising pattern emerged.

- Among women 18 to 35 years old, lust for chocolate, cake and other sweets outranked cravings for pizza and steak by two to one.
- Among women over age 65, ardor for meats and sweets was equal.
- Men, regardless of age, reported a clear, two-to-one preference for meat and other protein-rich entrées.

Evidently, men and women snack on opposite sides of a culinary divide. He wants beef jerky. You need a brownie. Why the difference? And will a yen for sweets fade as you age?

"Cravings are very complicated," says Dr. Pelchat. "Some researchers say carbohydrates subtly alter your brain chemisty and work like self-medication for depression or feeling blue. That could be caused by fluctuating hormones. Or," she continues, "you might need the nutrition in that food. Or you may want something simply because it's forbidden or because you haven't had it for a while."

Older women, she said, may simply crave sweets less because they grew up when food choices were somewhat limited—during the Depression and World War II—and therefore have developed different tastes than younger women who came of age during times of plenty.

Regardless of sex, the cravings men and women reported had one thing in common: Most were fairly high in fat. "No one said they were dying for a piece of fruit," says Dr. Pelchat.

THE SKINNY ON ARTIFICIAL SWEETENERS

Three artificial sweeteners are currently available in the United States—aspartame, saccharin and acesulfame K. They're 180 to 300 times sweeter than sugar, with virtually no calories. But are they the best way to subdue a ravenous sweet tooth without packing on the pounds?

Available in diet sodas, baked goods and candies and in powdered form, these sweet pretenders, researchers say, can help cut calories and contribute to successful weight loss and weight maintenance—particularly for women.

A case in point: Dr. Drewnowski tallied the calories consumed by 24 Parisian women and men who'd eaten a breakfast of *fromage blanc* (a mild, custardlike cheese) that was either sweetened (high in calories), plain or artificially sweetened (both low in calories). At the end of the day, the low-calorie group had consumed 300 to 400 calories less than the high-calorie group.

Interestingly, the low-calorie group reported feeling hungrier at lunch, and they ate slightly more at a midday buffet—but not to the point where they made up the calorie deficit from breakfast.

"If a woman is trying to lose weight and every calorie counts, then artificial sweeteners, when used in a responsible regimen with diet and exercise, may help," says Dr. Drewnowski. "The psychological benefit is that they make available foods like sodas and desserts that used to be out of reach for dieters."

In another study, Barbara J. Rolls, Ph.D., professor of nutrition at Pennsylvania State University in University Park, reviewed 13 artificial sweetener studies and found they never made people eat more.

The key to using artificial sweeteners judiciously? Avoid falling prey to the "diet soda and cheesecake" syndrome, warn experts.

"A diet soda won't neutralize the calories in a slice of cheesecake," says Dr. Drewnowski. "Diet foods are not 'negative calories' that let you eat excess calories somewhere else." In other words, don't assume that as long as you switch to artificially sweetened foods and beverages, you have license to eat whatever you want with impunity.

"From a weight-loss and nutrition standpoint, artificial sweeteners are a double-edged sword," notes Dr. Steelman. "If they displace sugary, fatty foods, that's helpful. If they displace nutritious fruits and vegetables and dairy products, they're not."

If you elect to use artificial sweeteners, there are a few things you need to know. A study conducted at the University of Washington in Seattle found that some people got headaches after drinking aspartame-sweetened beverages. And a small study at Northeastern Ohio Universities College of Medicine in Rootstown found that women and men with a history of depression felt more depressed and irritable and had more trouble sleeping after taking aspartame.

Also, according to the ADA, women diagnosed with phenylketonuria (a rare, genetic enzyme deficiency that affects 1 in 150,000 Americans) should restrict their intake of aspartame. To alert consumers who may be affected, some soft drinks that contain aspartame carry a notice warning of this link.

A number of laboratory studies found a higher incidence of bladder tumors in male rats exposed to high levels of saccharin. More than 30 follow-up studies on humans, however, found no connection between saccharin consumption and increased risk of bladder cancer. Therefore, the National Cancer Institute has concluded that there is no evidence of increased risk of bladder cancer with long-term use of saccharin. Nevertheless, saccharin-containing products carry a label warning of a potential hazard.

SWEETENER SAVVY

Nutritionists and doctors say there are healthy, satisfying ways to fulfill sweet cravings without gaining weight or sacrificing nutrition. One point they all agree on is this: Make sure you're eating for nutrition *before* you go for a sweet treat.

"Have at least five fruits and vegetables a day. Eat breakfast, lunch and dinner. The bonus food comes afterward," says Moag-Stahlberg. "If you're filled up, a little chocolate bar will do."

As for satisfying your sweet tooth, the experts offer these suggestions.

Make it natural. Guide your hand toward the fruit bowl first, suggests Dr. Steelman. Fruits that are sweet also supply nutrition you need, he says. "And the fiber delays the absorption of sugar into the blood-stream, so you don't get a rapid rise and fall of blood sugar."

Go for texture. Like your desserts cool and creamy? Try nonfat frozen yogurt, suggests Powers. Need something sweeter than a piece of fruit? Try sorbet (exotic new flavors include mango and tangerine). Comforting and creamy? Pudding made with skim milk may fill the bill, she says. "And it's a good source of calcium," she adds.

Have just a taste. "Sometimes the best thing to do is give in to the urge for something sweet," says Dr. Steelman. "The trick is to control the portion size."

So split that lemon cheesecake with your dining companions. If you must have rich, creamy ice cream, limit yourself to one scoop. If you crave chocolate, buy one or two small pieces. Or freeze chocolate kisses and satisfy your sweet urge with two or three—they melt very slowly in your mouth!

Pair sugar with protein. Eating a small sweet with a protein-rich meal or in combination with a protein—like fruit with low-fat cottage cheese—seems to diminish the craving for more sweets later on, Dr. Steelman says. In contrast, he says, "having something sugary by itself could make cravings worse later."

Reach for fat-free sweets. Powers suggests mixing your own low-fat, low-sugar treats. Try hot cocoa made with skim milk, cocoa powder and a little sugar, honey or artificial sweetener. Or have an ice pop. Make your own by freezing fruit juice in ice cube trays and inserting ice pop sticks, suggests Moag-Stahlberg.

For dessert, says Powers, consider the natural taste of fresh fruit or a cup of flavored coffee (regular or decaf) served with low-fat or skim milk if desired. Or for that gourmet taste, shake a little vanilla powder, cinnamon or sweet cocoa into your coffee.

Spice it up. Baking? Make creative use of cinnamon, nutmeg, cloves, mint, vanilla and almond—they're natural sweetness enhancers. Reduce the sugar in cookie and cake recipes and add a dash of extra nutmeg. Or sprinkle cut-up fruit with cinnamon instead of sugar. Buy plain low-fat yogurt and add a drop of vanilla flavoring.

Scrutinize low-fat labels. Low-fat foods often replace a few grams of fat with extra carbohydrates, like sugar, says Powers. As a result, some low-fat foods have the same number of calories (or more) than the standard version. So compare nutrition labels for sugar content.

Add fake sweetener last. Aspartame loses its sweetness in hot foods. If your hot drinks don't taste sweet, try adding the sweetener as late as possible—just before drinking, Powers says.

Use less. Some people find that saccharin, the sweetest of the three artificial types, can have a bitter aftertaste. If one sweetener doesn't meet your needs, try another or try using less. "A bitter taste might go away if you use a smaller amount," says Powers.

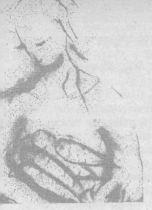

48

WEIGHT LOSS

What works for women

Nationwide surveys say that on any given day, one out of every three women is trying to lose weight. They fast, skimp on calories, count fat grams, join weight-loss programs, take supplements, pop diet pills and run, walk, bounce and swim in their quest for svelte and healthy silhouettes. They do lose weight, sometimes even lots of weight. Some lose it permanently, but many gain back some or all of the weight within a couple of years.

Terry C., who responded to our *Food and You* survey, is typical of women who've tried just about anything and everything in order to lose weight.

"I've tried various diets, prescription diet pills, Slim Fast, aerobics classes, liquid shakes, a doctor-supervised diet, Deal-a-Meal and the Rotation Diet," Terry told us. "They all worked—temporarily. The weight always came off, and I always gained it back."

STRATEGIES WOMEN USE—AND WHY THEY WORK

Still, our *Food and You* survey revealed plenty of weight-loss success stories—people who lost weight and kept it off for two years, five years—or forever. Why do some women succeed where others don't?

Of the women we heard from, those who reported lasting success at weight control used various strategies, from limiting fats in their diets to exercising regularly or making subtle changes in the way they viewed food. Many credit their success to a combination of simple but effective strategies.

Their triumphs over yo-yo weight patterns conform to what experts are finding about long-term weight loss. Strategies that succeed seem to have seven elements in common, according to John P. Foreyt, Ph.D., director of the Nutrition Research Clinic at Baylor College of Medicine in Houston, and G. Kenneth Goodrick, Ph.D., assistant professor of medicine at Baylor. Key strategies include:

- Realistic weight goals
- "Normalized" eating routines
- Exercise
- Social support
- Focus on health rather than appearance
- Enhancement of overall self-esteem
- Control of binge eating (sometimes through therapy)

Here's what worked for the women in our survey, with commentary by weight-loss experts.

MAKE FRIENDS, NOT COOKIES

Lorraine C., age 50, lost 40 pounds

Lorraine says that when she was a child, "my rotund Italian Grandma would pinch my cheeks and ask my mother in dismay, 'Don't you feed her?' "

Lorraine abhorred becoming a "skinny, flat-chested teenager" (as she described herself), and she responded by eating rich, fat-laden foods that gave her voluptuous curves. But at size 16, she found herself unhappy and unhealthy.

"In terms of food addiction, I 'bottomed out' after a holiday binge and a big-time New Year's depression," Lorraine told us. "I realized I was losing nearly everything but my weight.

Unfortunately, that's sometimes what it takes before we begin to take control to save our own lives.

"I had a support system," says Lorraine. "I had a friend, Jerry, who had lost weight and kept it off, whom I could phone when I needed support. I also had new friends who were in control of their lives. And I consulted professional advisers who specialized in weight loss. Following their recommendations, I decided that for me, the best thing was to eat small meals throughout the day. And I joined a gym that provided a personal trainer, plus workout equipment and instruction for how to use it."

Why it works: Lorraine is to be commended for taking control of a difficult problem, comments Peter D. Vash, M.D., Ph.D., assistant clinical professor of medicine at the University of California at Los Angeles. Lorraine's family, like so many other families, equated the extra pounds with robust and vigorous health, sex appeal and happiness.

For many women, says Dr. Vash, weight is an issue deeply rooted in childhood, entwined in genetics and firmly bound to family expectations and heritage. Lorraine set out on her own path, re-educated herself about food and managed to avoid turning to food as comfort when things got tough. In Jerry she found a role model she could emulate, rather than slipping back to food, her family's solution to every problem.

"When your family uses food as a psychological tool, you need to break the environmental pattern," Dr. Vash says. "To cope with your problems, start by confronting them directly. To solve problems, think them through. Food never solves anything."

HIGHER SELF-ESTEEM EQUALS FEWER BINGES

Krystal V., age 20, lost 40 pounds

Unlike Lorraine, Krystal's weight problem began in childhood, not adolescence. When other children made fun of her, Krystal found food to be a "great source of comfort and an unconditional friend."

As Krystal grew up, she fell into a pattern of starving and bingeing. Over the years, her self-esteem plummeted as her weight rose. Soon she was smoking, drinking, stashing candy bars in her car and living on food from convenience stores. "By the time I reached high school, I was five feet five inches tall and weighed 195 pounds," she told us.

"It finally got to the point where I decided to turn things around," she says. "First I quit flooding my body with drugs and other toxins. I started eating whole grains and four to five servings of fruits and vegetables each day. Now I eat mostly a vegetarian diet, with some low-fat dairy products and an occasional egg. I find that if I focus on the healthful foods and take time to eat them, I don't have cravings or binge.

"I'd always thought that if only I was thin, I could be happy," says Krystal. "But it's the other way around—if I'm happy, it's easier to stay thin."

Why it works: Krystal's destructive eating habits clearly had a psychological and emotional underpinning, which she was able to confront and conquer, says Maria Simonson, Sc.D., Ph.D., professor emeritus and director of the Health, Weight and Stress Clinic at Johns Hopkins Medical Institutions in Baltimore. "Why do we eat in the first place? We eat because we're hungry. But we also eat when we're happy, when we're sad, when we're angry or when we're frustrated, anxious or depressed." Krystal achieved success when she came to see that food, instead of comforting her, was punishing her body.

Krystal reached a point where she said, "I can do it, and I will do it." "That sense of determination and accomplishment gave her strength and hope and a future," says Dr. Simonson. About 80 percent of the people who seek help from the Johns Hopkins clinic have an emotional component to their overeating or undereating, she says. Many need professional help to understand and overcome the psychological as well as the physiological challenges to losing weight.

GET BUSY

Cass M., age 27, lost 14 pounds

"I seem to gain weight when I'm idle or depressed," says Cass. "The only times I have ever successfully lost weight and maintained that loss for more than a year was when I was not thinking about it. I had a negative body image and was very depressed over how I looked. Then I got busy with work and friends. About six months later, I was buying clothes and nothing fit. Everything was too big! I went home and found out I was down to my ideal weight.''

Why it works: Ironically, focusing too much on weight loss can itself undermine success, says Dr. Foreyt. Backsliding leads to blame, which can lead right back to overeating. One approach taken by weight-loss professionals looks at underlying issues rather than focusing solely on food. ''A large part of treatment should deal with improving self-esteem by focusing on other areas of life and helping people realize that self-worth is not dependent on appearance,'' says Dr. Foreyt. Cass stumbled upon that truth by herself, and found it worked.

EXERCISE, EXERCISE, EXERCISE

Regina P., age 40, lost 35 pounds

''I've lost my fat from being on a low-fat diet (15 percent of calories coming from fat) and exercise, exercise, exercise,'' says Regina.

Why it works: When it comes to maintaining weight loss, the evidence in favor of a low-fat diet plus a regular exercise plan is overwhelming. One reason, of course, is that you decrease the calories you eat and increase the calories you burn.

But researchers suspect there's an additional factor at work: Scientists at the University of Pittsburgh speculate that the magic may be in the flexibility of a diet-and-exercise regimen. A woman who only watches what she eats has only one option when it comes to compensating for slip-ups, and that is tightly reining in on food. If she eats right *and* exercises, she can step up her exercise in order to compensate for stepping slightly out of bounds at the buffet table. Exercise also may produce mood or appetite changes that make it easier to stick with healthy food choices, according to Nicolaas P. Pronk, Ph.D., formerly at the University of Pittsburgh School of Medicine and now with Health Partners, an HMO in Minneapolis.

EAT SMART, WALK MORE

Beth E., age 28, lost 20 pounds

"I weighed 200 pounds all through high school, and went up to 242 after I was widowed. Through the years, I have tried every diet, fasted, and even had my stomach stapled. I finally found out that, if you really want to lose weight, watching fat is where it's at!

"So much is mental," adds Beth. "For the first time, food is okay, as long as I watch what kind of food I eat. There are so many fat-free snack foods. I love eating, but I am still losing, slowly and consistently. And I'm walking at least three times a week."

Why it works: Indeed, studies affirm Beth's conclusion that "fat is where it's at" when it comes to losing weight. Each ounce of fat has at least double the calories of an ounce of nonfat food, according to weight-loss specialists at the Weight Management Program at the California Pacific Medical Center in San Francisco. They encourage people to lose weight "not by eating less but by eating smart."

As for walking, many physicians recommend walking (along with dietary changes) as a simple, inexpensive way to exercise while losing weight and particularly to maintain a healthy weight, according to Dr. Pronk. Beth's on the right track.

DIET AND EXERCISE BEAT GENETICS

Karen M., age 32, lost 25 pounds

The only one of ten siblings who is not now overweight, Karen found she could not lose weight until she understood her family's "genetic, emotional and physical health patterns." In the household where she grew up, "food meant good times," as in "a reward."

"When I moved out on my own for the first time, I wasn't very good at cooking," says Karen. "That turned out to be a blessing: My diet consisted of lots of fruit, raw veggies, rice and pasta. I was also very active and spent lots of time outdoors. I began to realize my body treated me well if I treated it well. I don't deprive myself of sweets. But they're the exception, not the rule. I take nutrition and health classes when

I can at local colleges. And when I shop for food, I read labels carefully.

"I'm proud to say that at the age of 32, with two daughters ages 4 and 2, I look and feel better than I did at 18," says Karen.

Why it works: With so many overweight brothers and sisters, there's a good chance Karen inherited her tendency toward overweight, says Dr. Simonson. She may have also inherited the eating and living habits that contribute to overweight. We inherit our families' faulty nutritional patterns as well as their genes, according to Dr. Simonson.

If both your parents are overweight, there's an 80 percent chance that you will be overweight, says Dr. Simonson. If one parent is overweight, the child has a 40 percent chance of being overweight. (In contrast, two normal-weight people have a 9 percent chance of having an overweight child, says Dr. Simonson.)

Moving away from home didn't alter Karen's genes, but it precipitated other changes—a less fatty diet and more exercise—that helped her overcome her tendency to gain weight.

BREAKING OLD HABITS

Michelle M., age 32, maintains a healthy weight

"My diet changed dramatically for the better when I had a roommate who only cooked healthy foods," says Michelle. "I adopted her diet and found my body preferred it to the diet I had grown up with (lots of meat and a few overcooked vegetables). I eat a low-fat, low-sugar, high-carbohydrate diet to maintain consistent energy levels and to fuel my sports-intensive lifestyle. I eat small, frequent meals throughout the day. Overindulging in rich (fatty or sweet) foods definitely makes me feel lethargic, sometimes queasy and generally unhealthy."

Why it works: By moving into a new household, Michelle snipped the ties to her family's poor eating habits, says Dr. Simonson. "Habit accounts for a great deal of poundage," she says. Michelle's roommate led her to an eating plan that makes scientific sense. Paradoxically, a roommate who has faulty eating habits can influence a woman for the worse, says Dr. Simonson.

Researchers in Britain found that carbohydrates act powerfully on people's perception of how "full" they feel. Adding a carbohydrate to your breakfast, for example, is likely to curb your hunger for two to three hours and reduces the likelihood that you'll crave a midmorning snack. Eating the same amount of a high-fat food with your breakfast produces no similar long-term feeling of fullness, called satiety.

Another study, published at the University of Minnesota, followed two groups of overweight women, one on a balanced low-fat diet that restricted calories and the other on a low-fat diet that advised them to avoid meat or eat only small amounts but let them eat as many complex carbohydrates as they wanted. The low-fat, high-carbohydrate group lost more weight than the restricted-calorie group. But perhaps more significant, the dieters who were allowed to eat unlimited carbohydrates consistently rated the diet as more pleasant, the food more tasty and their quality of life while on the diet better than those on the reduced-calorie plan. The researchers surmised that people who could eat plenty of carbohydrates "may have felt less deprived of food," since carbohydrates filled them up. Clearly, a dietary plan that is easier to live with has important implications in helping people lose weight and keep it off.

LESS FAT SPELLS SUCCESS

Carol P., age 47, lost 20 pounds

"I don't buy foods that aren't healthy or low-fat," says Carol. "Then when I raid the refrigerator or cupboards, at least my choices are healthier. Now if I eat a high-fat food—like a cheese steak, for example—my digestive system lets me know it. My mind and taste buds want it, but my body doesn't."

Why it works: Scientific evidence is mounting in support of the theory that it may be the amount of fat a person eats, not the amount of total food, that makes the difference in weight loss. A variety of studies have shown that people can lose weight by cutting fat, even when they are eating the same number of calories. Intriguing research from the University of

Minnesota hints that avoiding specific foods (hot dogs, beef, sweets, dairy products and french fries) may result in more impressive weight reduction than avoiding fats in general.

Carol's right, by the way, when she notices that heavy, fatty meals don't sit well with her anymore, says Robert Kushner, M.D., director of the Nutrition and Weight Control Clinic at the University of Chicago. Eating a lower-fat diet, with little or no meat, has conditioned Carol's stomach to expect healthy, reasonable portions, he says. When she suddenly eats a big beef sandwich, "her stomach gets distended because it's not accustomed to the high-fat load."

PORTION CONTROL WAS THE KEY

Jean L., age 41, lost 15 pounds

"After years of failed attempts to control my weight and eating habits, I consulted a nutritionist, who taught me the difference between a normal portion and what I was eating," says Jean. "I'm Italian. I come from a background where we eat large amounts of pasta, for example. It was a shock to me that a half-cup of spaghetti is considered a portion. So I started measuring everything.

"The nutritionist also showed me that what I was eating could use some improvement," says Jean. "I was avoiding vegetables and fruits because they're usually sprayed with pesticides, which I wanted to avoid. But I ended up eating mostly prepackaged foods and homemade baked goods."

Why it works: Experts have observed that people who carefully monitor their food intake—actually measuring their food portions and counting fat grams, for example—have greater success in dieting than those who guesstimate or do not keep track of quantities. And Jean's misjudgment of portion sizes is all too common. In a study conducted at St. Luke's–Roosevelt Hospital and Columbia University in New York City, people who said they were unable to lose weight even on restrictive diets were carefully monitored by researchers for two weeks while keeping their own records of their diets and activity levels. Unwittingly, the people who felt they were "diet-resistant" underreported the amount of food they ate by an

COMMERCIAL DIET PLANS
Should You Sign Up?

Among the women who responded to our *Food and You* survey, a fair number told us they'd tried commercial weight-loss programs such as Weight Watchers, Nutri/System, Jenny Craig, Diet Center and Optifast, among others. That corresponds to a national survey of more than 12,700 women dieters, which found that about one in ten had joined an organized weight-loss program.

Some women in our survey credited commercial weight-loss programs with long-term success on the scale.

"I lost 30 pounds eating healthy (not dieting) through Diet Center," says Mary M., age 31.

"About 18 years ago, I gained 40 pounds in six months," says Linda F., age 41. "Then I joined Weight Watchers and began to exercise faithfully. It took about a year and a half, but I lost the weight."

Other women tried commercial programs but dropped out, for various reasons.

"I need to lose weight on my own," says Sandi L., age 31. "When I have to report in weekly, I resent it and ultimately sabotage my efforts. Although weight comes off quicker through these programs, my way is less threatening."

"I went to Weight Watchers for 25 years, with limited success," says Roberta K., age 46. "At times it was humiliating. I also tried newer programs, including Jenny Craig, but their food was more expensive than grocery store food and, for me, not as tasty."

It seems that for every satisfied customer (like Mary or Linda) there is at least one unhappy individual (like Sandi or Roberta). And in fact, surveys suggest that dropout rates in the programs run as high as 70 percent in 12 weeks.

SHOP AROUND

Nevertheless, many people do lose weight (and keep it off) on these programs. Should you try a commercial weight-loss program? While there's no one answer—or program—

that's right for everyone, here's what experts say you should consider.

What can you eat? Programs that successfully encourage you to reduce your caloric intake and especially your fat intake while still meeting your nutritional needs are going to help you lose weight, says John P. Foreyt, Ph.D., director of the Nutrition Research Clinic at Baylor College of Medicine in Houston.

Does the program include exercise? Whether you're trying to lose or maintain your weight on your own or through a commercial weight-loss program, exercise and diet work best in tandem, says Dr. Foreyt. One without the other just won't give you the same results and won't help you keep the weight off.

What other elements make up the program? "Successful programs include classes offering behavior modification and encouragement," says Dr. Foreyt.

Does the program provide social support? Sometimes women lose weight through commercial programs because they offer structure and support for what can be a lonely and difficult endeavor, says Dr. Foreyt. That may include group problem-solving, one-on-one telephone calls or other encouragement.

What are the degrees and credentials of the staff members? Do they have degrees from accredited colleges or universities? They should be registered dietitians with an R.D. At the least they should have a bachelor's degree in counseling (better yet is a master's degree in counseling), advises Thomas A. Wadden, Ph.D., professor of psychology at the University of Pennsylvania School of Medicine in Philadelphia and director of the Weight and Eating Disorders Program.

How many people enrolled and stayed with the program? You're entitled to an accurate description of the program's clients and how much weight they lost over what period of time, according to the Institute of Medicine of the National Academy of Sciences.

How much does it cost? According to the Institute of Medicine, you're entitled to full disclosure of costs.

Are you willing to spend the money? Ironically, although some people complain about the cost of weight-loss programs, charging money may partially explain why they work, says Dr. Wadden.

"To be successful, you need to feel some commitment or obligation," he says. "For some people, money institutes a sense of motivation. Other people are motivated without paying money."

Will they return your deposit if you're not satisfied or if you drop out? Dr. Wadden adds that while cash might be a motivational tool, lots of cash should not be necessary to make you feel loyal to the cause. Studies indicate that programs that return deposits to people who stick to the program and adhere to its guidelines have been shown to improve weight loss more than those that hold on to your fee if you drop out.

---

average of 47 percent. They also overestimated their physical activity by 51 percent.

If you really want to lose weight, seeing a professional, as Jean did, is one way to go, says Dr. Simonson. Many times a professional, such as a registered dietitian recommended by your doctor, can point out hurdles to progress that we can't see in ourselves, she says.

Dr. Simonson recommends caution when selecting a nutritionist. "Many so-called nutritionists go to schools without proper professional training, just 'quick weight-loss methods,' or they just call themselves nutritionists. A registered dietitian (R.D.), licensed by the American Dietetic Association, is your safest choice," says Dr. Simonson. If you go this route, "it will cost you money, but it will be the best money you've ever spent," she says.

People's eating problems are not all the same, so it makes sense that the solutions should be individualized. Nutritionists' fees are often dependent on the weight of the individual, their state of health and several other special considerations. At Johns Hopkins, for example, the program is individualized to take into consideration such things as ethnic background, family health background, religious beliefs about food and social, psychological and environmental factors, as well as how much the client can afford to spend on food, among other factors.

SHAKE THE "DIET" MENTALITY

Joyce S., age 46, lost 45 pounds

"A few years ago I was depressed and sought counseling," says Joyce. "One of my problems was poor self-image. The therapist suggested I stay away from the scale and start walking for 10 minutes a day. As I walked, I did a lot of thinking. My 10-minute walks increased to 20, 30, then 40 minutes.

"I thought, why not try to eat healthy and see if I could reduce my cholesterol level? I read a pamphlet on controlling cholesterol and followed the suggestions. My cholesterol level dropped 84 points. As an added bonus, I lost 45 pounds!" says Joyce.

"Walking compensates somewhat for my indulgences—although I don't keep a lot of junk food around the house," says Joyce. "I don't think of myself as being on a diet, because then I'd think 'failure' and put myself down. My goal is to get healthy mentally and physically."

Why it works: Joyce got good advice from her counselor, says Dr. Foreyt. "Regular physical activity improves well-being, self-esteem and a sense of control. All of those components helped her stabilize her eating habits and put food in its proper perspective in her life. Exercise works, not only because of the calorie expenditure. It's the psychological component, changing your outlook," he says.

Joyce is also doing herself a favor by avoiding a "diet mentality," since experts say that "going on a diet" implies short-term deprivation that tends to give way to old eating habits. In fact, a study conducted at the University of Minnesota found that over a two-year period, women who were dieting *gained* weight when compared to co-workers who weren't actively trying to lose weight.

Dr. Simonson warns that diet pills or "fly-by-night diets" can be useless and yet harmful. "We can't stress strongly enough the dangers in these two modes of weight loss without professional review of some kind," says Dr. Simonson.

SLIM, TRIM AND SUGAR-FREE

Elizabeth C., age 32, lost 23 pounds

"Over two years ago, I made one major health decision: no more refined sugar. No candy, cola, cakes, cookies and so on," says Elizabeth. "About six months later, I decided to start walking. No dieting, no aerobics classes, no hunger. I've lost 23 pounds—slowly—but it's stayed off," she says.

"I finally feel in control of what I eat," says Elizabeth. "I feel great!"

Amy P., age 26, maintains "comfortable" 130 pounds

"I've found that sugary foods greatly increase my appetite and don't satisfy me, except momentarily," says Amy. "So I avoid them altogether. If I only allow myself 'real' foods (not treats), I know I am eating out of true hunger and true hunger alone.

"Weighing myself each day and writing it down is very helpful also," says Amy. "It is easy to rationalize or deny your eating habits. When you write it down it makes you aware, and to me, that's the biggest step in weight loss."

Why it works: Like Elizabeth and Amy, many people blame sugar for their weight problems. At Johns Hopkins, Dr. Simonson does a computer profile covering physiological, psychological and emotional factors to discover the real reason people crave sugar. And in fact, cutting out the sweet stuff seems to work for some people—it's a significant source of unneeded calories. And by cutting out sweets like doughnuts, pies and ice cream sundaes, you're also cutting out fat, another source of excess calories, says Dr. Simonson.

Evidence suggests that sweets as well as fats may stimulate opioid peptides ("feel good" receptors in the brain), and these foods are often associated with binge eating at times of stress or unhappiness, say Dr. Foreyt and Dr. Goodrick, although human studies have failed to confirm the connection.

Weighing yourself regularly and writing it down, as Amy did, is also effective, says Judith S. Stern, R.D., D.Sc., professor of nutrition and internal medicine at the University of California, Davis. "People who weigh themselves every day tend to be more successful at weight maintenance," says Dr. Stern. To avoid obsessing over your weight, however, Dr. Stern advises people to record their weight weekly, not daily.

A VEGETARIAN DIET WORKS FOR HER

Alice F., 46, lost 15 pounds

"I gave up meat, period," says Alice. "For me, vegetarianism works. For some reason, I can have the occasional piece of chocolate and not overdo it. But an occasional hamburger opens the floodgates, and I just keep eating.

"Also, I espouse the spiritual viewpoint that the body is the temple of the soul," says Alice. "Focusing on that philosophy helps me stick to my rule. For me, closing the door to fatty foods like red meat is easier than cutting back."

Why it works: Cutting out red meat automatically cuts out a primary source of fat (and calories) in the diet, accounting for Alice's success at weight loss after going vegetarian, says Dr. Vash.

Alice's hamburger-triggered eating binges aren't that atypical. Research suggests that eating fat does in fact stimulate the appetite. When it comes to fat, the more you eat, the more you want. Conversely, reducing "sensory" exposure to fats—not eating fatty foods or smelling them, for instance—reduced people's desire for them. Dr. Simonson adds that fat gives food its flavor, and we learn to like it and crave it. About two-thirds of the people who binge do so because of the fat alone. Even if they don't see it or smell it, they remember the taste, and that's what triggers them to binge.

To explain Alice's ability to resist hamburgers but not chocolate, Dr. Simonson acknowledges that different foods trigger temptation in different people. We all have our own likes and dislikes, says Dr. Simonson, and Alice is wise to recognize her danger zones. "Still, she needs to be sure her vegetarian diet is meeting all of her nutritional needs, especially for protein, iron and B vitamins," says Dr. Simonson.

SHE EATS THE SAME FOODS EVERY DAY

Barbara B., age 55, lost 60 pounds

"Every morning, I eat a half-cup of cooked oatmeal with a half-cup of skim milk," says Barbara. "I eat three prunes and drink a cup of green tea on my way to work. For lunch, I eat a salad, usually spinach, with onion, tomato, black olive slices, grated carrots and broccoli pieces. I dip my fork in the dressing and then stab the salad. I also eat about half a can of tuna in water, drained and mixed with several spoonfuls of low-fat cottage cheese and chopped onion. For dinner,'' says Barbara, ''I have either pasta and a vegetable or meat and one vegetable.''

Why it works: Like Barbara, a number of women who responded to our survey said that they managed to lose weight by eating the same foods each day, ordering the same foods at lunch and putting the same things in their grocery carts each week. Experts call this strategy ''sensory-specific satiety.''

If a rigidly structured diet is based on the food guide pyramid—emphasizing grains, fruits and vegetables and beans and going easy on meat, sugar and fat—it probably can be followed without unhealthy consequences, says George L. Blackburn, M.D., Ph.D., associate professor of surgery at Harvard Medical School and chief of the Nutrition/Metabolism Laboratory at Deaconess Hospital in Boston. ''And it can unquestionably lead to short-term weight loss,'' he says. ''That's because it's very boring. Food loses its appeal, so you don't overeat.''

According to Dr. Blackburn, the plan's victory through boredom is also its pitfall—few people could stay with such a plan for very long. As noted, when people feel deprived of food, they sometimes binge later. So this approach may work only for highly disciplined individuals.

LOW-FAT, NOT NONFAT, CAN WORK

Lois H., age 49, lost 7 pounds and maintains weight at 108

''Post-40 weight gain is for real,'' says Lois. ''So I try to stick to a low-fat and low-cholesterol diet, although I do allow myself certain liberties. I just can't make lasagna with fat-free ingredients,'' she says. ''Low-fat, yes; nonfat, no. And once in a while—on Sunday morning, especially—I treat myself to whole milk in my coffee.

'' 'Buddying' works for me, too,'' says Lois. ''When my friend (a co-worker) and I decided to diet at the same time, we ate lunch together every day and planned our evening meals together, even went shopping for groceries together.''

Why it works: Lois may worry that she is sabotaging her weight-control plan by slipping a little low-fat cheese into her lasagna or treating herself to real milk occasionally. But many diet experts believe that, for people like Lois, wavering now and then may actually boost weight maintenance in the long run. Few people have the unwavering discipline of Alice or Barbara, who succeeded by making no exceptions, ever. For Lois (and many others like her) a rigid, unrealistic eating plan is unlikely to last a lifetime, says Dr. Foreyt. ''The stronger the feeling of hunger and deprivation, the greater the urge to break the diet,'' say researchers at the University of Colorado.

And, like others who responded to the survey, Lois benefited from buddying up with a friend who shared her goal.

49

FOOD AND YOU: THE DIET PLAN

A program for losing 10, 20, 50 pounds or more

Our *Food and You* survey turned up a large number of dieters. Some wanted to lose as little as 5 pounds, some wanted to lose 50 pounds—or more. Their reasons varied as much as their goals—to look better, feel better, lower their risk of serious disease or simply be healthy. And, we found, these women are no different from women all across America. According to a survey conducted by the American Dietetic Association, one-third of those who responded reported that they were trying to lose weight—23 percent to look better, 43 percent to improve their health and 34 percent to look and feel better.

Many of the women in our survey had lost weight in the past, only to regain it in time. Their experience, too, corresponds to larger studies indicating that 95 percent of all dieters who lose weight eventually gain it back.

How can we lose weight—permanently—without the hunger, boredom and failure that too often accompany most weight-loss programs? We posed this challenge to Judith S. Stern, R.D., Sc.D., professor of nutrition and internal medicine at the University of California, Davis. The result is this program, based on what has been scientifically proven to work and tailor-made by Dr. Stern for *Food and You*.

The basic idea is simple, says Dr. Stern.

"You start out each day with two 'bank accounts,' " she says. "One tallies your intake of fat (in grams), and one tallies time spent exercising (in minutes). Your dual goals are to stay strictly within your fat-gram expense account and to meet (or even exceed) your exercise allowance. Remember, you've got to expend more energy than you take in in order to lose weight."

This plan is based on losing weight in increments of ten pounds each, with a special mini-plan for dropping five pounds quickly.

"With this plan, you can't *help* but lose weight," says Dr. Stern.

To make sure those pounds come off and *stay* off, the plan includes tips for modifying eating behavior that can derail the best-intentioned weight-control efforts.

WEEK ONE: THE KICKOFF

On this program, you won't start changing your eating habits or food choices just yet. Rather, start by taking stock of where you are and decide what you want to accomplish. To begin:

- Weigh yourself.
- Decide how much weight you want to lose.
- Choose a "weight-loss belt."
- Start a food diary.
- Assess portion sizes.
- Do ten minutes of toning exercises a day.

Here are the details.

Weigh in, and repeat daily. If you don't already have a reliable scale, buy one, says Dr. Stern. "We spend so much money on everything else; you should really treat yourself to a good scale," she says. "Say to yourself 'This is my present to me.' "

Dr. Stern suggests you weigh yourself around the same time daily, after voiding and in the nude. Don't be discouraged by fluctuations in your weight from day to day. This is why some plans tell you to weigh yourself only once a week. But Dr.

Stern's experience is that daily weighers stay more committed. "Make it a habit to step on the scale every day," says Dr. Stern. "People who weigh themselves regularly tend to be more successful at weight maintenance."

Decide how much you want to lose. To determine what weight is optimal for you based on your health profile, read chapter 44. Decide how many pounds you need to lose overall, but for now, concentrate on losing just ten.

"Losing the first ten pounds should take anywhere from a month to six weeks," says Dr. Stern, although she adds that the heavier you are at the outset, the faster the initial weight will come off.

Put on a snug belt. Measuring your waist and hips enables you to calculate your waist/hip ratio (WHR), one criterion of ideal weight. (See "How to Determine your Waist/Hip Ratio" on page 328.) If your WHR is 0.8 or higher, you need to shed some excess weight. And, says Dr. Stern, a good, snug belt can help you keep track of progress.

"This first week, take a belt that fits snugly," she says. "Make note of where it closes. Once a week, try on your belt so you can watch your waistline shrink as you move from one hole to the next," says Dr. Stern.

Record your weight weekly. To avoid becoming obsessed with your weight (or frustrated by minor daily weight fluctuations), record your weight once a week, on the same day at the same time, says Dr. Stern.

Keep a log. "Write down everything you eat," urges Dr. Stern. "For most people, seeing that information in black and white is amazing."

Discover true portion size. Overly generous food portions are as much responsible for weight gain as are too many fat grams and too little exercise, says Dr. Stern.

If you cook a lot, you may have a pretty good idea of what constitutes, say, one cup or eight fluid ounces. On the other hand, maybe you've been guessing wrong for years. To be certain, weigh and measure your food.

"Educate your eye," says Dr. Stern. "For low-fat, low-calorie foods, like greens, it doesn't matter if you're not all that precise. But for other foods, accuracy is critical. A three-ounce serving of cooked meat, fish or poultry, for example, should be about the size of a deck of cards."

Keep food out of sight. You've heard the old joke "I'm on the 'see-food diet'—I see food, so I eat it." It might seem obvious, but to avoid unconscious eating, get rid of those bags of candy in your desk drawer and those bags of chips or peanuts on the kitchen counter at home. "The idea is to make it harder to get to food," says Dr. Stern.

Exercise for at least ten minutes a day. That's *every day*, says Dr. Stern. "Most women are always ready to diet, but it's hard to get them to exercise." Yet the program *must* include exercise, she says, in order to preserve (or even increase) lean muscle mass, burn fat, keep your metabolism going, enable you to eat enough food to feel satisfied and help keep your weight off.

"Lean muscle mass is your body's metabolic engine," explains Dr. Stern. "It's the key to a slim, trim, calorie-burning physique."

Start your day with light exercise. If you're already exercising, keep it up, says Dr. Stern. "If not, start the day with some toning exercises for the abdominal area such as curls and leg raises as soon as you get out of bed," she says. Afterward, you can do toning exercises for your upper arms and waist.

"Toning exercises preserve and build muscle mass and lose fat," explains Dr. Stern. Since muscle is denser than fat, it takes up less room. So in time, you should see a difference in your body shape—you'll be slimmer, even if you weigh the same. "Depending on how many repetitions you do, toning exercises can also use energy and therefore promote weight loss," she adds. Do as many of the following exercises as you can comfortably perform in ten minutes.

To do curls: Lie flat in bed with your arms straight out at your sides, with the palms downward, and your knees together and slightly bent. Slowly curl your upper body forward, bringing your forehead close to your knees. Return to the starting position. Do ten repetitions.

To do leg raises: Lie on one side with your hips, legs and knees together and horizontal. Brace yourself with your arms so you remain on your side. Keeping your top leg straight and your toes pointed forward, raise your top leg, then lower it. Do not let the top foot touch the lower foot. Raise and lower your leg in one fluid motion; this is one leg raise. Do ten continuous repetitions without resting in between. Then turn over and do ten repetitions while lying on your other side.

Once you're out of bed, try chest stretches, arm curls and trunk rotations.

To do chest stretches: Stand and extend both arms to the sides at shoulder height, with your palms downward. Bend your elbows and bring your hands to your chest, keeping your palms down. Keeping your elbows bent, pull both arms back at the same time so you feel your shoulder blades squeezing together and your chest stretching. Do ten repetitions.

To do arm circles: Stand and extend both arms to the sides at shoulder height, with your palms downward. Make ten backward circles in the air. Keeping your arms extended at shoulder height, make ten forward circles.

To do trunk rotations: Stand and put your hands on your hips. Twist at your waist all the way to the right, then, in one continuous motion, twist back all the way to the left and return to the center. Do ten repetitions.

Take it easy. Aim for just ten repetitions of each exercise. "No matter how busy you are, most people can add ten minutes of exercise a day to their routine if it's done first thing in the morning," says Dr. Stern. Also, if it's been years since you've done any kind of exercise, it's a good idea to get a doctor's okay before you begin, she says. The same advice applies if you have diabetes or high blood pressure or take medication for a chronic condition.

WEEK TWO: THE FAST START

This week you will:

- Eat 1,000 calories a day.
- Set up your fat-gram and exercise-minutes accounts.
- Add ten minutes of walking a day.
- Drink three cups of skim milk a day.

"A lot of people want to start losing weight right away, and eating 1,000 calories a day will get them off to a fast start," explains Dr. Stern. As a general rule, weight-loss experts advise against routinely eating less than 1,200 calories a day. For the first week, this plan makes an exception—"to take advantage of your enthusiasm,'' says Dr. Stern. After two weeks, you'll be up to 1,200 calories a day, and you'll stick with that until you reach your weight goal, says Dr. Stern. This is for slow, steady weight loss; people who are extremely obese may require a faster, more restrictive plan, best followed under a doctor's supervision.

Limit calories from fat to between 20 and 25 percent of calories. At 1,000 calories per day, that means 26 fat grams per day—not very many at all. So you need to read food labels and pay attention to your daily total. Do that, and those pounds will soon be slip-sliding away, according to Dr. Stern.

"Every morning, imagine that you wake up with 26 fat grams in your 'bank account,' " says Dr. Stern. "You can consume those fat grams any way you want, but when they're spent, that's it! If you choose to blow most of your fat grams on a piece of chocolate cake for lunch, for example, you have to limit yourself to fat-free foods like steamed vegetables for the rest of the day. It's a good idea to try to 'bank' some fat grams for the end of the day. Whatever you do, don't borrow fat grams from the following day."

Invest in a fat-gram counter. Pocket-size fat-gram and calorie counters, often sold in bookstores, can help you calculate your fat intake. To give you an idea of various ways you can choose to "spend" your fat grams, consult the following list. *Each item on the list contains 26 fat grams*, an entire day's allotment.

- Six ounces of canned white tuna with two tablespoons of full-fat mayonnaise
- One cup of premium vanilla ice cream
- One cheese Danish pastry
- Two ounces of dry-roasted peanuts
- Two tablespoons of olive oil
- Three ounces of pork spareribs
- Three one-ounce homemade brownies with nuts
- Eight slices of bacon

At the other end of the spectrum, certain foods are so low in fat that you'd have to eat gargantuan amounts to even come close to spending your allotment. To get the same 26 grams of fat, you could have:

- 11 cups of egg noodles
- 44 pounds of iceberg lettuce
- 30 ounces of broiled halibut
- 43 cups of strawberries
- 65 cups of cooked spaghetti squash
- 52 cups of orange juice

No one eats that much, of course. The point is, you need to balance out high-fat foods—in reasonable portions—with those that contain very little or just a trace. In other words, says Dr. Stern, spread your 26 fat grams and 1,000 calories evenly throughout the day.

Start with breakfast. Think of your day's meal plan as a series of mini-meals and healthy snacks, beginning with breakfast. According to C. Wayne Callaway, M.D., an obesity specialist at George Washington University in Washington, D.C., people who skip breakfast burn about 5 percent fewer calories than people who eat three meals a day or more.

Dr. Stern says that a typical breakfast should consist of one cup of ready-to-eat, high-fiber cold cereal, such as raisin bran (a good source of fiber, and the raisins add texture and sweetness), eight ounces of skim milk (half as a beverage and half poured on the cereal; you can also use some in your coffee or tea) and coffee or tea, if desired.

Help yourself to a midmorning snack. Have half a banana—it's a great way to get your potassium, needed for regular heart rhythm.

Make lunch lean. Even on just 1,000 calories a day, you don't need to skip meals (nor should you). Make yourself half a sandwich with two ounces of turkey or chicken (skinless) on one slice of whole-grain bread (or a small whole-grain roll), layered with lettuce and tomato and spread with mustard or fat-free mayonnaise. On the side, have one cup of fresh strawberries (a terrific source of vitamin C).

Down it all with an eight-ounce glass of skim milk. Dr. Stern emphasizes that women need to drink three eight-ounce glasses of skim milk a day to get a plentiful supply of its bone-building calcium. "The first health crisis for women is weight; the second is osteoporosis," she says. Skim milk addresses both concerns, says Dr. Stern. "It has 300 milligrams of calcium per cup, vitamin D to help the body utilize the calcium, and zero grams of fat, plus some protein, phosphorus and magnesium, making it the perfect ready-to-drink health beverage,'' she says.

The colder, the better. To give skim milk extra taste appeal, drink it icy-cold, says Dr. Stern. Freeze skim milk in an ice cube tray and plunk a couple of cubes into your milk to make it even colder; it's especially delicious on a warm day.

Or get your skim-milk fix at a coffee bar. Order a large latte made with skim milk; about half of it will be milk, the other half coffee. (Order decaf, if you prefer.) You can also try a 50-50 split with a tea-and-milk combo.

Snack on some carotenoids. At just 1,000 calories a day, every food needs to contribute to your daily intake of vitamins or minerals. Otherwise you set yourself up for critical deficiencies. Today have some raw carrot sticks. They're a concentrated source of beta-carotene and similar substances, called carotenoids, that, when consumed regularly, protect your health. So you don't want to miss out.

Dine well. Plan your evening meal around three ounces of fish or very lean beef and generous amounts (one to two cups) of steamed vegetables, such as broccoli or brussels sprouts. Add a small green salad drizzled with fat-free salad dressing or balsamic vinegar, fresh fruit (such as a peach) and a zero-calorie beverage, such as mineral water or diet soda.

Make milk your nightcap. For a relaxing late-night beverage, add a couple of drops of almond extract to an eight-ounce mug of hot milk, says Dr. Stern. Bedtime is a good time to drink milk, because the body uses calcium for bone-building while you sleep, and the vitamin D helps your body utilize the calcium. Drink skim milk in a coffee mug or a colored or nonclear glass if the milk's color looks unappetizing.

Toast a slice of raisin bread. It goes great with milk. The raisins add sweetness, so you can eat it plain and not miss the butter, says Dr. Stern.

Tally your fat and calories. Total grams of fat for Day One is 13, and the approximate number of total calories is 985. Keep track of your daily fat-gram expenditures, says Dr. Stern. Daily fat-gram totals should average 26 for the following six days; daily calories should average 1,000.

In total, your diet should consist of six servings of bread, cereal, rice and pasta; three or more servings of vegetables;

two servings of fruit; three servings of skim milk, yogurt or other fat-free or low-fat dairy products, and two servings of lean meat, poultry, fish or cooked beans.

Continue to keep a food diary. Write down everything you eat and the fat-gram total for each food.

Walk briskly for ten minutes a day, at least five days a week. This is *in addition* to your 10 minutes of morning toning exercises, says Dr. Stern. In other words, you're now exercising for a total of 20 minutes a day—10 minutes of toning and 10 minutes of walking.

Brisk walking is aerobic—that is, it uses the large muscle groups of your legs, buttocks and back, burning calories in the process, explains Dr. Stern. "Walking also preserves lean muscle mass and, if done briskly, improves cardiovascular fitness."

Swing your arms. To maximize the number of calories you burn as you walk, swing your arms as you go, urges Dr. Stern. For now, don't worry about how fast you can walk. Just do it as many days a week as you can manage, wherever it's convenient for you to walk.

Try hand weights. "You'll burn even more calories and tone your muscles further if you use hand weights when you walk," says Dr. Stern. The added weight provides resistance, making your muscles work harder and grow larger. Muscle burns more calories than fat, plus you burn more calories walking with light weights than walking without them, says Dr. Stern. For the beginner, two-pound weights may be too heavy, and you could drop the dumbbells as you walk. She recommends Heavyhands—light weights with handles for a secure grip—instead.

Try ankle weights for your morning leg raises. To turn your morning toning exercises into resistance training exercises, climb out of bed and strap a one-pound ankle weight to each leg, then do your usual repetitions. These are best done on carpeting or another firm but padded surface.

Tally your "exercise account." As with your fat-gram account, you will now be setting up your exercise-minutes account. At the start of every day, you've got 20 minutes to play with. Be sure to "spend" them all each day, divided between aerobic work (like walking) and toning or resistance exercises.

A SAFE WAY TO DROP FIVE POUNDS FAST—
And Keep Them Off

A fair number of women who responded to our *Food and You* survey were generally happy with their weight. Occasionally, a few said they wished they could drop five pounds fast—in time for summer or their high school reunion, for example.

It *can* be done—and in as little as two weeks, says Judith S. Stern, R.D., Sc.D., professor of nutrition and internal medicine at the University of California, Davis. Best of all, you needn't shortchange yourself nutritionally in the process.

"By cutting back on food in general and fat in particular, you can follow a healthy, 1,000-calorie-a-day diet and lose five pounds in two weeks," says Dr. Stern. At least a couple of those pounds will be water, she notes. "When you complete this program, it's important not to go back to your original eating habits; otherwise, you'll regain the weight you lost."

Here's what a quick-weight-loss menu looks like, says Dr. Stern.

BREAKFAST

½ cup ready-to-eat cereal
8 ounces skim milk (part on cereal, part to drink)

LUNCH

6¼ ounces water-packed tuna with fat-free
   mayonnaise, greens or tomato slices and sprouts
2 slices melba toast or a small whole-grain roll
1 piece fresh fruit
8 ounces skim milk

SNACK

Carrot sticks or other raw veggies

DINNER

Green salad with fat-free dressing

3 ounces poached, broiled or baked skinless chicken or a 200-calorie frozen entrée

1 piece fresh fruit

8 ounces skim milk

To help ensure success, Dr. Stern adds the following advice.

Don't skip meals. Whatever you do, "don't eat fewer than 800 calories a day," says Dr. Stern. "Very low calorie diets pose significant health risks, such as heartbeat irregularities and mineral imbalances, which can be life-threatening."

Take a multivitamin/mineral supplement. For the duration of your two-week weight-loss blitz, Dr. Stern also recommends a daily vitamin/mineral supplement. "You won't get all the nutrients you need eating 1,000 calories a day. Even at 1,200 calories a day, it's hard," says Dr. Stern. But the supplement will help bridge the gap. (For details on selecting a supplement, see chapter 43.)

Exercise. Speedy weight loss is virtually impossible without moving that body. "What's more, exercise helps preserve lean body mass, so you lose fat, not muscle," says Dr. Stern. Plan on a regular workout these next two weeks—and then some, she says.

"Aim for 30 minutes a day of walking, starting with 15 minutes a day if necessary, and work your way up. Gradually work on increasing your speed or intensity (or both). You can swing your arms or carry weights as you walk," advises Dr. Stern.

If you don't have the time for a full half-hour session each day, you can split it into two 15-minute walks and get the same benefit.

Before you proceed, think twice. This weight-loss program is not for pregnant women, who should not be trying to lose weight at this time, says Dr. Stern. Also, if you have a chronic condition, such as diabetes, heart disease or high blood pressure, you should check with your doctor before beginning any weight-loss plan.

WEEK THREE: MORE FOOD, MORE EXERCISE

With the plan in full swing, you'll now move up a notch. On the third week of the plan, you'll find out how to:

- Eat 1,200 calories a day.
- Change "automatic" eating habits.
- Exercise for a total of 30 minutes a day (including 20 minutes or more of brisk walking or other form of aerobic exercise).

Add 200 calories a day to your basic diet. "Adding a little more food feels good, and it makes good nutritional sense because it gives your meals more variety," notes Dr. Stern. How to "spend" your additional calories? Not on a pint of premium ice cream. "Add more grain—an extra slice of whole-grain bread, a serving of brown rice or couscous at dinnertime, and certainly some extra vegetables and fruit," she says.

Shoot for 30 fat grams a day. From here on in, consider 30 fat grams a day your magic number. Or, Dr. Stern says, have 20 to 25 percent of calories from fat per day.

Eat slowly. "If you are a fast eater, you'll eat less if you slow down," says Dr. Stern. "Time yourself. If breakfast takes less than five minutes to eat and lunch takes less than ten, you're eating too fast. Consciously try to extend each meal by a few minutes. Midway through the meal, for example, stop eating for two minutes. If you're with other people, pause to talk."

Chew. Swallow. Repeat. Make sure you never have food in your mouth and food on your fork at the same time, says Dr. Stern. And don't start to cut your food while you're still chewing. Over the course of this plan, eating slowly will become a habit.

Consider some indoor exercise equipment. "If you can manage the expense," says Dr. Stern, "you might want to invest in a treadmill. If you use a headset, you can walk on the treadmill and talk on the phone at the same time." Or consider a stationary bike "with a comfortable seat—you may have to buy your own from a bicycle store," says Dr. Stern. The exercise variety keeps you from getting bored, she says.

Increase your exercise to 30 minutes a day. This week, boost your daily 20 exercise-minutes account by 10. Again, use your minutes during the day as you see fit—a brisk 30-minute walk after dinner, for instance, or a 20-minute walk coupled with 10 minutes of resistance training. Aim for as close to a seven-day-a-week schedule as possible.

Check your target heart rate. To derive the maximum heart fitness from your workout, says Dr. Stern, you need to work within your target heart rate—about 60 percent of your maximum heart rate—for at least 20 minutes.

First determine your heart rate at rest. Before you begin to exercise, take your pulse at your neck or wrist, using your middle finger. Count for 10 seconds and then multiply by six, or count for 30 seconds and just double the figure, says Dr. Stern. The average person has a resting heart rate of about 70 to 80 beats a minute. Typically, the fitter you are, the lower your resting heart rate, says Dr. Stern.

To determine your maximum heart rate, subtract your age from 220. (Are you 45? Then your maximum heart rate is 175.) After five or ten minutes of exercising, take your pulse again to see how close you've come to your target heart rate. Your goal is to work hard enough to raise your heart rate from its resting rate to approximately 60 percent of the maximum, but no higher. To determine the 60 percent, multiply your maximum heart rate by 0.6. (If you're 45, your target is 105 beats per minute.) If your heart rate is higher, slow down. If it's lower, pick up the pace.

The exact calorie-burning potential of your workouts depends on individual factors, such as previous activity level, degree of overweight and general cardiovascular condition. Generally, though, you don't necessarily have to work harder to burn more calories, says Morris B. Mellion, M.D., medical director of the Sports Medicine Center in Omaha, Nebraska. The key is duration and frequency.

Twenty minutes is not long enough to enhance your calorie-burning capacity, says Joanne Curran-Celentano, R.D., Ph.D., associate professor of nutrition and food sciences at the University of New Hampshire in Durham. You need to increase your exercise time to between 30 and 45 minutes, with 45 minutes being optimal, to gain both cardiovascular protection and calorie-burning capacity.

Don't overdo it. Pay attention to how you're feeling, and don't overexert yourself, says Dr. Stern, "If you feel pain or shortness of breath as you exercise, stop." You should be able to carry on a conversation comfortably.

Balance your account. Keep jotting down what you "withdraw" from your daily fat-gram account and what you deposit into your exercise minutes account.

WEEK FOUR: PUMP UP YOUR CALORIE-BURNING WORKOUTS

This week focuses on ways to burn more calories and speed up your weight loss. You will:

- Consider buying a pedometer.
- Add stair-climbing to your exercise routine.

Buy a pedometer. To keep track of the distance you're covering in your daily walks, Dr. Stern strongly suggests you buy a pedometer (under $20 in many sporting goods stores). "Overweight women, who are usually sedentary, average about two miles per day as part of their daily activity. But you should be aiming for at least four miles a day."

If you go on vacation, pack your pedometer along with your walking shoes. Holidays often mean added indulgence, so try to increase your walking to offset the extra food, says Dr. Stern. If you're at the beach or in the country, you'll have lots of opportunities for outdoor walking. But even if it's a city vacation, you can cover plenty of ground visiting museums and other sites of interest.

Walk up a flight of stairs. Climbing about 15 to 20 stairs counts as part of your 30 minutes a day. (If you have hip, joint or cardiac problems, Dr. Stern advises that you check with your doctor before walking up more than a flight of stairs.)

Figure out what time of day is best for you to exercise, and stick to it. According to one study overseen by Dr. Stern, many women who regain their weight practice what she calls "escape/avoidance." They say, "I'll do it later," but later never comes, says Dr. Stern. The study, which involved over 100 women, showed that women who succeed in keeping their weight off deal with their problems directly instead of pro-crastinating.

Be creative in sneaking in your daily exercise. "Did you know that, during a typical half-hour TV show, there are be-tween eight and ten minutes of commercials? Use that time," says Dr. Stern. "When a commercial comes on, get up off the couch and walk around the house. Every time you do that, you get in an extra few minutes of exercise. You notice I'm not telling women to stop watching TV; just make the most if it. The idea is to build good habits. The hope is that, when ex-ercise opportunities—like taking stairs—present themselves, you'll automatically take advantage of them."

Do a midday fat-gram and exercise check. Dr. Stern says that you should check yourself midway through the day to be sure you're pretty close to using up your exercise minutes *and* that you've "banked" enough fat grams to see you through dinnertime. "Remember," she says, "by the end of the day you want fat grams left over, but you *don't* want exercise minutes left over."

Record your weight at the end of the week. Also slip on your weight-loss belt to see how much you've lost from your waistline.

WEEK FIVE: SPICE UP YOUR MENUS

This week, the focus reverts to food. You will learn ways to:

- Vary your meals.
- Cut back on meat (and eliminate it at least once a week).

At this point, it's important that you build variety into your menus. Otherwise you'll get bored and yield to the siren call of the nearest bakery.

Rethink breakfast. If the cereal-and-milk routine is getting tiresome, try a fruity, frosty shake instead, says Dr. Stern. The night before, slice half a banana and freeze it. In the morning, toss the sliced banana into a blender with about a half-cup of sliced strawberries, a cup of skim milk and, if you like, some artificial sweetener. (A blender will make a smoother shake than a food processor.) A drop or two of lemon or a sprinkle

SLIMMING STRATEGIES AT 40-PLUS

You're digging through the back of your closet, searching for the circa 1972 fringed leather miniskirt that's inexplicably back in vogue. Then it suddenly dawns on you: There's no way the thing will still fit. You've gone up four dress sizes since you wore it in high school.

Sound familiar? If so, you're not alone. Most of us are carrying a few extra inches by the time we turn 40, and we're having a tough time taking them off.

"The decade of the greatest weight gain for women *and* men is between ages 30 and 40," says James M. Rippe, M.D., director of the Center for Clinical and Lifestyle Research, affiliated with Tufts University School of Medicine in Boston.

Where do the pounds come from? Inactivity, for starters. Sure, we're *busier* than ever. By age 40, we may still have kids at home and more obligations at work. But there's less time for physical activity, says Michael Hamilton, M.D., director of the Diet and Fitness Center at Duke University in Durham, North Carolina. We exercise less and burn off fewer calories. Yet most of us continue to eat the way we did at 20, so we gain weight, says Dr. Hamilton.

You might get away with slacking off exercise in your twenties—for a while. But as you approach 40, says Dr. Hamilton, inactivity starts to take a toll on muscle mass. Underutilized, our muscles start to shrink. Since muscle is the most metabolically active tissue in our bodies, our metabolic rates take a nosedive, making it even easier to pack on pounds and even more difficult to unload them, he says.

Then, as women approach menopause, hormonal changes magnify the problem. Not only do our ovaries start producing less estrogen, they cut back on production of testosterone, too. This not-for-men-only hormone is partly responsible for maintaining muscle tone, explains Donald Robertson, M.D., medical director of the Southwest Bariatric Nutrition Center in Scottsdale, Arizona. So fat takes over.

INSIDE TIPS FOR MIDLIFE DIETERS

Take heart, ladies: There's hope for that fringed miniskirt yet. Research suggests we can minimize muscle loss and metabolic slowing—and vanquish after-40 weight gain—by eating a low-fat diet and exercising, says Dr. Hamilton.

The benefits are more than cosmetic. Data from the Harvard University Nurses' Health Study (an ongoing study of 115,000 women considered a landmark source of evidence regarding women's health) indicates that even modest weight gains—an accumulation of just 20 pounds between heading off to college and packing our children off to college 20 years later—can double a woman's risk of heart attack. Other research suggests weight gain after 30 increases a woman's risk of developing breast cancer.

Here's some expert advice on lowering your health risks by dropping that extra weight and keeping it off.

Shoot for 20 percent of calories from fat. If you don't have a weight problem, eating a diet that gets no more than 30 percent of calories from fat—as recommended by the American Heart Association and other medical authorities—may be low enough to maintain your weight. But at 40, you may need to cut the fat further, says Dr. Robertson.

At 40, your metabolism inevitably slows to some degree, so you'll probably need fewer calories even if you stay active, says Dr. Hamilton. Cutting fat is the best way to cut calories without feeling hungry or deprived.

Red-flag red meat. After menopause, you don't need as much iron in your diet. So substitute a low-fat protein source like beans or tofu for steak, chops and burgers—you save on fat *and* calories, Dr. Hamilton says.

Sidestep "invisible" fat. A fair amount of fat is hidden in foods like yogurt, nuts and eggs. Check the labels on foods you eat frequently. You may be surprised by what you find, says Dr. Robertson.

Watch portions. If you eat king-size bags of low-fat chips and cookies, bowl after bowl of fat-free frozen yogurt and several slabs of fat-free coffee cake, you'll still gain weight, says Dr. Rippe. Foods that don't contain fat still contain calories. If you want to lose weight, pay attention to serving sizes, says Dr. Rippe.

Exercise every day. To fight fat, says Dr. Hamilton, enlist the dynamic duo—aerobic exercise (like brisk walking) and weight training (like lifting dumbbells and using ankle weights). You burn more calories during an aerobic work-out than during a weight-training session. But resistance training builds more muscle than aerobic exercise does, and muscle burns calories faster than any other kind of tissue—all day long.

"A reasonable approach is to do some aerobic training every day and some weight training every other day," Dr. Hamilton says. To hold the line on midlife weight gain, he recommends 20- to 40-minute sessions of aerobic exercise and 10- to 20-minute sessions of weight training. (An easy, at-home resistance regimen is included in this chapter.)

---

of cinnamon gives the shake an extra flavor kick. If you forget to freeze the banana, you can still blend it, but add an ice cube to the blender. If you use peaches instead of strawberries, you may want to add a pinch of cinnamon. "This works well with just about any fruit in season, except oranges," says Dr. Stern.

As yet another alternative, oatmeal makes a healthy, hearty breakfast, says Dr. Stern. If time is short, use the quick-cooking kind that you can microwave. Dr. Stern prepares hers from scratch, with a half-cup of skim milk, then pours another half-cup onto the cooked cereal. You can cook a few raisins with it also. "On cold mornings, it's very satisfying," she says.

At midday, soup is super. A study done by Harry Kissileff, Ph.D., at the St. Luke's-Roosevelt Hospital Obesity Research Center in New York City, showed that when people have soup for lunch, they eat less at that meal and feel more satisfied. "Eating soup gives your body a chance to say 'I'm full,'" says Dr. Stern.

Homemade soup is ideal, but canned soup is fine, provided you check the label to make sure fat-gram counts are low, says Dr. Stern. Prepared soups are often packed with sodium but, says Dr. Stern, "unless you have high blood pressure and are also salt-sensitive—most people are not—there's no need to be overly concerned. In fact, when you're on a calorie-restricted diet, you need electrolyte minerals like sodium."

Serve meat with plenty of vegetables and grain foods.
Dr. Stern's favorite accompaniments for flank steak include
steamed snow peas with minced ginger and garlic and a small
serving of rice, plus a large green salad with parsley. Think
of vegetables as the entrée and meat as the accompaniment.

Add beans for variety without the fat. Dr. Stern urges
you to make sure to have at least one vegetarian dinner a week,
and certainly more if you like. "Concentrate on high-quality
protein such as beans (especially bean-and-rice combinations,
such as chili and rice), low-fat tofu and fat-free cheeses. And
cheese pizza, for example, is a wonderful vegetarian meal
when made with part-skim mozzarella and whole-grain pita or
whole-grain dough."

Weigh in—again. Don't forget to exercise faithfully and
weigh in at the end of the week.

WEEK SIX: TIPS FOR MAINTENANCE

This week you'll be:

- Making sure you're still on track.
- Giving yourself a weight-loss reward.
- Deciding whether to maintain your weight or keep going.

If all has gone according to plan, by now you should have
lost about ten pounds, says Dr. Stern. Here's what to do next.

Reward yourself. If you've reached your first goal, a gift
is definitely in order, says Dr. Stern, "But try not to celebrate
with food," she says. Instead, she says, "buy something nice
for yourself—a blouse, jewelry, even an offbeat pair of socks.
You don't have to get something expensive. Anything that
makes you feel good will work."

**If you've reached a plateau, exercise for a few extra
minutes a day.** Sometimes you hit a weight-loss plateau because your body is stabilizing at its new weight, which may
be a signal to increase your exercise, says Dr. Stern.

Eat more food. If you decide you're happy with what
you've lost so far, focus on maintaining your new weight.
"Slowly add food back to your diet, concentrating on grains,
vegetables and fruits," says Dr. Stern. Each week add 100 to

200 extra calories a day, until your daily total reaches about 1,800 calories (including 45 fat grams). Your target should always be between 20 and 25 percent of calories from fat. If you target 25 percent, you will likely keep your fat total under 30 percent. Food is not precise, adds Dr. Stern.

Weigh yourself. If you neither gain nor lose weight, stick to 1,800 calories a day, says Dr. Stern.

Continue to exercise. A study done at Rockefeller University in New York City found that, after you lose weight, your metabolism slows and you need fewer calories to maintain that lower weight. The study, published in the *New England Journal of Medicine*, involved 18 obese women and men and 23 who had never been overweight. They were examined at their usual body weight and after certain weight changes—either a 10 to 20 percent reduction or a 10 percent increase. The researchers found that metabolism slows in proportion to the amount of weight lost and increases in proportion to the amount of weight gained, making it difficult for most people to maintain a weight loss.

What this means, says Dr. Stern, is that if you want to maintain your weight after you've lost, exercise isn't optional—it's mandatory.

"You're going to have to counteract your metabolism's tendency to slow down after weight loss," says Dr. Stern. How? "Exercise!" Otherwise, the six weeks you've invested will be for nothing—you'll regain the weight.

THE NEXT 10, 20 OR 50 POUNDS

If you decide to drop additional pounds, cut back to 1,200 calories a day and exercise for 30 minutes or more per day—in essence, repeating the core elements of Week Three of the program. Continue to weigh in weekly and to limit your intake of fat to 30 grams a day. You can expect to lose about two pounds a week. Dr. Stern adds that when you repeat the core elements of Week Three of the program, you need to maintain the 30 minutes a day·of exercise or even up it to 40 minutes a day. She says it takes from six to eight weeks before you begin to "love" to exercise. To maintain interest and motivation, Dr. Stern offers the following advice.

Get acquainted with more low-fat foods. Experiment with new low-fat or fat-free foods and recipes, says Dr. Stern. Above all, "continue to be a fat-gram mathematician," she says.

Try new forms of exercise, like swimming or cycling. The more varied your activities, the less likely you are to get bored and give up.

Recruit a friend. The support of a close friend, significant other or family member can play a key role in keeping you motivated over the long haul, says Dr. Stern. The two of you can swap low-fat recipes, exercise together or simply call each other as needed (such as when you need someone to steer you away from that late-night snack).

Think in ten-pound increments. "If you have a lot more weight to lose, continue to do it in ten-pound increments," says Dr. Stern. "Breaking your long-range goal into mini-goals prevents you from getting overwhelmed." Small losses, if maintained, improve your health. If you weigh 160 pounds and want to lose 16 pounds, lose the first 10 as a mini-goal and then lose the next 6, she adds.

PART 5

FOOD AND YOUR
MEALTIME STRATEGY

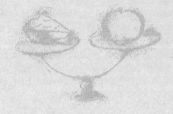

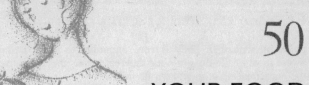

50

YOUR FOOD PERSONALITY

**Passions and preferences
that shape your eating habits**

Are you outgoing? Shy? Flamboyant? Reserved? Believe it or not, your personality may be a big factor in how you approach mealtime.

And no matter what kind of personality you have, you might even have a separate *food* personality. Your eating routine, your favorite foods, your beliefs about what constitutes good nutrition and other factors all help to mold your food personality.

Take 36-year-old Sue R., for instance. In response to our *Food and You* survey, she told us that Monday through Friday, she eats a varied, low-fat diet, even during frequent business lunches with clients. Come the weekend, she splurges on her favorite ice cream with whipped cream "not just once, but sometimes twice." Sue plays racquetball regularly, is in good health and in 15 years, she's barely deviated from her usual 130 pounds (a good weight for her height). "During the week I have fairly strict food guidelines, and if I stick to them, I do what I like—within reason—on weekends."

According to Susan Olson, Ph.D., a clinical psychologist and consultant to the Southwest Bariatric Nutrition Center in Scottsdale, Arizona, "Sue is what I call a Fitness Fan. These women are conscious of exercise, nutrition and health—what's

413

going on with their body is very important to them. Being aware most of the time of what they eat means they can have the occasional splurge without harm."

Another respondent to our survey, Lisa McG., is what Dr. Olsen calls a Human Do-er. At home, Lisa loves to cook. Whenever possible, "I eat very healthfully," she says. "Very little red meat, lots of vegetables, everything low-fat." But her job is pressure-packed. Nine-to-five, she lives on coffee and salad-bar fare—which, she says (alluding to the fried and oil-soaked items frequently found in today's salad bars), "doesn't necessarily mean healthy food." Plus, she also enjoys dining out. Lisa says she's pretty satisfied with her present weight, but adds, "If I had more time, I'd eat better."

"Women like Lisa are the Type-A people—always on the run, always juggling many things at once," says Dr. Olson. "It's vital that they tune into their surroundings; otherwise, they might just head for the vending machine because it's *there*. But they can do well with their eating if they understand nutrition and make smart choices."

THE FOOD PERSONALITY QUIZ

Office workers aren't the only women struggling with a schizophrenic eating style. From dog groomers to restaurant managers, women's passions, preferences and personal health goals impact on their food personality. Sue and Lisa exemplify two of seven food personalities identified by Dr. Olson, who works closely with health organizations and fitness clubs. Your food personality will determine how successfully you maintain a reasonable body weight, how energetic you feel when you wake up in the morning and even how often you catch cold. So any sound nutritional plan needs to start with a reality check about your style of eating as well as what you eat.

Enter the Food Personality Quiz that follows. This quiz is unlike generic diet questionnaires that you're apt to encounter elsewhere. Based on client interviews conducted by Dr. Olson, this quiz goes beyond the standard questions about age, weight and medical history. There are no right or wrong answers; it's a guideline to reveal clues about your personal style.

"Having a client fill out a questionnaire helps me know where she is, where she's been and where she wants to go in terms of her health and weight," explains nutritionist Judy E. Marshel, R.D., director of Health Resources in Great Neck, New York, and former senior nutritionist for Weight Watchers International. "But in addition to asking about her typical food intake, I look at her weight history and her previous diets, her food preferences, her overall health, her lifestyle habits, any medications she may be taking and her family's health and weight history. All of this information will help us put together a plan of action."

Savvy nutritionists have discovered that handing out a generic "diet sheet" doesn't work; customized plans do.

"It's hard to overhaul somebody's eating habits if what you're asking her to do doesn't fit into her lifestyle," adds Mindy Hermann, R.D., a nutrition counselor in Mount Kisco, New York. "By asking questions, you know what she's already doing and where changes can be made to keep her in some kind of regular routine."

Once you've filled out the quiz, use your responses to shape a smart mealtime strategy for life, based on your food personality and health goals.

Part I
Your Food Personality

Given my normal eating patterns, I would describe myself as a:

☐ **1. Feeler:** I often eat in response to my emotions, both positive and negative. Turning to food when I feel happy, depressed, bored or angry is a very comfortable and common reaction.

☐ **2. Human Doer:** I eat on the go, and I often eat before I think. Frequently I eat without thinking, and when I'm asked to follow a strict eating routine, I usually have difficulty following through.

☐ **3. Thinker:** I'm highly critical of myself, and I can be compulsive in my behavior. I tend to think in all-or-nothing terms, so if I believe I've made an eating mistake, it will often turn into an all out binge.

☐ **4. Food Hedonist:** For me, food is very sensual. I love the look, the smell and especially the taste of food. I enjoy reading food magazines and trying recipes the way some people get into music or art.

☐ **5. Dreamer:** I want to reach my ideal weight or eat the perfect diet for me. But I get easily discouraged and tend to fall back into counterproductive eating habits.

☐ **6. "People" Person:** Friends and family mean the world to me. I love nothing better than to go to a party or have lunch with a friend at a nice restaurant. But I'm always afraid I'll lose control of sensible eating in social situations.

☐ **7. Fitness Fan:** My body and my health are very important to me—I'll do anything I can to learn how to feel and look better. You'll never catch me looking for an excuse to not exercise or eat right. Sometimes I can be too compulsive about eating and/or exercising.

Dr. Olson offers tips for each of her seven food types.

Feelers need to recognize and express their feelings in healthy ways such as screaming, hitting a pillow, listening to a sad country song or calling a friend. They should try to control and defat their environment as much as possible.

Human Doers must make sure their eating style fits into their lifestyle. Grazing is okay, as long as it's healthy. They should learn the healthy choices—and stop feeling guilty if they don't eat the way others do. The simpler the better: Simplicity works well for these folks. They should generally cut fat and keep simple foods—such as bagels, cut-up carrots and fruit—available for snacks. Chapters 2 and 53 may be helpful.

Thinkers have to be gentler on themselves and keep their life balanced. They should be sure to plan fun things so they don't get too obsessive about eating or anything else. Some suggestions include taking 10 to 20 minutes over lunch for a meditation tape or a walk or buying a coloring book and coloring outside the lines.

Food Hedonists can help themselves to rechannel their passion for food into other areas, whether it's reading, crafts, music—even relationships. They should find lots of hugs or get massages or hug a teddy bear. If they love to cook, they can get creative with low-fat recipes. Chapter 52 will be of specific interest to those with this food personality.

Dreamers need to find a positive image of themselves, their own uniqueness and positive attributes. They should specifically picture whatever makes them feel good—wearing an attractive dress or managing a diet-related health problem—and mentally focus on their goals. Chapter 6 will help.

"People" People are most successful when focusing on the human connection; the food is secondary. Avoiding interactions until they are at their weight goal won't work for these people. And they need to learn nutrition so they can select healthy food while in social situations. Chapters 7, 53 and 56 will be of special interest for this food personality.

Fitness Fans are at an advantage—they exercise to burn calories and to relieve tension, and they probably wouldn't deliberately eat something that would harm their health. The trick is not to become overly obsessive about calories, exercise or avoiding other parts of their life, as pointed out in chapter 9.

Dr. Olson points out that you might be a combination of two or more food types. Above all, she urges women to use this self-analysis "to help you recognize certain tendencies without being judgmental or striving for perfection. There are many ways to accomplish the same goal."

The quizzes in Part II and Part III are based on actual client questionnaires compiled by nutritionists Marshel and Hermann and Angela Miraglio, R.D., who heads AMM Nutrition Services in Chicago.

PART II
Medical, Weight and Lifestyle Factors

---

1. My weight:_____   Today's date:_____

2. One or more of my immediate family members had/has the following health problems (check all that apply):

   ☐ Obesity   ☐ High blood pressure
   ☐ Heart disease   ☐ Stroke
   ☐ Diabetes   ☐ Cancer
   ☐ Other (specify)_____

3. I am on a special diet (check all that apply):

   ☐ Salt-restricted   ☐ Diabetic
   ☐ Lactose-free   ☐ Weight-loss
   ☐ Low-fat/low-cholesterol ☐ Vegetarian
   ☐ Macrobiotic   ☐ Other; specify:
                              _____

4. The nutritional supplements (vitamins, etc.) I take on a regular basis are

   _____

5. I smoke cigarettes: ☐ Yes   ☐ No

6. I exercise approximately _____ minutes/hours a week

7. My goal(s) now is/are to (check all that apply):

   ☐ Lose weight (_____ pounds)
   ☐ Gain weight (_____ pounds)
   ☐ Maintain weight (_____ pounds)
   ☐ Lower my cholesterol
   ☐ Lower my blood pressure
   ☐ Control my diabetes
   ☐ Cure my anemia

☐ Relieve my constipation/hemorrhoids/irritable bowel
syndrome
☐ Minimize allergic reactions
☐ Eliminte my migraines/headaches
☐ Control my hypoglycemia
☐ Protect against osteoporosis
☐ Improve the look/condition of my skin
☐ Ease tooth and gum problems
☐ Relieve bloating/water retention
☐ Minimize yeast and/or urinary tract infections
☐ Feel more energetic

8. I am allergic to (or have trouble digesting or tolerating)
the following foods:_____

PART III
The Way You Eat

---

1. I usually eat my meals/snacks in the following locations
(examples: at home, school/work cafeteria, at your desk, in
your car, at a fast-food place, and so forth). Fill in:
Breakfast_____ Lunch_____
Dinner_____ Daytime snack_____
Nighttime snack_____

2. I usually eat my meals/snacks with the following individ-
uals (examples: co-workers, spouse, family, others). Fill in:
Breakfast_____ Lunch_____
Dinner_____ Daytime snack_____
Nighttime snack_____

3. When eating either meals or snacks, I usually do the fol-
lowing (examples: watch TV, read, talk on the phone,
other). Fill in:
Breakfast_____ Lunch_____
Dinner_____ Daytime snack_____
Nighttime snack_____

4. I generally eat meals and snacks for the following reasons: (examples: hunger, food looks/smells good, boredom, other). Fill in:

Breakfast_____   Lunch_____

Dinner_____   Daytime snack_____

Nighttime snack_____

5. I normally eat (how many?) meals a day_____

6. I normally skip (how many?) meals a day_____

7. I normally eat (how many?) snacks a day_____

8. Each week, I use (how many times?):

_____ Alcoholic beverages   _____ Caffeinated coffee, tea or soft drinks

_____ Artificial sweeteners   _____ Diet sodas

9. I usually drink six to eight glasses of water each day:
   ☐ Yes   ☐ No

10. Most of the food shopping is done by:
    ☐ Myself   ☐ Other(s)

11. At my house, most of the cooking is done by:
    ☐ Myself   ☐ Other(s)

12. Each week, I eat (how many times?):
    _____ At a fast-food restaurant
    _____ At other restaurants
    _____ Take-out food from a deli, pizzeria, salad bar or others
    _____ Convenience foods (frozen meals)
    _____ Other (specify):_____

13. I generally prefer preplanned meals and menus (as opposed to spur-of-the-moment meals): ☐ Yes   ☐ No

14. I often overeat to the point of feeling stuffed:
    □ Yes   □ No

15. Whenever I eat anything, I'm very conscious of how it may or may not affect my weight: □ Yes   □ No

16. When I eat spur-of-the-moment meals or snacks, it's usually for some emotional reason (depression, loneliness, anger, sadness, other): □ Yes   □ No

17. I have specific food cravings, and they often lead to my overeating/bingeing on those foods: □ Yes   □ No

18. I usually crave (check all that apply):

    □ Sweets   □ Cheese
    □ Meat   □ Breads and/or other
                          starches
    □ Fatty foods   □ Salty foods
    □ Crunchy foods   □ Other; specify:
                        _____

19. The worse thing about my eating habits is
    _____

20. The best thing about my eating habits is
    _____

Part IV
Your Typical Meals

For three full days out of a week, write down whatever you eat and drink. Include everything from sit-down dinners to those hit-and-run encounters with food while preparing the kids' lunch, for instance, or while driving home from work. Carefully note how much you consume and the time of day you tend to eat. Also make sure to include a weekend day, when food patterns and quantities are often quite different from your Monday-through-Friday routine.

WHAT YOUR ANSWERS REVEAL

Now take some time to review your responses. No doubt much of this information will be very familiar to you. But it's likely that some of it will come as an eye-opener. Do you really eat that much high-sodium snack food on an average day? Could that be why your "low-sodium diet" doesn't seem to be helping to control your blood pressure? Are you relying on take-out food more than you thought you were? Could it be that you eat nearly twice as much when you read a book at lunchtime as when you get together with friends?

While recording the data above may have jolted you, that's precisely why this quiz works, say nutritionists who lent their expertise to its design.

"In order to make intelligent changes in your meals, you've got to first be *aware* of what you're doing now," says Miraglio. "Some women for example, sample the whole time they're preparing a meal. Then they say 'I never eat dinner.' That's because they've eaten beforehand!" It avoids confusion—and, adds Marshel, denial. "People don't always readily see the connection between what they're eating and their health or their weight," she says. "I have clients who tell me 'I can't understand why I'm overweight! I don't eat between meals.' But in truth, their portion sizes may be much larger than normal, or they consume much more fat than they realize."

So review part III carefully. What are your patterns, passions and preferences? Too much high-calorie nibbling in front of the TV, leading to that bulging middle? Too much high-fat fast food, causing fat-packed arteries? Too little fiber, resulting in constipation?

Perhaps smart dining at home is a cinch for you but eating in restaurants or when traveling is a lot trickier. Or maybe it's a case where someone else in the family does most of the cooking, and you're not *quite* sure what's in that casserole dish.

Use this quiz to become your own mealtime detective, and

make adjustments accordingly. (Be sure to read the chapters devoted to your particular health concerns, as well as the strategies that follow in this section.)

One last word of advice: Just as with psychological personalities, food personalities don't change overnight. "Don't plan on making sweeping changes all at once," says Miraglio. "Everyone wants a magic bullet, but you should start with what you're already doing and go slowly. Small steps are always more effective and long-lasting."

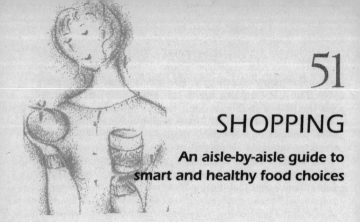

51

SHOPPING

An aisle-by-aisle guide to smart and healthy food choices

Want to stay slim, get your fill of all the vital nutrients your body needs, protect yourself against disease, *and* delight your taste buds—all on a busy schedule? Sounds like a tall order. But you can do it.

Like clothes shopping, grocery shopping can be either satisfying or bewildering. By following a few key guidelines, you can turn every visit to the supermarket into an opportunity to load your basket with the foods women need most.

"Smart supermarket shopping strategies are the key to eating well at home," says Bonnie Tandy Leblang, R.D., author of the nationally syndicated column "Supermarket Sampler" and six cookbooks, including *Grains, Rice and Beans*. "To eat healthy, you need to buy healthy."

DRAWING YOUR NUTRITIONAL TREASURE MAP

The average supermarket sells thousands of items, from fruit to Froot Loops, eggnog to eggplant and fig bars to DoveBars. "Some foods are good for you, some aren't, and some are in between," says David Schardt, associate nutritionist at the Center for Science in the Public Interest in Washington, D.C., and author of *Eating Leaner and Lighter*. And the right choices aren't always obvious. "The key is knowing what to buy and what to pass up."

Nutrition counselors we talked to shared the following practical strategies for filling a shopping cart with the absolute best in each major food category.

Study the layout. The better you know the territory, the faster you can make the right choices, says Densie Webb, R.D., Ph.D., editor of the *Environmental Nutrition* newsletter and author of *The Complete Brand-Name Guide to Choosing the Lowest Fat, Calorie, Cholesterol and Sodium Foods.* "If you don't know your way around the supermarket very well, you'll have a hard time making healthy choices," says Dr. Webb. "Today's megasupermarkets have everything; the choices are tremendous. If you familiarize yourself with what's available, you'll have more options."

One woman who really knows her supermarket is Carol S., who responded to our *Food and You* survey.

"I always shop at the same store week after week," Carol told us. "I don't jump around from store to store, even when another one has sales," she says. "I know where everything in my store is located, which makes getting around easier."

List what you need, aisle by aisle. Experts say that pre-planning your trip helps you stay focused, minimizing high-fat, high-calorie impulse buys and helping to ensure that you'll come home with what you were looking for, says Schardt.

"I set up my shopping list by aisle," Carol continues. "After five years of going to the same place, I don't have to keep backtracking for something I've missed. I can zip right through."

PRODUCE TOPS THE LIST

"The best place to start is in the produce department—it's usually the section closest to the entrance," says Judy E. Marshel, R.D., director of Health Resources in Great Neck, New York, and former senior nutritionist for Weight Watchers International, who conducts supermarket tours for health professionals and health-conscious consumers.

Think five a day. "Buy enough produce to provide at least five servings of fruits and vegetables for each day's menu,'' says Marshel. Gareth E., a busy mother of three who responded to our *Food and You* survey, has been shopping with her eye on the produce prize for years. ''When I go to the market, I nearly fill my basket with fresh produce, and I plan my menus around what's in season,'' she says. ''It's not unusual for me to buy five different vegetables and three different fruits, and I can plan four meals around them.''

Reach for green and gold. Marshel urges women to concentrate on dark green and deep yellow fruits and vegetables, the ones that are full of beta-carotene, the antioxidant that is ''important because it protects against heart disease and certain types of cancer,'' she says. Her top picks are: kale, spinach, carrots, sweet potatoes, apricots and cantaloupe.

Dr. Webb urges women of childbearing age to eat sufficient quantities of green leafy vegetables for another reason: to fulfill a critical need for folate, a B vitamin that protects against spinal cord defects in developing fetuses. ''The first ten days after conception, the baby's neural tubes develop, and there could be neural tube defects if the mother hasn't been getting enough folate all along,'' explains Dr. Webb. ''Folate comes mainly from green leafy vegetables, and not that many women get green leafy vegetables on a daily basis.'' Top sources of folate, she says, are spinach, collard greens, broccoli and brussels sprouts.

Mix it up. ''The Nutritional Top 40'' on page 428 ranks produce that's tops in terms of total nutrient value. But it's crucial that you vary your selections from one shopping trip to the next, says Marshel, since some foods are higher in particular nutrients than others.

While bananas don't appear on our Top 40 list, for example, they certainly provide excellent nutrition, with plenty of potassium to help regulate high blood pressure and PMS symptoms, says Marshel. And although parsley didn't make the Top 40 list, the bright green sprigs are a good source of cancer-fighting vitamin C, folate and iron, to head off iron-deficiency anemia, she says.

Save time—buy prewashed. Mindful of time constraints at home, nutritionists like Leblang are big fans of fresh, prewashed, bagged vegetables found in supermarkets. ''This is a convenience that's worth the extra money,'' she says. ''Men and women alike should be eating many more fruits and vegetables, to help reduce the risk of heart disease and certain cancers,'' she explains.

Don't shun the canned-goods aisle. Or the freezer case. If you shop every other week, back up your fresh purchases with canned fruit or frozen vegetables, say nutritionists. ''Canned and frozen vegetables are acceptable alternatives,'' says Marshel. Although you lose some nutrients, it's better to eat frozen or canned vegetables than no vegetables at all, according to Marshel. ''The loss of nutrients is negligible in frozen vegetables but is significant in canned vegetables,'' adds Suzanne Havala, R.D., a nutritionist in Charlotte, North Carolina, and author of *Shopping for Health*. Nevertheless, they still count toward achieving your daily quota of five or more servings a day, says Marshel.

BREAD, CEREAL AND BEAN TERRITORY

Some experts say the healthiest choices are often found around the refrigerated periphery of the supermarket. And to some degree, that's true. The exceptions are legumes and grains—canned or dried beans, brown rice, whole-grain breads and cereals and whole-wheat pasta, which are often found in interior aisles of most stores. They're a major source of fiber, of which we need 20 to 30 grams a day, according to the National Cancer Institute.

Follow the two-for-one rule. ''When it comes to bread, look at fat and fiber content,'' says Janis Jibrin, R.D., a nutrition consultant in Washington, D.C. ''Otherwise, they don't vary significantly.'' Her nutrition rule of thumb: Buy bread (including English muffins) with about two grams of fiber and no more than one gram of fat per slice, with about 65 or 70 calories. Possible exceptions are mini-pita loaves and ''lite'' breads, some of which are as low as 40 calories per slice.

Opt for whole-wheat over white. To boost your fiber intake, says Jibrin, ''look for whole-wheat flour as the first ingredient. Even if the package is marked 'wheat bread,' it may be made with white flour, not whole-wheat flour, or contain a small quantity of whole-wheat flour.'' Oat-bran bread products are usually good nutritional choices, says Jibrin.

THE NUTRITIONAL TOP 40

To make trolling the produce aisle a breeze, consult the following shopping lists for vegetables and fruit. Selections are based on how well these foods satisfy the Daily Values (DV) for key nutrients and fiber. (Unless otherwise noted, nutrient analysis for vegetables is based on a half-cup of cooked vegetables.)

A single check mark ✓ indicates that a food provides 10 to 25 percent of the DV; a double check mark ✓✓ indicates that a food provides more than 25 percent of the DV.

VEGETABLES

Vegetable	Fiber (g.)	Beta-Carotene	Vitamin C	Folate	Iron
Asparagus (4 spears)	1.26	✓	✓	✓	
Broccoli, raw	1.32	✓	✓✓		
Brussels sprouts	3.35	✓	✓✓	✓	
Cabbage, shredded	2.10		✓✓		
Carrot, raw	2.16	✓✓	✓		
Cauliflower	1.67		✓✓		
Collards, chopped	1.28	✓✓	✓		
Kale	1.30	✓✓	✓✓		
Kohlrabi	0.90		✓✓		
Peas, edible pods	2.24		✓✓		
Peas, green	4.40		✓	✓	
Peppers, chili, raw	1.39		✓✓		
Peppers, sweet, green, raw	0.90		✓✓		
Peppers, sweet, red, raw	1.00	✓✓	✓✓		
Potato, with skin	4.66		✓✓		✓✓

Vegetable	Fiber (g.)	Beta-Carotene	Vitamin C	Folate	Iron
Rutabaga, cubed	1.53		✓✓		
Spinach	2.16	✓✓	✓	✓✓	✓
Squash, butternut, cubed	N/A	✓✓	✓✓		
Sweet potato	3.42	✓✓	✓✓		
Tomato, raw	1.35	✓	✓✓		

FRUITS

Fruit	Fiber (g.)	Beta-Carotene	Vitamin C	Folate	Potassium
Apricots (3)	2.54	✓✓	✓✓		
Banana	2.74		✓		✓
Blackberries (½ cup)	3.60		✓✓		
Blueberries (½ cup)	3.92		✓✓		
Cantaloupe (1 cup cubed)	1.28	✓✓	✓✓		✓
Casaba (1 cup cubed)	1.36		✓✓	N/A	✓
Cherries, sweet (1 cup)	3.34		✓		
Grapefruit (½)	1.32		✓✓		
Grapes (1 cup)	1.60		✓✓		
Honeydew (1 cup cubed)	1.02	✓✓	N/A	✓	
Kiwifruit	2.58		✓✓	N/A	
Orange	3.14		✓✓		
Papaya	5.47	✓	✓✓	✓✓	✓
Pear	3.98		✓		
Pineapple (1 cup diced)	1.86		✓✓		

FRUITS

Fruit	Fiber (g.)	Beta-Carotene	Vitamin C	Folate	Potassium
Plum	0.99		✓		
Raspberries (1 cup)	8.36		✓✓		
Strawberries (1 cup)	3.43		✓✓		
Tangerine	1.93	✓	✓✓		
Watermelon (1 cup diced)	0.80	✓	✓✓		

Put cereal on the list. Breakfast cereal is one of the best ways to meet your daily fiber quota and get your fair share of B vitamins, says Jibrin. "There are some super-high-fiber cereals, some with as many as 13 grams of fiber per serving. If you like the taste, go for the highest-fiber ones you can get—at minimum, one containing 4 grams of fiber per ounce."

Read before you buy. When it comes to cereal, you need to read labels carefully, says Jibrin. Traditionally packed with fat, granola cereals are now available in fat-free versions, for example. But many are loaded with sugar, making their calorie counts sky high, she says.

"Some consumers find the Nutrition Facts labels confusing, because they count natural sugar, such as is found in fruit, in with added sugar as part of the total grams of sugar," says Marshel. "Read the label for raisin bran, for example, and it appears to be high in sugar. But raisins, not added sugar, account for the total. So you have to read the ingredients listed and note what order they're in. If sugar, fat or sodium is high on the list, avoid that cereal."

For some people, says Jibrin, a *little* sugar is a worthwhile tradeoff. "If the only high-fiber cereal you like is sweetened, then buy it, but count that toward your day's sugar allowance," says Jibrin. "Still, calories rise with the addition of sugar and fat," she adds. "Avoid cereals with a sugar content

BEANS AND GRAINS: A SHOPPER'S CHECKLIST

In most supermarkets, you'll find beans and grains conveniently located in the same aisle, or near each other. This handy guide will help you make your selections when planning meatless meals—high in fiber and key minerals and low in fat. (Unless otherwise noted, values are based on a half-cup of cooked beans, grains or pasta.)

A single check mark ✓ indicates that a food provides 10 to 25 percent of the Daily Value (DV); a double check mark ✓✓ indicates that a food provides more than 25 percent of the DV.

BEANS

	Calories	Fiber (g.)	Folate	Magnesium	Iron	Zinc	Copper
Adzuki beans	147	N/A	✓✓	✓	✓	✓	✓
Black beans	114	7.48	✓✓	✓	✓		
Broad beans (fava beans)	94	4.59	✓				✓
Chick-peas (garbanzo beans)	134	N/A	✓✓		✓		✓
Cowpeas (black-eyed peas)	100	5.59	✓✓	✓	✓		✓
Cranberry beans	120	N/A	✓✓	✓	✓		✓
Great Northern beans	104	6.16	✓	✓	✓		✓
Kidney beans	112	6.51	✓✓		✓		✓
Lentils	115	7.82	✓✓		✓		✓
Lima beans	108	6.58	✓	✓	✓		✓
Mung beans	106	7.68	✓✓	✓			
Navy beans	129	N/A	✓✓	✓	✓		✓
Pink beans	125	4.45	✓✓	✓	✓		✓

	Cal-ories	Fiber (g.)	Folate	Mag-nesium	Iron	Zinc	Copper
Pinto beans	116	7.31	✓✓	✓	✓		✓
Small white beans	128	N/A	✓✓	✓	✓		
Soybeans	149	5.16	✓	✓	✓		✓
Split peas	116	8.13	✓				
White beans	125	5.67	✓	✓	✓		✓
Yellow beans	127	N/A	✓	✓	✓		

GRAINS AND PASTAS

	Cal-ories	Fiber (g.)	Folate	Mag-nesium	Iron	Zinc	Copper
Amaranth	367	14.90	✓	✓✓	✓✓	✓	✓✓
Barley, pearled	97	3.00					
Buckwheat groats	91	N/A		✓			
Bulgur	76	4.10					
Couscous	101	1.26					
Millet	143	1.56		✓			
Oat bran	44	N/A		✓			
Oats	303	N/A	✓	✓✓	✓	✓	✓
Quinoa	318	5.02	✓	✓✓	✓✓	✓	✓✓
Rice, brown, long-grain	109	1.76		✓			
Rice, white, enriched	100	0.35					
Triticale	323	N/A	✓	✓✓	✓	✓	✓
Wheat germ (¼ cup)	104	3.83	✓	✓	✓	✓	✓
Wild rice	83	1.48					
Macaroni, enriched (2 oz.)	99	0.91					

	Cal-ories	Fiber (g.)	Folate	Mag-nesium	Iron	Zinc	Copper
Spaghetti, enriched	99	1.19					

that's more than 25 percent of the total carbohydrates and more than two grams of fat per ounce.''

Buy the king-size box of oatmeal. Don't ignore that perennial cold-weather favorite, oatmeal, which is low in fat and high in soluble fiber to help slash cholesterol.

Add a box of cream of wheat. If you tend to run low on iron, try cream of wheat, a serving of which provides 42 percent of the Daily Value for iron.

Don't run out of rice. Like breads and cereals, whole grains like brown rice are high in fiber, says Jibrin. ''So the more whole grains you buy—like brown rice and whole-grain pasta—the better. To avoid getting bored, experiment with interesting varieties of rice, such as Texmati and Jasmati rice.''

Pair up with beans. Nutritionally, beans and grains differ in their nutritional makeup: Beans contain a generous amount of protein and fiber. Grains (rice, pasta, bulgur and the like) contain a generous amount of complex carbohydrates but less protein. Beans are high in fiber, and most contain little fat (except for soybeans). Together, beans and brown rice are a low-fat, high-fiber duo that experts say is nutritionally preferable to meat.

''If you have beans two to three times a week, you'll be doing a lot to increase your fiber level, and you'll also be getting an excellent source of vegetable protein,'' says Schardt.

Canned beans spell instant meals. Dried beans require long hours of soaking and cooking, and they tend to lose flavor and moisture in the process, so many cooks prefer to buy canned beans. Nutritionists like Marshel give canned beans their blessing. ''If time is short, canned beans and lentils are pretty good. If you're worried about the sodium content, rinse them before eating—it reduces the sodium by about one-third.''

Seek out soybeans. Soybean guru Mark Messina, Ph.D., who has done extensive research on the subject of soy products, extols the virtue of soy in all its incarnations but particularly the soybean itself, which is loaded with isoflavonoids, substances that have been shown in studies to slow the growth of cancer cells. What's more, soy has been linked with relieving menopausal symptoms, thanks to its abundance of phytoestrogens, estrogen-like substances that are found in some plants. Dr. Messina says four ounces of tofu or eight ounces of soy milk a day seems to be helpful. He cautions however, that soyburgers are not a good source of isoflavonoids because they are made with soy concentrate that has been processed in a way that removes the isoflavonoids.

Soy products share some of the same virtues as other bean foods, so the smart shopper can't go wrong adding soy foods to her shopping cart, says Jibrin.

"You're finding more and more soy products in supermarkets now," says Jibrin. "They've really moved into the mainstream. Soy foods are also available at health-food stores, farmer's markets and Asian grocery stores."

Conveniently, beans and grains are frequently shelved near each other in the supermarket.

IF YOU BUY MEAT, GO LEAN

If meat is on your shopping list, you'll probably find the meat case along the refrigerated periphery of the store. While most of us will want to limit consumption of meat to control intake of saturated fat, "women of childbearing age need iron, and lean red meat is a rich source," says Dr. Webb.

Stick to lean cuts. This is Marshel's advice. "If you compare heavily marbled meats (like a Porterhouse steak or pork chop) with lean meat (like a top round of beef or boneless center pork loin), you'll see that when the fat is ingrained in the meat, rather than around the edge, it's much harder to trim off, and you'll end up eating more fat."

For a list of meat and poultry cuts that are lowest in unwanted fat and calories, see the table on page 435.

A MEAT-LOVER'S GUIDE TO SELECTED CUTS

The following list will help you select cuts of meat and poultry that supply easily absorbable iron yet offer limited quantities of saturated fat. (Unless otherwise noted, values given are based on three-ounce servings of trimmed meat or skinless poultry, cooked.)

Meat	Calories	Total Fat (g.)	Saturated Fat (g.)	% Saturated Fat
Turkey breast	115	0.63	0.20	2
Chicken breast	142	3.07	0.87	6
Turkey wing	98	2.06	0.66	6
Beef, top round, select	144	3.15	1.08	7
Turkey (leg meat)	135	3.21	1.08	7
Veal leg	126	2.88	1.04	7
Chicken drumsticks (2)	151	4.98	1.30	8
Beef, eye of round, select	136	3.40	1.23	8
Pork tenderloin	139	4.09	1.41	9
Beef, bottom round, select	167	5.78	1.96	11

NOTE: Values based on U.S. Department of Agriculture data.

FISH: CHOOSE FRESH, FROZEN OR CANNED

Ocean fish (like cod), seafood (like lobster) and lake fish (like pike) are low-calorie sources of cell-building protein, says Marshel. And the omega-3 fatty acids found in fish are thought to reduce triglycerides, inhibit growth of breast cancer and prevent gallstones. For recommended choices, see ''Fish Picks'' on page 437.

Splurge on salmon. Fattier fish are a bit higher in calories, but they're even richer in omega-3 fatty acids. So nutritionists say you may want to include these fish in your menu: three ounces of cooked Atlantic herring (173 calories and 1.7 grams of omega-3's), canned pink salmon (118 calories and 1.4 grams of omega-3's) or cooked Atlantic mackerel (223 calories and 1 gram of omega-3's). To get the benefit of fish oil, fresh or canned will do.

Pack in some tuna and sardines. Less glamorous but equally nutritious is good ol' canned tuna, a pantry staple from the canned fish aisle. Low-sodium, water-packed albacore tuna is a terrific low-calorie source of protein. And three ounces of canned sardines with bones provides about the same amount of calcium as a cup of skim milk. Canned salmon is a close second. Throw it into your cart with a package of whole wheat crackers, some vegetables and fresh fruit, and you have the makings of a perfect lunch.

BONE-BUILDING CHOICES FROM THE DAIRY CASE

"Women who need to stock up on good sources of calcium will find much of what they need in the dairy case," says Schardt. Choose from low-fat dairy products, skim or 1 percent milk, low-fat or nonfat cheese, fat-free ricotta, reduced-fat cheese, nonfat yogurt and the like.

Count fat grams, not percents. As with buying cereal, reading milk labels is critical, says Marshel. "Whole milk has eight grams of fat per cup. By comparison, 2 percent milk isn't low-fat—it has five grams of fat per cup. One percent milk is considered low-fat (although it contains three grams of fat per cup). Skim milk, on the other hand, has only a trace of fat. So if your goal is to get your calcium from foods lowest in fat, grab a carton of skim," says Marshel.

Pick up some cottage cheese. Apply the "grams, not percent" rule to cottage cheese. A tub of creamed cottage cheese contains five grams of fat per half-cup serving. In contrast, the same amount of 2 percent contains just over two grams of fat, and 1 percent has about one gram. With the two reduced-fat versions, you get about 70 milligrams of calcium with a fraction of the fat.

Take home a substitute. The dairy case is also home to eggs and refrigerated cholesterol-free egg products. (Frozen egg substitutes are in the frozen foods section.) Egg substitute

FISH PICKS

Try using this handy chart when you shop for fish, you can serve fish twice a week and not repeat a meal for weeks. To benefit from omega-3 fatty acids (which seem to reduce blood levels of triglycerides and bestow other possible health benefits) without going overboard on calorie intake, alternate between low-fat species (like haddock) and fattier choices (like salmon). (Unless otherwise noted, values given are for three ounces of fresh fish cooked with dry heat, such as broiling.)

Fish	Calories	Total Fat (g.)	Saturated Fat (g.)	Omega-3 Fatty Acids (g.)
Bass, fresh-water	124	4.02	0.85	0.65
Bluefish	135	4.62	1.00	0.84
Catfish	89	2.42	0.63	0.21
Crab, Alaskan king (moist heat)	82	1.31	0.11	0.35
Crab, Dungeness	140	1.57	0.21	0.50
Flounder or sole	99	1.30	0.31	0.43
Grouper	100	1.11	0.25	0.21
Haddock	95	0.79	0.14	0.20
Halibut	119	2.50	0.35	0.40
Herring, Atlantic	173	9.85	2.22	1.71
Mackerel, Atlantic	223	15.14	3.55	1.02
Perch	99	1.00	0.20	0.28
Pike	96	0.75	0.13	0.12
Salmon, Coho	118	3.66	0.90	0.90
Salmon, canned	118	5.14	1.30	1.41
Sardines, canned (2)	50	2.75	0.37	0.23
Snapper	109	1.46	0.31	0.27
Swordfish	132	4.37	1.20	0.70

Fish	Calories	Total Fat (g.)	Saturated Fat (g.)	Omega-3 Fatty Acids (g.)
Trout	128	4.95	1.38	0.84
Tuna, fresh	156	5.34	1.37	1.28
Tuna, light, canned in water	99	0.70	0.20	0.23
Tuna, white, canned	115	2.09	0.56	0.60
Whitefish	146	6.38	0.99	1.38

will save about half the calories and all of the cholesterol and fat you'd get eating whole eggs, notes Marshel.

SWING BY THE OIL SECTION

Nutritionists advise steering clear of solid fats like butter, lard and margarine found in the dairy case. Butter is two-thirds saturated fat, which seems to drive up blood levels of cholesterol. Lard is about 40 percent saturated fat. Margarine is a significant source of trans-fatty acids, which have been implicated as contributing to heart disease.

Seek out bottled vegetable oils. Instead of seeking out margarine and other spreads, says Marshel, wheel your shopping cart down the oil aisle and go for the cooking and salad oils that are highest in monounsaturated and polyunsaturated fats (olive, canola and safflower, for instance). While they still contain about 120 calories and 14 grams of fat per tablespoon, liquid oils are lower in saturated fat and higher in monounsaturated and polyunsaturated fats, which are less harmful and may even protect against heart disease. Vegetable oils also supply vitamin E, one of the antioxidants that seems to protect against heart disease.

So while you want to keep your intake of fats and oils low to stay slim and keep your heart healthy, says Marshel, the right types of oils, when used judiciously, can have their place on your shopping list.

A WOMAN'S GUIDE TO LOW-FAT DAIRY FOODS

The table below can serve as a guide to the very best low-fat sources of calcium in the dairy case, to help you avoid osteoporosis without piling on too many calories. Values vary from brand to brand, so read labels when you make purchases.

A single check mark ✓ indicates that a food provides 10 to 25 percent of the Daily Value (DV); a double check mark ✓✓ indicates that a food provides more than 25 percent of the DV.

CHEESE

Food	Portion	Calories	% Fat	Calcium
American, singles, fat-free	1 slice	30	0	✓
Cheddar, fat-free	1 ounce	45	0	✓
Cheddar, reduced-fat	1 ounce	80	8	✓
Monterey Jack, reduced-fat	1 ounce	80	8	✓
Mozzarella, fat-free	1 ounce	45	0	✓
Mozzarella, light	1 ounce	60	5	✓
Mozzarella, part-skim	1 ounce	90	9	✓
Ricotta, fat-free	¼ cup	60	0	✓✓
Ricotta, light	¼ cup	75	6	✓

MILK

Food	Portion	Calories	% Fat	Calcium
Buttermilk	1 cup	99	20	✓✓
2%	1 cup	137	32	✓✓
1%	1 cup	119	22	✓✓
Skim	1 cup	100	6	✓✓

YOGURT				
Fat-free, fruit	8 ounce	100	0	✓✓
Low-fat, fruit	8 ounce	225	10	✓✓
Low-fat plain	8 ounce	144	22	✓✓
Skim, plain	8 ounce	127	3	✓✓

Buy an oil or two and make it last. Among oils most commonly sold in supermarkets, these are your best choices, ranked from lowest levels of saturated fat to the highest.

1. Canola oil
2. Walnut oil
3. Safflower oil
4. Sunflower oil
5. Corn oil
6. Olive oil
7. Sesame oil
8. Soybean oil
9. Peanut oil

HUNTING THE "TROPHY" JUICES

Wending your way through the juice section, you'll encounter towering shelves of juices, juice drinks and juicelike drinks. Here's a quick guide to what merits purchasing.

Shoot for the Big Three. Stock up on orange, grapefruit and prune juice. They pack the biggest punch of vitamins and minerals. Apple juice is at the bottom of the list.

Buy a week's supply of OJ. "Of the five servings of fruits and vegetables in your diet, one should be orange juice, a very concentrated source of folate," says Jibrin. "Few other foods are as rich in folate."

Say yes to 100 percent juice. "If the label says anything besides 100 percent, odds are the drink has been diluted with sugar water," says Marshel.

Round out your selections with vegetable juices. Carrot, tomato and mixed-vegetable juices supply lots of cancer-

TAKE THIS CODE SHEET TO THE SUPERMARKET

Nutrition Facts labels make it easy to compare various brands of supermarket items and make the right choices in terms of calories, fat, sodium and key nutrients. But what about those *other* key words and phrases on labels? Just as authorities such as the Food and Drug Administration and the U.S. Department of Agriculture set strict guidelines for those Nutrition Facts labels, they also have set criteria for other labeling language. Here's how to decipher the label lingo.

Sugar-free: Contains less than 0.5 gram of sugar per serving.

Calorie-free: Contains fewer than five calories per serving.

Low-calorie: Contains 40 calories or less per serving.

Reduced-calorie: Contains one-fourth fewer calories than the regular product.

Fat-free: Contains less than 0.5 gram of fat per serving.

Low-fat: Contains three grams of fat or less per serving.

Reduced-fat: Contains no more than 75 percent of the fat found in a comparable food.

Low in saturated fat: Contains one gram or less of saturated fat per serving, and no more than 15 percent of the food's calories come from saturated fat.

Reduced saturated fat: Contains no more than 75 percent of the saturated fat found in a comparable food.

Cholesterol-free: Contains less than two milligrams of cholesterol per serving and two grams or less of saturated fat per serving.

Low-cholesterol: Contains 20 milligrams or less of cholesterol per serving, 2 grams or less of saturated fat per serving and 13 grams or less of total fat per serving.

Reduced-cholesterol: Contains 75 percent or less of the cholesterol found in the regular food and two grams or less saturated fat.

Sodium-free: Contains less than five milligrams of sodium/salt per serving.

Low-sodium: Contains 140 milligrams or less of sodium per serving.

Very low-sodium: Contains less than 35 milligrams of sodium per serving.

Reduced-sodium: Contains no more than 75 percent of the sodium found in the regular food.

High in . . . : One serving provides 20 percent or more of the recommended Daily Value of this nutrient.

Good source of . . . : One serving provides 10 to 19 percent of the recommended Daily Value of this nutrient.

Light or "lite": Contains one-third fewer calories or half the fat of the regular food. It could also apply to a "low-calorie" or "low-fat" food that contains 50 percent less sodium than the regular food. In all other cases, the package must specify whether the word "light" refers to color, texture or other qualities.

Fresh: Food that is raw and has not been processed, frozen or heated and contains no preservatives.

Freshly: May be used with "baked" if the food has been made recently.

fighting plant substances known as carotenoids, which are found in fruits and vegetables, says Jibrin. Just be sure to check labels for juices with extra-high sugar levels. "Know that when you're drinking certain juices, like grape juice, it's similar to drinking soda in terms of calories."

HEALTHY CHOICES IN THE SNACK AISLE

Not all snacks are junk foods, say the pros. When chosen carefully, they can actually be a low-calorie, low-fat way of helping you get your nutrients.

Crackers count. Low-fat crackers, says Jibrin, will help you achieve the daily fiber quota recommended by experts. Jibrin recommends crackers that contain about 2 grams of fiber per half-ounce, with zero to four grams of fat. "They're a really good way to get a lot of fiber, especially if you can develop a taste for those Scandinavian or German-type brands such as Wasa and RyKrisp. Even some brands of whole-wheat matzoh have 11 grams of fiber per half-ounce serving."

Graham is good. Graham crackers are generally low in fat and provide some iron and riboflavin, earning them a spot on your shopping list.

SLASH FAT AND SAVE CASH

Think changing your diet to lower your cholesterol will inflate your grocery bills? Well, think again—you'll actually save money, says Thomas Pearson, M.D., Ph.D., professor of epidemiology and medicine at the Columbia University College of Physicians and Surgeons in New York City and Bassett Hospital in Cooperstown, New York, who conducted a five-year study of more than 300 people who were attempting to reduce their cholesterol levels by reducing their dietary fat intake to 30 percent of calories. The results? The low-fat diet cost about a dollar less per day per person than a high-fat diet.

"It's a myth that a low-cholesterol diet costs more," says Dr. Pearson. "In fact, we found that those people who changed their diet the most also spent the least money to buy those foods. If you have bread and fruit for lunch instead of meat and cheese, for example, you tend to spend less."

Saving a dollar a day may not sound like a lot, says Dr. Pearson. "But for a family of four, that translates into $1400 a year." (And that's not even counting the money you'll save on doctor bills.)

Reach for the unsalted and fat-free nibbles. Marshel's top picks: unsalted whole-grain pretzels, corn or rice cakes, and baked fat-free potato or tortilla chips.

"Some of these snacks are good sources of fiber, and you should use the same rule of thumb you would with crackers: Try for two grams of fiber per half-ounce," says Jibrin.

Check for sugar. One caveat; Marshel reminds us not to be seduced by every label marked "low-fat" or "fat-free." "The first ingredient listed on a package of low-fat and fat-free cakes and cookies is usually sugar—which means it may be high in calories."

Try more than one brand. "Some of the fat-free baked chips taste rather bland, and some are not so bad, particularly with salsa, so you've got to experiment," says Jibrin.

DELI AHEAD: PROCEED WITH CAUTION

If you should happen to head for the checkout counter without stopping at the deli, you'll probably save money, fat *and* calories. Should you stop at the deli, proceed with caution, says Marshel. Few of the items you'll see here sport nutrition information, she says, so it's advisable to approach this tempting display of variety meats, cheeses, prepared salads, barbecued chicken and other delicacies carefully. Here are some guidelines for buying the best and leaving the rest.

Be specific. Think about what you want and be very specific when you order, says Marshel. "If you're asking for turkey, for example, ask for 100 percent turkey rather than turkey roll, which is higher in sodium because it's been processed."

Limit your choices to unprocessed foods. Some processed deli foods may have added sugar, says Marshel. And the prepared salads often contain too much mayonnaise, which means lots of fat. The more you stick to unprocessed foods, such as sliced turkey or chicken, the better off you'll be. If you're buying cold cuts at all, you might want to buy the low-fat packaged kinds found in the refrigerator case. "There you're able to read the labels, which you often can't do behind the deli counter. Many of those products are also high in sodium and sugar," notes Marshel.

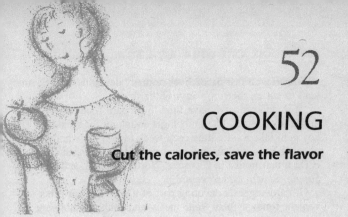

52

COOKING

Cut the calories, save the flavor

If you're like most women, you eat about 21 meals a week—
and you prepare most of them yourself. Even if you work
outside the home, a fair percentage of your meals originate in
your kitchen—with you at the kitchen controls.

That handy-dandy room with all those pots and pans and
gizmos has the potential for being the healthiest room in your
house—*if* you make the most of your time there. And, as
you're about to learn, it doesn't take a whole lot of time to
cook healthfully. "Women today don't have time for recipes
with 15 ingredients. Cooking healthy meals can be done fast,
easily and using readily available products," says Gloria Rose,
author of *Cooking for Good Health* and director of the Gourmet Long Life Cooking Schools, with headquarters in Spring-
field, New Jersey.

A SMART START

Smart cooking begins with a plan, says Judy Gilliard, author
of *The Guiltless Gourmet* and other cookbooks, who started to
cook healthier when she was diagnosed with diabetes.

445

"Women with fast-paced lives or many demands on their time tend to eat on the run," says Gilliard.

"We don't always have time to prepare food, so we make unhealthy choices, like grabbing a doughnut for breakfast. The key is to take a little time each week to preplan what we'll be cooking for ourselves and our family," says Suzanne Havala, R.D., a nutritionist in Charlotte, North Carolina, and author of *Simple, Lowfat and Vegetarian*.

Gilliard suggests devoting part of a weekend (or other convenient time) to plan your meals and make a shopping list. Select healthier recipes you'd like to try. That way, mealtime becomes a snap.

To motivate yourself and make cooking easier, Gilliard suggests you "make your kitchen a fun place in which to spend time." Here's how.

Reorganize your pantry. If your foods aren't where you can easily find them, you'll waste time hunting when you could be cooking, says Gilliard. "Group your canned tomato products—tomato sauce, tomato puree, stewed tomatoes and the like—in one logical, convenient place, for instance. Do the same with canned beans, grains, oils, condiments and so forth."

Out with the old. Go through your refrigerator, cabinets and pantry and clean them out, says Gilliard. "Get rid of high-fat items and old items. The average shelf life for spices is about one year; it's three months for flour, for example."

Check your tools. Make sure you have a full complement of accurate measuring cups and spoons, says Jim Fobel, chef and author of seven books, including *Jim Fobel's Big Flavors*. "I weigh everything," says Fobel. "Measuring everything I eat helped me lose over 100 pounds, and it ensures that recipes will turn out right."

FAT-SPARING TECHNIQUES FROM PRO CHEFS

Doctors advise women who need to cut their fat consumption to limit their intake of vegetable oil to a total of three tablespoons a day, including what they use for cooking. The ideal percentage of calories from fat, say experts, is 25 to 30 percent or less, most of which should come from unsaturated vegetable oils, not butter, meat or dairy products.

When it comes to cutting fat, then, the logical place to start is with the dishes you prepare yourself. Gilliard and other experts offer the following strategies.

Sauté in droplets, not pools. Rose urges her cooking students (many of whom come to her schools at their doctors' recommendations following heart attacks and other medical problems) to limit themselves to a half-teaspoon of fat per person, per recipe. "That should automatically keep you at the 15 to 20 percent of calories from the fat level I recommend in my classes," says Rose, who believes that sautéing in oil is simply wasting your daily quota of it.

"Oil should be used only as a condiment, to add flavor to a dish, not as an ingredient," says Rose. "If a recipe calls for oil, butter or margarine in the first five ingredients of the list, nine times out of ten it will be used for sautéing. Use less, or sauté in broth or stock instead, and you will save a tremendous amount of calories from fat."

"There's no need to sauté food in a quarter-cup of fat—unless you're making a dish for 20 people," says Marian Burros, who writes the "Eating Well" column for the *New York Times* and is the author of ten books, including *Eating Well Is the Best Revenge*. "You'll get the same taste using much less fat."

The way to spray. By now many of us have discovered the joys of nonstick cooking sprays—with one 1¼-second spray, you can cover as much cooking area as with one tablespoon of oil, for a mere 7 calories (as opposed to 100 calories). Even so, says Rose, you shouldn't get too carried away. "If you spray a skillet, turn it sideways and see liquid running down it, you've used too much," she says.

Paint, don't pour. If you prefer to use bottled oil instead of a spray, says Rose, you can minimize the amount of oil you use by lightly "painting" the surface of your saucepan, skillet or cookie sheet with a small, clean pastry brush or paintbrush. To lend additional flavor, add cumin, garlic or whatever other flavor you prefer to the oil.

Turn up the heat. Burros shares a similar fat-sparing technique that makes browning foods a snap. "Start with the best-quality nonstick pan you can afford," she says. "Heat it until

WOMEN WHO LOVE TO COOK

Hate to cook? Here are a few lessons in learning to love preparing food.

"Cooking is fun for me because when I'm using fresh ingredients, chopping, looking at the food, smelling the nice aromas and knowing I'm about to put something healthy into my body, it's all very nurturing," says Judy Gilliard, author of *The Guiltless Gourmet*.

Some people are born to cook—others are less than enthusiastic. If you're having trouble getting motivated to pick up a ladle, read what other converts have to say. Here are some insights from women who responded to our *Food and You* survey.

LAURA H., AGE 33

Tapped Her Creativity
"I like the act of preparing food—I find it very satisfying," says Laura. "Planning the menu, cutting the vegetables, creating something—I find it all creative. I don't do gourmet cooking, but I don't think you have to. A simple chicken-and-pasta dish can be very exciting." Among her friends, Laura is well-known for hosting "theme nights." "Sometimes it will be Italian night, and I'll cook an Italian dish and play Italian music as loud as I can; other times it will be Mexican or Spanish night. Even if I'm having just one guest, I'll do it."

CHRISTINE M., AGE 27

Two's Company
"It's enjoyable having somebody else cook with you," says Christine. "My husband doesn't have to actually be *helping* me; I find it nice just to have him sit there while I'm cooking and tell me about his day. The companionship is fun."

KELLY W., AGE 34

Likes the Challenge
"I challenge myself to experiment more," Kelly told us. "I've made a New Year's resolution to try new recipes from new

> cookbooks. I recently made a low-fat peach crisp that was out of this world! I make a point of trying out a new recipe about twice a month. Pushing myself to be more creative makes cooking more enjoyable. Otherwise, you get bored with the same things all the time."

it's very hot but not smoking, then reduce the heat to medium-high. That way, you can get away with using just a *little* oil—like one to two teaspoons—to get a really good browning effect on things like potatoes and chicken breasts.'' Burros notes that pans that are heated to high temperatures for lower-fat browning tend to wear out earlier, but in her view, the trade-off is worth it.

Bread one side only. Love the taste of batter-sautéed fish fillets and chicken cutlets? Want to save calories and fat grams? You can, says Fobel. ''Bread just one side. Dip one side in egg white and bread crumbs, and place that side down in a little oil in a nonstick skillet. Brown it really well, turn it over and finish cooking it.'' Then serve it breaded side up.

Bake, don't fry. Another way to ''fry'' chicken without traditional ingredients like butter is to dip skinless chicken pieces in skim milk or egg white and crushed low-fat, unsweetened cereal and bake it on a cookie sheet sprayed with cooking spray, says Rose. ''Or, for a Tex-Mex flavor, you can buy flavored fat-free tortilla chips, crush them and use them instead of bread crumbs.''

Baste with broth. When roasting turkey, says Gilliard, glaze the top with chicken broth instead of oil, then sprinkle with oregano and garlic powder. ''It's lower in fat than glazing with oil, but your turkey will still have nice, crisp skin.''

Make savory soup without pork fat. Most recipes for split pea or lentil soup call for ham hocks or other animal fat, adding unwanted calories from fat. Burros suggests using a roasted pepper or some smoked turkey instead of a ham hock or other smoked pork product to get that smoky flavor without the fat.

Make meatless chili. One way to cut fat (and increase your intake of fiber and important vitamins and minerals) is to use less meat, says Havala. Begin by making minor adjustments to your current favorites. ''One change I made long ago was to take the meat out of chili and turn it into a colorful multi-bean chili, using chick-peas, kidney beans, pinto beans and others," says Havala. "It smells good and looks beautiful, and it's much higher in fiber and lower in fat than chili con carne."

Nuke your fish. Sarah Schlesinger, author of 500 *Fat-Free Fruit and Vegetable Recipes*, prefers cooking fish in the microwave, sprinkled with herbs. If you like tartar sauce on the side, says Rose, you can make it nonfat by blending two parts of no-salt-added prepared sweet relish to one part fat-free mayonnaise.

Use fresh herbs and spices. If you cook with little or no fat, says Gilliard, the rest of your ingredients must be super-fresh. "If the herbs, spices and other ingredients you use are stale, your food will taste stale. If they're fresh, your food will taste wonderful—and still be healthy."

"When I buy herbs and spices, I write the date on the packages," says Fobel. Experts say that while buying the freshest ingredients may cost more, they're worth it because they help you adhere to a healthy diet.

Buy a cheese grater, and use it. "I love grating fresh Parmesan or Romano cheese," says Gilliard. "When you grate it yourself, you get so much more flavor than if it's pregrated, so you don't need to use as much."

VEGETABLES WITH FLAIR, NOT FAT

Nutritionists say that for women, vegetables are a must—they're key sources of vitamins and minerals that women need but tend to fall short in. Here's what professional chefs suggest.

Steam it up. "If you sauté or stir-fry vegetables in less oil, the vegetables may come out dry," says Fobel. "To compensate and add moisture, add a few tablespoons of water and cook over very high heat. Cook until the vegetables are tender, adding more water if necessary."

Turn on the juice. "Depending on the dish, I like to play with a variety of juices when I'm steaming or sautéing," says Schlesinger, who revamped her cooking style when her husband had a heart attack in his thirties. "I use tomato juice thinned down with water, or citrus juices."

Flavor while you steam. "Instead of topping cooked vegetables with butter or margarine, add lemon juice and garlic to the water you use for steaming vegetables,'' suggests Schlesinger. ''The flavor permeates the food even better than flavoring vegetables after they're cooked, and you infuse your cooking with some wonderful and exotic flavors while slashing fat.'' Schlesinger often steams broccoli in a pineapple juice/water mixture, for example. Other times, she'll also add water chestnuts, ginger or garlic. ''To give food a strong tropical or Asian flavor, I sauté in pineapple juice,'' she says.

Unbutter those carrots. Carrots are about the best thing you can eat, says Judith S. Stern, R.D., D.Sc., professor of nutrition and internal medicine at the University of California, Davis. To season carrots without butter or margarine, says Rose, mix two tablespoons of undiluted apple juice concentrate with cinnamon, allspice and orange peel and warm. As the mixture heats, add arrowroot and water and let it thicken. Pour it onto your steamed carrots and, says Rose, ''they become a gourmet delight.''

Braise, don't fry. Yet another cooking option is braising—browning ingredients in a small amount of oil and then cooking them in seasoned liquids. ''I like to braise foods because it tenderizes food and seals in the natural flavors and nutrients,'' says Sam Okamoto, a food consultant in Vancouver, British Columbia, and author of *Sam Okamoto's Incredible Vegetables*. Okamoto says that braising is generally used for cooking hard root vegetables, such as potatoes and carrots. An even quicker braising method, using less liquid, is best for cooking leafy or other soft veggies. One of Okamoto's specialties: beta-carotene-packed spinach, braised for five minutes with tofu in a blend of Asian flavorings, including mirin and low-sodium soy sauce.

Microwave your spinach. Use your handy-dandy microwave to help retain nutrients in grains and veggies, as well as to save time, urges Jim Fobel. ''I like the microwave for cooking spinach,'' he says. ''I just put some wet leaves in the microwave, turn it on and watch them collapse.''

Precook your onions. Schlesinger prepares onions for the soups she makes by first ''sautéing'' chopped onion in her microwave. ''Instead of cooking the onion in oil in a pan, I'll put chopped onion in a microwave-proof bowl along with the onion with a little liquid—juice or water with some garlic.

Then I'll stick it in the microwave for 1½ minutes to soften the onion—it's like sweating them. Just as sautéing releases the flavor of food, the same thing happens in the microwave."

Schlesinger cooks other vegetables in the microwave, too. "The microwave doesn't require or even welcome the presence of fat," she says.

Make every soup vegetable soup. The quickest way of all to get vegetables on the menu: If you're making soup, dump half a bag of frozen veggies into it while it simmers, suggests Havala.

Consider a pressure cooker. "To cook more healthfully, speed is essential," says Mardee Haidin Regan, a cookbook and kitchen-equipment writer and former columnist for *Food and Wine* magazine. "When you cut down on the time, you cut down on the loss of nutrients. Your goals are twofold: one, to preserve as many vitamins and minerals as you can, and two, to avoid making healthful eating a cumbersome project."

Regan is a pressure-cooker fan. "After the microwave, the pressure cooker is the most efficient way of cooking food quickly," she says. "With a pressure cooker, none of the nutrients escape when you're making soups, stews or roasts. I recently tested 10 or 12 different models, and they are foolproof, if you follow the directions."

Grill it. "I use a $20 stovetop grill, and it's great for vegetables, chicken and fish," says Burros. "Food tastes so wonderful when prepared on the grill—especially if you have good-quality ingredients to begin with—and you don't even have to do very much. It's a delicious way to cook without fat."

FASTER (AND FAT-FREE) RICE, POTATOES AND PASTA

"The key to optimal health—not just weight loss, but disease prevention—is to design your meals around carbohydrates— fruits, vegetables, grains, grain products and legumes," says Kathie Swift, R.D., nutritional director of the Canyon Ranch Spa in Lenox, Massachusetts. Here are tips for putting carbs on the table.

Presoak rice. A half-cup of cooked brown rice has 1.7 grams of fiber—eight times as much fiber as white rice. But it also takes longer to cook. To reduce cooking time of regular brown rice, Burros soaks it overnight. Then, the next day, it cooks as quickly as white rice. "And," she adds, "nutritionists have assured me that this method doesn't cause nutrients to leach out into the water."

Rice 'n' easy. One of Gilliard's favorite kitchen gizmos for preparing quick, healthy meals is her rice cooker. "Even when I don't have much time, it lets me make a great, one-dish meal," she says. "I'll use brown rice and lentils cooked in a little bit of chicken or vegetable broth, maybe mixed with some sautéed onions, mushrooms and green peppers. Occasionally I'll also add some chicken to it."

Micro-bake your potatoes. "I suggest partially cooking potatoes in the microwave," says Fobel. "Cook them halfway, then finish them off in the oven. Precooking saves time, and you don't have to heat up the kitchen. But the potato will still have a nice, crispy skin."

Mashed potatoes? Skip the salt. While some physicians suspect salt may not be the primary culprit in high blood pressure, salt restriction seems to be appropriate for at least some people. To meet the health needs of their customers, many professional chefs have devised creative ways to minimize the need for salt content in their recipes. One is Peter De Marais, executive chef of the Sheraton Palace Hotel in San Francisco.

"Try my rutabaga/mashed potato recipe," suggests De Marais. "Boil rutabagas in chicken stock flavored with bay leaf and herbs, like rosemary or thyme. Then mash the rutabagas with cooked potatoes. Add grated orange rind and some fresh cracked pepper. You don't need salt, cream or butter—and it's delicious."

A grown-up use for baby food. One of the women who responded to our *Food and You* survey found creative and nutritious uses for baby food. "I love to put pureed carrots on a baked potato," says Gareth E., mother of three children. "It tastes really good—like a sweet-potato soufflé."

"Pureed carrots are a good way to add beta-carotene without the fat," says Janis Jibrin, R.D., a nutrition consultant based in Washington, D.C.

A leaner way to make stuffing. Gilliard recommends using chicken broth instead of butter or margarine to moisten bread stuffing.

A WEEK'S WORTH OF SALADS

So much for cooking the main course and side dishes. Gilliard suggests the following Monday-to-Friday menu of salads to work greens, fruits and vegetables into your menu and complement the main course when you're pressed for time.

Sunday is wash day. On the weekend, wash a couple of heads of greens—Romaine and butterhead lettuce, spinach and raddichio or red cabbage—then dry the leaves in a salad spinner or pat dry between absorbent towels. Store them in an airtight container in the fridge. (In a pinch, says Gilliard, you can buy prewashed, precut greens.)

"Properly washed and stored, salad greens will keep for four to five days," says Gilliard.

Add pears and walnuts. For added fiber, says Gilliard, top your greens with some canned sliced pears (drained) and a few walnut pieces and toss with a dressing of pear nectar and rice wine vinegar with a little water.

Have a midweek bean salad. Toss a half-cup of canned black or white beans (rinsed under cold water to remove the sodium) in with your greens, along with some cut-up veggies, says Gilliard.

Use leftover chicken. For a main meal salad, says Gilliard, add julienned strips of turkey or chicken breast along with shredded carrots, chopped red cabbage and pepper strips.

Top it off with tuna. Add chunks of drained, canned tuna, cucumber slices and tomato wedges and toss with a dressing of balsamic vinegar blended with a little honey, some mustard and a bit of water, says Gilliard.

Toss in some avocado. Toss one-eighth of a cubed avocado with sunflower seeds, fresh chopped tomato and romaine lettuce and sprinkle with rice wine vinegar. That amount of avocado is just enough to make this a real treat without adding too much fat, says Gilliard.

Try Marian's dressing. "My greatest coup," says Burros, with pride, "is perfecting my low-fat salad dressing. It's one part balsamic vinegar, one part olive oil and one part honey mustard. If you use a teaspoon of each, you end up with one tablespoon of dressing all together, enough for two servings of salad. The flavor is wonderful—much better than bottled dressings, I think."

Drizzle, don't drench. Whatever dressing you choose, says Burros, go easy. "I've seen salads with so much dressing that the lettuce slips off the plate," she says. Use just enough to flavor the greens, not drown them.

SNEAKING IN EXTRA NUTRIENTS

There's more to healthy cooking than cutting fat and saving time. Every meal is an opportunity to get your daily quota of beta-carotene, fiber, folate, iron, calcium and other nutrients women need. Dietitians and other cooking experts offer their advice for adding nutrients to your meals.

Looks count. "Healthy food looks *and* tastes appealing," says Rose. The key to a tantalizing presentation? "Color!" says Rose. "If you have a dish that calls for green peppers, for example, use yellow, red or orange pepper strips, too. They make a stir-fry, paella or stew vibrant and irresistible." (Not to mention the extra nutritional boost it gets from that rainbow of vitamin C-rich veggies.)

Try vegetable lasagna. For an extra dose of beta-carotene in your home-baked lasagna, layer it with some cooked spinach or shredded carrots, says M. J. Smith, R.D., author of *The Miracle Foods Cookbook.*

Make a veggie pizza. Pile your homemade or frozen pizza with veggies like red and green peppers (both packed with vitamin C), mushrooms and onions (both good sources of fiber), says Smith.

Go for beta, not bologna. To add fiber to your diet, make a pita sandwich stuffed with shredded cabbage, sliced tomatoes and sliced radishes, says Smith. For extra folate (a B vitamin that's essential before and during pregnancy), add romaine lettuce or spinach leaves, Smith says.

Top taters with salsa. Give your baked potatoes a vitamin C boost: Top them with tomato-and-green-pepper salsa, suggests Smith.

Supplement with dry milk powder. Boost your daily calcium intake by preparing hot cereals with four tablespoons of nonfat milk powder per serving and sprinkling six tablespoons of nonfat milk powder into each pound of lean hamburger meat, suggest nutritionists at the Calcium Information Center at the Oregon Health Sciences University in Portland. What's more, by adding four tablespoons of nonfat milk powder to each cup of skim or low-fat milk you drink, you double your intake of calcium and riboflavin from milk.

Whip up some eggplant and lentil spread. Known as baba gannouj, (*bah-BAH ga-NOOSH*), this Middle Eastern eggplant spread is low in fat and high in fiber and is a low-fat substitute for sour cream dip. If you add lentils, as Burros suggests, you double your intake of folate and iron and increase potassium by 50 percent.

YOU CAN DO IT

A word of advice from Sarah Schlesinger: If healthy cooking is new to you, take it one step at a time.

"You may be gung-ho about transforming yourself into a healthy cook *par excellence*," says Schlesinger. "But be realistic, too, so you don't sabotage yourself. Stick to food you're most likely to eat, with ingredients that are not too difficult to find or prepare. Your cooking style needs to fit your lifestyle, or you won't keep it up.

"When I changed my way of preparing food for the sake of my husband's health and my own," she says, "my feeling was that it was exciting to control our destiny, to play a part in preserving our health. Cooking is an important way of taking care of yourself. Make it a priority."

53

DINING OUT

Making the most of away-from-home meals

What do you say we go out to dinner?''

Do those words conjure up visions of fine food (that you *don't* have to cook yourself!), relaxation (no dishes to wash!), a dash of ambiance and catching up on news with a special friend or loved one? Sounds great in principle. But then you start to worry: Will you blow your diet? Scarf down enough cholesterol to permanently clog your arteries? Eat more than you should because you can't (or shouldn't) let food go to waste?

These days, eating out is practically unavoidable. No longer limited to special-event occasions, the average American eats out 198 times a year, which translates to nearly four times a week. In fact, 44 cents of every food dollar go to ''meals'' away from home: The hot dog with the works from a street-corner or ballpark food stand or the snack shack at the beach. Take-out cartons from your favorite Chinese restaurant. Coffee and a-bagel-with-a-shmeer from the corner deli on the way to work in the morning. Yes, food service, as those in the business call it, is big business—and, for better or worse, it's a major factor in your nutritional status.

THE ULTIMATE TREAT

The reasons we enjoy dining out are as varied as the foods we order. For many, it's the ultimate treat. Who among us doesn't get just a *tiny* thrill upon walking into a restaurant, even the simplest diner or deli?

"I eat out about three times a week, and for me, it's always an indulgence," says Lisa McG., one of the respondents to our *Food and You* survey. "It's a chance for me to loosen up my usual eating habits, to have whatever strikes my fancy on the menu. My husband and I go to a lot of different ethnic restaurants, and I always like to try new foods."

Others have less pretentious tastes. "I'd eat Whoppers and Kentucky Fried Chicken every day if I could—they're my favorite foods," says another woman we heard from—new mom Debbie W., who was only slightly apologetic. "In fact, I can't think of one fast-food place I *don't* like! I go about once or twice a week, and I really have to fight myself to not go more often."

For some diners, the food is secondary. Why else would anyone spend a week's worth of grocery money on a week's worth of fat and calories in one sitting? Forty-one-year-old Beryl M.'s reasons for eating out three times a week are typical: "I hate to cook and I hate to do dishes," she told us. "It's just my husband Ray and me—we have no kids—so it's easy for us to go to one of the many restaurants in our neighborhood; every imaginable type of food is within a block of where we live."

Time is another, equally compelling factor for Beryl and others. "Ray and I each work more than one job, and we're always trying to find time to be together. Going out to a restaurant feels like a date. It rejuvenates the relationship—the ambiance of the restaurant grounds us again after a crazy week of dashing around."

Mary McH. echoes those sentiments. "It's a treat to get dressed up and go out to eat with my husband," says this survey respondent. "It's very romantic. Earl and I spend the time appreciating each other, saying nice things about each other—the kinds of things we used to say when we were dating. It's not like being at home over the dinner table, rehashing the issues of the day."

THE PSYCHIC REWARDS OF DINING OUT

If you feel guilty about indulging in meals away from home, rest assured—dining out is a bona fide form of stress therapy. "It's good to dine out," says David A. Levitsky, Ph.D., professor of nutrition and psychology in the Division of Nutritional Sciences at Cornell University in Ithaca, New York. "The act itself is relaxing and beneficial, just as taking a vacation is relaxing and beneficial. Putting yourself in a different context, such as a restaurant, relieves much of the anxiety accrued through daily interactions. We come into a meal burdened with all the problems of the day. But with the change of venue, the memories fade," he says.

To illustrate his point, Dr. Levitsky cites research on the dining habits of college students. When the students surveyed heard lectures in one room and were then tested in another room, they didn't do as well as when they were tested in the lecture room. "That's because information learned in one place is more easily retrieved in the place where it's been obtained. So," he says, "if you've had an argument with the kids and you eat dinner with your husband at home, the memories of that argument with the kids will be stronger than if you were to dine away from home."

Not only does eating out improve your mood, it also improves your relationships. "Eating out is a fantasy—it removes you, at least for a little while, from the reality in which you live. And the more removed from your everyday life you can get—with the help of music, candlelight, tablecloths and china—the more conducive it is to interacting with people in a meaningful way," says Dr. Levitsky. "You're not talking about the electric bill. It lets you focus on the other person."

What's more, eating out is a solid ego-booster, according to Dr. Levitsky. "All day long you do things for others," he notes. "But when you eat out, people are doing things for *you*, which is good for your self-image and your self-esteem."

NOT JUST FOR BIRTHDAYS AND ANNIVERSARIES

All that recharging of your emotional batteries—for the price of a hamburger. And yet, as we well know, that hamburger—or whatever it is you eat—can take a serious toll on the way

THE FINE ART OF DINING SMART

In the supermarket, the Nutrition Facts label tips you off to what's in a box, jar or carton of food. On restaurant menus, key words and phrases are tipoffs. Once you learn the lingo, dining out is easier. The following guidelines are based on information from the American Heart Association and Hope S. Warshaw, R. D., author of *The Restaurant Companion: A Guide to Healthier Eating Out.*

"YES" FOODS

- Broiled, charbroiled, grilled, roasted, braised or baked
- Steamed or poached
- Lightly stir-fried
- In broth or in wine
- Florentine (spinach)
- Primavera (with vegetables; fine as long as it's not in a cream sauce)
- Marinara (tomato sauce)
- Stuffed with vegetables (or herbs)

"NO" FOODS

- Au gratin, escalloped, in a cheese sauce, with parmesan or au fromage
- Creamed, in a cream sauce or Hollandaise
- Crispy, sautéed, fried, pan-fried or deep-fried
- Breaded, dipped in batter, batter-fried or tempura
- In butter sauce or buttery
- Bisque
- In gravy
- A lá mode (topped with ice cream)
- Alfredo (butter-and-cheese sauce)
- Carbonara (butter-and-cheese sauce plus bacon)
- Casserole (could contain undetermined—and often rich—sauces or other fatty ingredients)
- Stuffed with cheese (or meat)
- Large, extra-large, jumbo, piled-high or stacked
- All you can eat

you feel from the neck *down*. When people ate out once in a blue moon, nutritional vigilance wasn't too important. Eat several meals a week away from home, however, and the wrong choices can jeopardize your health goals.

"Twenty years ago, when people went out to eat, it was a splurge—it almost didn't matter what you ate. But now that people are spending nearly half their food dollar in restaurants, it *does* matter, particularly when it comes to calories, fat and sodium," says Jayne Hurley, R.D., senior nutritionist with the Center for Science in the Public Interest, a non-profit consumer group in Washington, D.C., that's known for its nutritional "report cards" on Chinese, Italian, Mexican, delicatessan and seafood restaurants. Hurley insists that the public is as hungry for solid nutrition information as it is for great restaurant food.

People don't have to stop eating at restaurants, ethnic or otherwise. But now they have the information they need to make smarter selections.

THE BIG FAT PROBLEM

So what exactly is the problem with eating out?

According to Hope S. Warshaw, R.D., author of *The Restaurant Companion: A Guide to Healthier Eating Out*, there are actually three: the aforementioned fat and calories, large portions and undue emphasis on protein (meat).

"First of all, restaurant meals are high in fat, and that fat comes in a variety of choices, whether it's from salad dressing, from a 'special sauce' or from cheese, avocado, bacon bits, olives and so forth. Whatever form fat takes, it all adds up to more calories," says Warshaw.

Think about the way we really eat: "Americans are having an Egg McMuffin for breakfast, a Big Mac and french fries for lunch, fettuccine Alfredo for dinner and popcorn at the movies," says Hurley. "Because of that kind of diet, one in three adults today is seriously overweight. As many people die from bad diet and lack of exercise each year as they do from smoking."

RESTAURANT OPTIONS
More Choices Than You Think

Even at your favorite surf and turf palace with plates the size of trampolines, you can slash fat, reduce serving sizes and focus on body-healthy foods.

AMERICAN-STYLE RESTAURANTS

Instead of	Have
A double cheeseburger with large fries	A small cheeseburger with small fries and a side salad
Caesar salad with anchovies and egg	Spinach salad with mushrooms and vinegar (dressing on the side)
Any sandwich on a croissant	A sandwich on whole-grain bread or a roll
Cheesecake	Frozen yogurt

CHINESE RESTAURANTS

Instead of	Have
A whole entrée and one bowl of rice	Half an entrée and one bowl of rice
A whole protein-based entrée	Half the entrée and a side order of steamed vegetables
Kung Pao chicken	Chicken with vegetables, chicken chow mein or szechuan shrimp

FAST-FOOD RESTAURANTS

Instead of	Have
Combo meals, double or triple cheeseburgers	Sandwiches without the extras, single hamburgers

FAST-FOOD RESTAURANTS, continued

Instead of	Have
Sandwiches with "special sauce" and/or mayonnaise	Sandwiches with mustard or ketchup
Side order of french fries	Small side salad or fresh veggies from the fixings bar
Chicken McNuggets	Grilled chicken sandwich
Wendy's single burger	Wendy's chili
Fast food as a between-meal snack	Fast food as a meal

ITALIAN RESTAURANTS

Instead of	Have
Fettuccine Alfredo or lasagna	Pasta topped with tomato sauce, red or white clam sauce, meat sauce or meatballs
Garlic bread	Plain Italian bread without butter
Salad with mystery house dressing	Salad with reduced-calorie dressing or a little oil and vinegar

MEXICAN RESTAURANTS

Instead of	Have
Shrimp, vegetable or chicken fajitas with the works (sour cream, guacamole and refried beans)	Fajitas without the extras or, if available, nonfat sour cream and beans made without added oil
Chicken burrito with sour cream and cheese	Grilled chicken or a chicken burrito made with nonfat sour cream and reduced-fat cheese

MEXICAN RESTAURANTS, continued

Instead of	Have
Side order of refried beans	Side order of beans made without added oil, or rice
Guacamole as a dip	Salsa as a dip
Tortilla chips	Soft flour tortillas dipped in salsa

SEAFOOD RESTAURANTS

Instead of	Have
Fried fish	Broiled, grilled, blackened or steamed fish
Stuffed fish or fish in cheese, cream or tartar sauce	Simple fish dishes
French fries	Baked potato with sour cream on the side
Biscuits	Rolls without butter or very lightly buttered

SOURCES: Hope S. Warshaw, R.D., Jayne Hurley, R.D., and Marion J. Franz, R.D.

HOW EUROPEANS KEEP THEIR FIGURES

The large portions often served in restaurants spell trouble, says Sachiko St. Jeor, R.D., Ph.D., director of the Nutrition Education and Research Program at the University of Nevada School of Medicine in Reno.

"We overeat because too much is served," says Dr. St. Jeor. "When it's there, we eat it. When it tastes so good, it's hard *not* to finish the whole serving."

Martha Rose Shulman, author of *Provençal Light* and other healthy cookbooks, lived in France for 12 years and thinks European restaurants can teach us a thing or two about appropriate serving sizes. "When Americans go out to dinner, they will, in general, eat what's put on their plate, especially if they're paying for it," she says. "I don't think that much food needs to be served. In Europe, diners are accustomed to smaller portions, yet you don't hear them complaining."

The third contributing factor is entrées that focus on protein—specifically animal protein, says Warshaw. "Even in a Chinese or Thai restaurant, where vegetable and grain dishes are plentiful, most people sit down to dine, open the menu and say, 'Pork or beef, shrimp or chicken?' It always comes down to the protein. A lot of people are on automatic pilot when they order protein as their main dish."

IN SEARCH OF NUTRITIONAL *AND* CULINARY BLISS

So yes, dining out is tricky. That doesn't mean you can't enjoy yourself and stay within healthy-eating parameters. How? By learning to love—or leave—particular food items (or at least eat less of what you order). Here's what the experts say you should do.

Pass up the fat. Weed out the worst choices—the broiled flounder is lots better than the duck. Ask how the dish you're considering is prepared—make sure it's not deep-fried or slathered with butter, cheese or a cream sauce, says Hurley.

Ask yourself if fettuccine Alfredo tastes four times better than spaghetti with meat sauce—because you're getting four times the fat, notes Hurley.

Dress it yourself. Have any sauces or dressings served on the side. "Salad dressing is the largest source of fat in a woman's diet. Few people realize how fattening dressing is," says Hurley.

Stick to fresh fruit or sorbet for dessert. You don't have to say no automatically when the dessert cart is wheeled over, says Warshaw. "Depending on the restaurant, you can opt for various sweets that are heart-smart and kind to your waistline. Try sorbet (often available in a rainbow of colors and exotic fruity flavors). Or lemon ice, offered in some Italian restaurants." Other options, says Warshaw, are fresh raspberries or strawberries with a bit of liqueur. "Also, some family-style restaurants offer low-fat frozen yogurt," she adds.

Make a side dish your entrée. As Warshaw points out,

most restaurant menus emphasize protein and fat; grains, carbohydrates and vegetables (like rice, potatoes and greens) are
an afterthought. Warshaw advises diners to be creative. "Don't
feel that you *have* to order an entrée. Take advantage of ap-
petizers and side dishes. Share several dishes among your-
selves." If, say, the minestrone is wonderful, why not have
that as your main course, along with some crunchy bread and
a green salad?

If you don't see it, ask for it. "Don't be afraid to make
special requests," says Carole Livingston, a frequent
restaurant-goer and author of *I'll Never Be Fat Again*! "For
example, if you don't see a simple pasta dish on the menu but
you *do* see that the restaurant serves other dishes that contain
pasta or tomatoes or vegetables, ask for pasta prepared with
vegetables in a tomato-based sauce. Ask the chef to put things
together. Often, the better the restaurant, the easier it is to
make alternate choices."

And ask nicely. The trick to being assertive without being
unpleasant is to be polite and specific, says Eric Asimov, a
New York Times restaurant critic and author of *$25 and Under:
A Guide to the Best Inexpensive Restaurants in New York*. "I
think people often don't feel confident in a restaurant situation,
and so they fear making their needs known," observes Asimov, who eats out about 40 times a month in the line of duty.

With a little ingenuity, you can even use dining out as an
opportunity to *improve* your diet.

In fact, sometimes it's easier to eat nutritionally in restaurants than at home. Says Mary: "I don't eat vegetables at
home—they're too much trouble to prepare. So when I dine
out, I always make a point to order vegetables—usually a
salad—and I look forward to it. I like grilled tuna on top of a
bed of greens, for example."

Pay attention. "Salad bars can be healthy or unhealthy,
depending on what you choose," says Warshaw. "The same
is true for salad entrées: You can order a grilled chicken salad,
feeling virtuous for having ordered a salad but 'forgetting' that
it comes with avocado, grated cheese, bacon bits and blue
cheese dressing. In that case, you can ask the server to hold
the cheese and serve the dressing on the side, then add just a
little bit for taste. Also, get some vinegar on the side to water
down the dressing.

BEFORE YOU HEAD OUT TO EAT . . .

Part of the fun of dining is the element of surprise—trying a new restaurant or a new dish. But that doesn't mean you're at the mercy of the menu. Here are ten steps you can take before you step out of the house to help ensure wise eating.

1. Wear something nice—but a little form-fitting. There's nothing like a precision-fitted waistband to remind you to practice portion control.

It sounds crazy, but it works, agrees Susan Olson, Ph.D., a clinical psychologist and consultant to the Southwest Bariatric Nutrition Center in Scottsdale, Arizona. "Your focus shifts from the sensations of the taste, smell and sight of the food and to your body and how you want to look. It's also a good delay tactic: Being aware of how your clothes fit gives you time to think about your food choices."

2. Add your two cents. When the topic of "Where should we eat?" arises, suggest places you know are apt to accommodate your wishes.

3. Have a little something. Yes, it's perfectly okay—in fact, it's smart—to have a low-cal snack or beverage at home; it will tame your hunger pangs so you don't gorge later on. Good choices include a few crackers with low-fat cheese or a small green salad with a bit of fat-free dressing. In essence, you have your first course at home, and skip to the entrée at the restaurant.

"This technique works on the same principle as not going into the grocery store hungry," says Dr. Olson. "If you eat a little before you leave the house, you'll be able to make rational choices in the restaurant instead of just eating out of hunger."

4. Visualize yourself eating wisely. Hope S. Warshaw, R.D., author of *The Restaurant Companion: A Guide to Healthier Eating Out*, says that part of her predining-out strategy is to mentally rehearse what she will order. Do the same, she says, and you'll be much more likely to make healthful selections at the restaurant.

"Imagery is a very powerful tool," agrees Dr. Olson. "What you put in your mind is what your brain will follow.

If you 'rehearse' a scene, you can 'see' yourself succeeding and set yourself up for success."

5. Call ahead. What's on the menu? You'll have far fewer unpleasant surprises—and will be able to plan accordingly—if you make a quick call ahead.

"Before you pick up the phone, think about what you want, then ask," suggests Judy E. Marshel, R.D., director of Health Resources in Great Neck, New York and former senior nutritionist for Weight Watchers International. "Then you'll know ahead of time if they can prepare broiled fish or simple baked potatoes or alter the menu for a low-sodium or low-fat diet."

6. Learn from your mistakes. Think back to your last restaurant meal. Were there any surprises? (Did the fish come swimming in butter?) The next time you dine out, anticipate how your meal *might* go—and clarify menu descriptions up front.

"Learning from your mistakes is a mastery process," says Dr. Olson. "It's one of the most important ways you can master weight loss and healthy eating. You're going to make mistakes, but anything you regret in the past you can turn into a lesson now to help you improve your skills and your decision-making."

7. Work off the calories. If you know there's a bigger-than-usual meal in your future, exercise will help burn those extra calories. A bonus: If you take your brisk stroll or quick run before dining out, you'll remember the effort that went into the workout and you'll be less likely to overdo it at mealtime.

An added bonus: "Exercise can curb your appetite, so you may end up eating less at the restaurant," notes Marshel.

8. Jot down tomorrow's menu today. Think of a restaurant or dinner-party meal as an opportunity, one of the 21 healthy meals you expect to eat this week. To help you see this meal in perspective, write down what you plan to eat tomorrow—and realize that you're not going to be happy having to cut back tomorrow's food because of today's splurge.

"If you want to lose weight or eat more balanced meals, you need to think things through very specifically—what you're going to do—and write them down," says Nathaniel Branden, Ph.D., author of *The Six Pillars of Self-Esteem* and director of the Branden Institute for Self-Esteem in Beverly Hills.

9. Focus on the chatting, not the chewing. Talking more and eating less is the secret to enjoying your meal without overindulging, says Dr. Olson.

10. Think about the trip home. How are you going to feel later as you're daubing your lips with your napkin and getting up from the table? Happy and satisfied, knowing you enjoyed pleasant surroundings, interesting dining companions and a delicious, good-for-you meal? Or will you be full of bad food (and regret), sounding like the man in that old Alka-Seltzer commercial who moaned, "I can't believe I ate the whole thing!"? Either scenario is possible; the choice is obvious.

"Watching what you eat in restaurants is not just for weight control but for your overall health and enjoyment as well," notes Martha Rose Shulman, author of *Provençal Light* and other healthy cookbooks. "It's unenjoyable to walk away from a table feeling full and wake up with a food hangover the next morning."

"Assess the whens, wheres and whys of the ways you typically eat out," says Warshaw. If you're serious about changing your behavior, you've got to really look at what you're doing when you polish off that bread-and-butter basket, or when you find yourself at a fast-food drive-up window five nights a week. Pinpoint the behavior—then fix it.

Eat a third less of what you're served. If you leave some food on your plate, you can still eat foods you enjoy while keeping a lid on your fat intake, says Faye Berger Mitchell, R.D., spokesperson for the Washington, D.C., Dietetic Association.

Eat half now, half tomorrow. "In most of the restaurants we surveyed, we found enormous portion sizes," says Hurley. "A Chinese restaurant may have three to four cups per serving. The same was true for many Mexican and Italian restaurants. Many restaurant meals have 1,000 calories or more—almost half an average person's daily allotment—in a single serving.'' The solution is simple: ''Ask for a doggie bag,'' she says. ''Eat half now and take the other half home for lunch or dinner the next day.''

Share. ''Another way to get around huge portions is to split dishes,'' says Warshaw. ''In Asian restaurants you typically split things. I do this all the time. At one typical restaurant meal, for example, three of us shared two different dishes.''

Remember: You're in charge. When it comes to dining out, remember that you have choices.

If you think of eating out as a ''special occasion'' and you do it four times a week—which is true for the average American adult—it's *not* a special occasion; it's your way of life.

54

SNACKING

Between-meal nibbles that nourish

For Laurie M., a busy mother, wife and teacher in her early forties who struggles with her weight, snacks are an ongoing, everyday issue.

"It's so unfair! My husband can—and does—eat anything, while I have to really work at keeping my weight down," she commented in her response to our *Food and You* survey. "If I could, I'd snack all day long, but I gain weight easily. I try to plan ahead. I take nutritious, low-calorie snacks to work with me so I'm not tempted by the vending machine in the teachers' lounge.

"But some days," she confesses, "I just don't want them. I want M&Ms, and nothing else will do."

Barbara B., on the other hand, has disciplined herself to avoid all sweet snack temptations. In her midfifties she is determined to maintain the weight loss that accompanied the stress of her recent divorce.

"Snacks have always been my biggest food issue, because I love sweets and I've been a binge eater much of my life," she says. "I have almost eliminated sugary treats from my diet. It takes a great deal of discipline. I feel deprived. But it's the only thing that works for me."

Laurie and Barbara have plenty of company in their strug-

471

gles with the snack monster. Like many women, they do well eating healthy meals but feel guilty about their snack habits.

FACING OFF WITH THE SNACK MONSTER

Temptation is everywhere—from buttery popcorn at the movies to the snack cart at work. Every supermarket and convenience store devotes ample space to quick, tasty finger foods, most of them high in sugar, fat and sodium and devoid of real nutrition.

Yet nutritional experts assure us that resisting these diet-derailing land mines *is* possible. How? By planning healthy snacks that are full of nutrients and fiber and low in fat and calories.

But if incorporating snacks into daily nutritional goals is so basic, why do women like Laurie and Barbara struggle so, and why are snacks the downfall of so many? According to the experts, the answer is rooted in the psychology of snacking.

"Too many of us won't accept healthy foods as snacks," says Alice K. Lindeman, R.D., Ph.D., associate professor at Indiana University in Bloomington. "We grew up with snacks as treats. Our mothers gave us cookies and milk after school, so that's what we want now. If we try to eat broccoli because we know it's good for us, we won't be satisfied. We'll feel deprived, and that can lead to binge eating."

Denying ourselves rarely works, agrees Margo Denke, M.D., associate professor of internal medicine at the Center for Human Nutrition at the University of Texas Southwestern Medical Center in Dallas and a member of the American Heart Association's Nutrition Committee. One thing that does work, she says, is cutting back on how often we snack as well as on how much we eat when we do snack. Also, she adds, don't assume that every single snack you eat has to be nutritious.

"Some can be just for fun," Dr. Denke advises. "It's the overall diet that counts in terms of nutrition. The problem is not our choices, it's that people eat too much for the activity they do."

That trade-offs are possible may be good news for some

people, but what about the concern that eating a sugary snack will trigger a desire for more sweets?

Research does not support this fear, according to Barbara Rolls, Ph.D., professor of nutrition at Pennsylvania State University in University Park. "We have no data to indicate that sugar acts as a trigger, so that if you begin to eat something sweet, you then eat more," she says. "In fact, one study showed that people given a sweetened drink then ate fewer sweets. The bigger issue is how people perceive their snack choice."

FALLING INTO THE LOW-FAT TRAP

In her own study, Dr. Rolls and her colleagues analyzed the impact of low-fat snacks on women's eating behaviors. They served both high- and low-fat yogurt to four groups of women a half-hour before lunch. They revealed the fat content of the yogurts to the first two groups, but told the second two groups nothing at all. Then they observed how much food the women ate at lunch. The women who chose low-fat yogurt ate a larger lunch than usual, while the others ate normal amounts.

"We concluded that thinking a food is low-fat can be a trap because we may believe it gives us license to overindulge in other areas," says Dr. Rolls.

In another study, Debra Miller, a Ph.D. candidate working with Dr. Rolls, witnessed similar results. A group of men and women was given both regular and fat-free, reduced-calorie potato chips. Some of them were told which chip was which, and some were not.

The men and women who were kept in the dark about what they were eating consumed the same amount of both types of chips. The most striking finding among those who knew what they were eating was this: People who had identified themselves as concerned about their weight ate significantly higher amounts of the fat-free chips.

Miller's conclusion?

"Weight-conscious people may overeat a product they think is lower in fat," she says. "This helps explain why people can gain weight even when they eat low-fat versions of some of their favorite snacks. Those products sometimes have high calorie counts from the sugar or other ingredients.''

Food manufacturers know that taste is the most important criterion in selecting snacks, according to Audrey Cross, Ph.D., associate clinical professor of public health at the Columbia University Institute of Human Nutrition in New York City.

"Manufacturers will make what sells, and if it's full of fat, sugar and sodium, then that's what they're going to market," she says. "Even if an item is healthy, they'll talk about taste before they talk about nutrition."

How we view taste is a product of our upbringing, says Dr. Cross. Most of us reach for snacks that we identify as "comfort" foods. "Fortunately, you can find many snack items like cookies, cake and ice cream in low-fat, low-sugar, low-sodium versions," she says. "By choosing these—in moderation—our snack urge can be quelled without disastrous nutritional consequences."

Even better, she adds, many people successfully learn to retrain their taste buds and lose interest in these foods.

Does that mean that we can learn to appreciate the color and crunch of a green pepper as much as the gooey richness of a Snickers bar?

"Yes. But for most of us, it's not easy," she warns. "It takes time. You may fall off the wagon occasionally, but you can do it."

TRAINING TO BEAT THE SNACK ATTACK

So how exactly do you get to where you can enjoy healthy snacking? How can you learn how to snack with pleasure and without guilt? Here's what the experts recommend.

Plan for moments of temptation. "Take your own snacks to work so that when everyone else is selecting an item from the snack cart, you have dried fruit in your desk or nonfat yogurt in your lunch bag," advises Dr. Cross. "That way you get something to eat, too."

Allow for an occasional indulgence. "If you really want to share one of those midmorning sugary doughnuts with your office mates, plan to do it just once a week," says Dr. Cross.

"That way you don't feel completely deprived, and you're more likely to be good the rest of the week."

Look for healthier substitutes. If you crave a salty snack, for example, and are used to appeasing that desire with a bag of potato chips, look for the new low-fat brands, says Dr. Lindeman. Just be careful not to eat more than you used to. An even better choice would be pretzels. "The big Dutch pretzels take a while to eat and can satisfy that desire for salt and for crunch," she says.

Think before you reach. In order to satisfy your taste buds, what you must learn to do is to intellectualize snack choices, advises Barbara Whedon, R.D., a dietitian at Thomas Jefferson University Hospital in Philadelphia.

"Often we grab what's near. We feel hungry so we hurriedly select something from the vending machine or have one of the cookies served at a meeting, with no thought about what we feel a need for," she says. "Further, cravings vary, and to deny them may lead to overeating later. The key is to satisfy them in an acceptable way."

According to Whedon, categories of snacks include such classifications as chewy, crunchy, smooth, creamy, cold, sweet and salty. Often, she says, "we want a combination. For example, if you crave something creamy and sweet, yogurt might be perfect. If you desire cold and crunchy, try slices of green pepper. An ice pop will take care of cold and sweet, while Gummi Bears are chewy and sweet."

Choose low-fat options. If only ice cream will do, be sure to choose the nonfat kind, cautions Whedon.

"Those grams of fat add up quickly," she explains. "I tell my clients that eating 40 to 60 grams of fat a day is reasonable. Dropping much below that greatly restricts your diet and is difficult to maintain. Then, depending on your height and body build and whether you're trying to lose or maintain your weight, you must make a decision about how many fat grams you should consume in a day and how many of them you can devote to snacks."

Don't be fooled. Just because the label says "low-fat" doesn't mean you can stuff yourself, however. A little math reveals why low-fat snacks can be a trap. Thirteen reduced-fat-mini chocolate-chip cookies may add up to only 130 calories. But if you eat the whole 7.5-ounce box, you've taken in an amazing 910 calories. It's awfully easy to do that while watching a favorite television show.

And those low-fat tortilla chips let you have 22 chips for 110 calories. Sounds great, but if you eat the entire seven-ounce package, you've also sucked down 770 calories.

Eat hearty at mealtime. Because food provides the body with necessary energy, if we don't consume enough at meals we may try to make up for it with snacks, says Miller. That's the reason people often feel so hungry by midmorning or mid-afternoon. One study in the Netherlands concluded that people who ate light lunches compensated for their reduced energy intake with snacks.

Think nutrition. In planning your daily nutrition goals, factor in snacks.

"Think of snacks as food eaten between meals instead of as treats or rewards," Whedon suggests. "Make your snack an extension of your meal. For example, plan to have soup, salad and fruit for lunch. Only don't eat the fruit. Save it for your snack. The same with your dinner dessert or bread or your breakfast juice or muffin. Some people regard this as having a number of mini-meals and no snacks instead of three meals and three snacks a day."

Don't stock up on snack food. If Barbara B. feels the need to have sweets in the house because she's going to be entertaining, she buys exactly what will be consumed and gets the items just before company arrives so she won't be tempted to snack on them. Do your shopping when you don't feel hungry.

Be selective. Supermarkets carry special lines of dietetic foods that offer a variety of snack choices. Health food stores also carry many snack items that are nutritious and low in calories and fat.

Plan ahead. "Understand that snacking can be a spontaneous behavior and be prepared," says Dr. Lindeman. "Keep some items like rice cakes, dried fruit or cereal mix in a desk drawer, or find a vending machine with healthy selections."

Practice damage control. Don't fall for the notion that if one tastes good, two taste better. Filling a small bowl with potato chips instead of diving into a full bag helps willpower do its work.

50 LOW-FAT SNACKS AT 100 CALORIES OR LESS

Run amok with snacks, and you'll gain weight. But experts say that an occasional indulgence won't hurt. And an occasional treat may actually help by preventing feelings of deprivation. The secret to successful snacking, say nutritionists, is to be selective. Instead of snacking mindlessly, think about your choices. Here are 50 indulgences that, when eaten in the portions listed, can help keep eating fun without packing on the pounds. More often than not, you should select nutrient-dense foods (like apricots and carrots) over all-sugar foods (like candy corn).

These items are available at most supermarkets. Individual brands can vary, so be sure to read package labels. Items listed as having no fat have less than one gram per serving.

Food	Portion	Calories	Fat (g.)
Apple	1 medium	81	0
Applesauce, unsweetened	½ cup	53	0
Apricots, dried	5	83	0
Apricots, fresh	3 medium	51	0
Bagel	½	81	0
Banana	1 medium	100	0
Blueberries	1 cup	82	0
Bread, sourdough	1 slice	70	1
Butterscotch candy	4 pieces	88	1
Cantaloupe	½ cup	57	0
Carrot	1 medium	31	0
Celery	1 stalk	6	0
Cereal, frosted wheat	4 biscuits	100	0
Cottage cheese, low-fat	½ cup	81	1
Cucumber	1 medium	16	0
Devil's food cookies, low-fat	1	50	0
Fruit roll candy	1 roll	81	1

Food	Portion	Calories	Fat (g.)
Gummi Bears candy	3 pieces	20	0
Fig bars, fat-free	2	100	0
Fruit juice bar, frozen	1	25	0
Grapefruit, pink or white	½ medium	37	0
Grapes	1 cup	58	0
Honeydew melon	1 cup	60	0
Jelly beans	8 large	83	0
Life Savers candy, all flavors	1	9	0
Orange, navel	1 medium	65	0
Peach, dried	1	62	0
Peach, fresh	1 medium	37	0
Pecan cookies, low-fat	1	70	3
Pepper, bell	1 large	20	0
Potato chips, fat-free	30	110	0
Saltines	5	60	1
Whole-grain crackers, fat-free	5	60	0
Whole-wheat crackers	6	96	3
Pickle, dill	1 medium	12	0
Pineapple	1 cup	77	0
Popcorn, caramel, low-fat	1 cup	100	0
Popcorn, light	1 cup	45	3
Pretzels, thin	10	70	0
Pretzels, whole-wheat	1 small	51	0
Pudding cup, chocolate	1 (4 ounces)	100	0
Raisins, seedless	⅛ cup	55	0
Rice cake, plain	1	21	0
Strawberries	1 cup	45	0

Food	Portion	Calories	Fat (g.)
String cheese, low-fat	1 piece	60	3
Tortilla chips, baked, low-fat, with salsa	10	90	1
Tuna, light, packed in water	2 ounces	65	0
Yogurt, nonfat	½ cup	60	0
Yogurt bar, frozen, nonfat	1	45	0

Avoid temptation. Boredom can lead to snacking. Nutrition experts advise keeping busy when you feel like having a snack. Food commercials and being around people eating can also trigger the urge to indulge. Laurie M. often leaves the room when her thin husband reaches for an evening snack. Dr. Cross bypasses the supermarket aisles loaded with finger foods and the checkout lanes with candy bars.

Take slip-ups in stride. Pick snack foods that won't do great harm if you overindulge, suggests Miller. Too many pretzels is very different from too much chocolate cake. If you do overindulge, forgive yourself, forget about it, and get back on course.

Treat yourself every once in a while. "If you're counting calories, save enough of them to give yourself an occasional treat," says Whedon. "That way you won't feel deprived, and that vastly increases your chances of success."

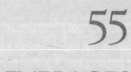

55

BEVERAGES

Drinkable feasts

Milk and cookies. Cake and coffee. Hot dogs and lemonade. Somehow, food and drink go together like a good book and a hammock on a lazy summer day.

Hot or cold, sweet or tart, plain or flavored, beverages are more than bit players in a healthy diet. They can (and should) supply needed fluid and vital nutrients. Yet most pack at least a few calories—a fact that, if forgotten, can wreak havoc with the best-laid weight-loss plans.

Everything a woman drinks affects her nutritional status—for better or worse. Here's what the experts have to say about what to drink, when—and why.

EIGHT GLASSES A DAY KEEP DEHYDRATION AT BAY

To perform the myriad essential tasks it performs every day, your body uses an average of two to three quarts of water, says John Peterson, M.D., a family practitioner and assistant clinical professor of medicine at Indiana University in Muncie. If you don't keep getting refills, it gets dehydrated.

Dehydration can cloud your thinking and sap your strength. And extreme dehydration can kill you, explains David Edelberg, M.D., director of the American Holistic Centers in Chicago. You have to drink to maintain your water stores.

As it turns out, maintaining those stores is a special challenge for women, says Felicia Busch, R.D., a nutritionist in St. Paul, Minnesota, and a fellow of the American Dietetic Association. That's because water is stored primarily in muscle rather than in fat, and women generally have less muscle than men do.

To stay hydrated, experts suggest you drink at least eight eight-ounce glasses of fluid every day. Water, or milk or juice—which are mostly water—will all do the trick.

Under certain circumstances, you'll need more than two quarts of fluid a day. Here's the lowdown on how to gauge your supply and demand for fluid.

Working out? Cooped up? Hydrate! Hot weather and physical activity—even moderate exercise like housework or gardening—make your body sweat more.

Since you lose water when you sweat, you need to drink extra to make up the deficit. While exercising, drink at least 16 extra ounces of fluid each hour. If you have a wristwatch with an alarm, set it to go off every 15 minutes or so to remind you to take a few swallows.

Indoor heating and mechanical air-conditioning can dry you out and increase your need for water, too. And flying—in arid, recirculated aircraft cabin air—can dehydrate you at jet speed. So drink an extra glass of fluid every hour you're on the plane, says Pittsburgh dietitian Pat Harper, R.D.

If you're sick, drink up. Fever, diarrhea and vomiting can make you lose water, too, says Busch. So you need to drink more when you're sick.

WATER WORKS

Although beverages like juice are mostly water, your best bet is to get a lot of the real thing in its purest form.

"Water is a nutrient—the most important nutrient," says Busch. Water is naturally low in sodium and contains no fat, no cholesterol, no caffeine and, best of all, no calories. (It's all too easy to consume a lot of calories in other beverages— you'll get 150 in a 12-ounce can of soda, for instance.) "So you should really try to get most of your eight glasses a day in the form of water," says Busch.

Here are a few watering tips from the experts.

Wake up with water. Drinking a glass of water as soon as you roll out of bed replenishes the fluids you lost while asleep, says Busch.

Keep it handy. Buy a 64-ounce container and fill it up every day. Keep it nearby—on your desk at the office or on the kitchen table at home—so you can see how much you're drinking. Take a sip now and then even if you don't feel thirsty. If you wait till you're parched, you're probably already down on fluid by a couple of cups, Busch says.

Chill and serve. For an all-day supply of refreshing chilled water, freeze a partially full plastic bottle of water overnight and add more water the next day, Busch suggests.

Fill 'er up before meals. Because water makes you feel full, it's a great weight-loss aid, says Busch. Take the edge off your appetite by having a glass of water instead of a snack or before a meal.

Scope out those labels. Carbonation gives club soda and seltzer water a pleasant, tingly appeal. But if you're counting calories or watching your sugar intake, read labels: Soda water, some flavored seltzer waters, and tonic water may contain sugar—and calories.

MILK FOR ALL IT'S WORTH

"Milk has a place in every woman's diet," says Liz Applegate, Ph.D., a lecturer at the University of California, Davis, and author of *Power Foods*.

And it's an important place, at that. For starters, milk is a good source of protein, riboflavin, vitamins A and D, phosphorus and magnesium. And it's one of the best sources of calcium going. Doctors and nutritionists suggest you get at least 1,000 milligrams of calcium every day—1,500 milligrams if you're past menopause and aren't on hormone replacement therapy—to protect your bones. A single eight-ounce glass of skim milk provides 300 milligrams of calcium.

Make it skim. Nutritionists recommend skim or 1 percent

milk—both are lower in fat than whole milk, says Dr. Applegate. One cup of skim milk has only a trace of fat, compared to five grams in 2 percent milk and eight grams in whole milk.

Reach for milk at mealtime. Even if you suffer from lactose intolerance (difficulty digesting milk sugar due to inadequate production of the enzyme lactase), you may not have to make do without milk. Drinking it with meals can help, since the other food in your stomach will help dilute the lactose and mute its unsettling effect.

Try lactase. You might also try adding lactase drops. Added to milk ahead of time, they break down the lactose for you. Brands like Lactaid are sold at most pharmacies.

Soy milk: yet another option. Made from soybeans, soy milk offers many of the nutrients found in cow's milk. It's higher in iron, niacin and thiamin but lower in calcium and vitamin A. It's also a good source of substances called phytochemicals, naturally occurring plant substances that appear to protect against cancer and heart disease.

Drink it c-c-c-cold. Some like milk icy cold, says Dr. Edelberg. Keep frosted mugs in the freezer, then add an ice cube or two and drink up.

Treat yourself to cocoa. For delicious hot cocoa, heat a cup of milk, then stir in a couple of tablespoons of unsweetened cocoa powder and a teaspoon or so of sugar or honey, Dr. Edelberg suggests.

Make a fruity milkshake. Cold milk mixed with fruit juice and nonfat yogurt makes a tasty milkshake, says Dr. Applegate. "One cup contains more calcium than a glass of milk. Plus, if you use yogurt with active lactobacillus acidophilus cultures, you may boost your immune system and fight off yeast infections," she says.

JUICES: JAM-PACKED WITH NUTRIENTS

Replete with vitamins, minerals and cancer-fighting substances of their own, fruit and vegetable juices are also good picks from the beverage lineup.

One caveat: Juice contains calories. Ounce for ounce, fresh apple cider has about the same number of calories as soda, for example. But it gives you far more in the way of nutrients than the soda does.

Here are some juicy suggestions.

Drink OJ once a day. Orange juice is a top source of vitamin C, a nutrient that acts as a potent antioxidant—it seems to offer protection against cancer and coronary artery disease by blocking the formation of free radicals, which are created as cells oxidize with age and exposure to pollution.

Orange juice fortified with calcium is a particularly good choice, says Dr. Applegate. One glass gives you the same amount of calcium you'd get in a glass of milk. What's more, you get the vitamin C and a bit of fiber—extra fiber if you choose juice with pulp, she says.

Go grape. Grape juice offers a bonus: Heart protection. Grapes are rich sources of a group of phytochemicals called flavonoids. Also found in red wine and berries, flavonoids are natural compounds in plants that keep blood platelets from clumping, helping to prevent clots that could lead to strokes and heart attacks.

"In our studies, we find that grape juice has anti-clotting ability," says John D. Folts, Ph.D., director of the Coronary Thrombosis Research Laboratory at the University of Wisconsin in Madison.

Try new combinations. You'll find a wide variety of fruit blends at your grocery store, from apple-cranberry to strawberry-kiwi. "That's good, because you get exposure to a greater variety of nutrients if you drink a wider variety of juices," Dr. Edelberg says. For even more variety, buy several different juices and mix them up in a pitcher at home.

Whip up a fruit smoothie. Dr. Edelberg offers a recipe for a nutrition-packed fruit smoothie: Blend together two bananas, a small can of pineapple tidbits packed in their own juice and a little bit of apple or other juice. For a more complete mini-meal, add protein powder, he suggests.

Treat yourself to a fruit slush. Pour fruit juice into ice cube trays, Dr. Edelberg suggests, then toss the frozen cubes into a blender with whole fruit to make a slush.

Make your own. You can make your own delicious and healthful juice concoctions with a juicer, says Dr. Applegate. A blender won't work—you'll end up with a pulpy mess.

Buy the real thing. No time to squeeze your own juice?

Shop for real juice made from real fruit, not "juice drinks" made with sugar (which adds calories but no nutrients).

"What you want is 100 percent fruit juice," says Dr. Edelberg. As always, you need to check the labels.

Concentrate is okay. Juice concentrates are acceptable alternatives to fresh juices, says Dr. Edelberg. But some contain added sugar, so you need to read labels.

Mix as you go. If you're using concentrates, prepare just enough juice to last two or three days, Dr. Edelberg says. "The fruit that goes into concentrate is usually picked at peak ripeness, so it contains a lot of vitamins and minerals. But once the juice gets exposed to light and air—either sitting in your refrigerator or on the table or counter—it starts to lose nutrients."

Make sugar-free lemonade. Skip store-bought mixes and try Dr. Edelberg's recipe for homemade lemonade: Blend two whole lemons (after removing the peels and most of the white) with a little bit of water. Sweeten to taste with white grape juice.

Treat yourself to carrot juice. You'll get beta-carotene, another powerful antioxidant. If you don't like the way carrot juice tastes straight, mix it with pineapple juice for a sweeter, more complex flavor and extra vitamin C.

Add v-r-o-o-o-o-m to vegetable juice. Add lively seasonings—a squeeze of lemon or a couple of drops of Tabasco—to bottled vegetable juice cocktail (like V-8) for a taste treat, Dr. Edelberg suggests, or buy tangy commercial versions. Or make a virgin Mary: Mix tomato juice or vegetable juice cocktail with a little pepper and celery seed, pour it into a tall glass and top it off with a stalk of celery. For a delicious chunky juice, blend vegetable juice with a whole tomato or watery vegetables such as cucumbers, peppers or yellow squash or zucchini.

POP PUTS ON POUNDS

At 150 calories per 12-ounce can, soda can add a lot of unwanted poundage without adding any nutrients.

"Sodas have absolutely no nutritional value," Dr. Edelberg says. "And they contain enormous amounts of sugar."

Colas also contain phosphoric acid, an additive that adds a slightly tart taste. Unfortunately, too much phosphoric acid is bad news for your bones. If you drink more than a cola or two a day, your body can't use calcium efficiently, say researchers. A study conducted at Harvard School of Public Health, for example, compared girls who drank at least eight ounces of cola a day with those who drank it infrequently. They found that the cola drinkers were three times more likely to suffer bone fractures than others. The researchers conclude that high cola consumption, coupled with low calcium consumption, puts teen-age girls at risk for osteoporosis later in life.

If you enjoy soda, nutritionists offer the following suggestions.

Ration yourself. A cola or two a day won't hurt you, Harper says. But you're putting your bone density on the line if you're guzzling six-packs of the stuff (particularly if you're not getting a lot of calcium in your diet).

Make your own "soda." For a bubbly drink with fewer calories, less sugar and a respectable amount of vitamin C, says Busch, mix a can of frozen lemon, lime or orange juice concentrate with four to six cans of sparkling water.

THE PROBLEM WITH DIET SODA

You've seen the ads: A tall, lanky (read: slim) woman walking down the beach drinking diet soda is admired by onlookers. A tall, lanky woman lolling by the pool drinking diet soda is admired by onlookers. A tall, lanky woman playing volleyball sips a diet soda and is admired by onlookers. The message seems to be "Drink what I drink, and you'll look like this, too."

Thanks to sweet-tasting but calorie-free substances like aspartame and saccharin, artificially sweetened sodas taste sweet but save calories—about 150 per 12-ounce can—compared to regular soda. If you have diabetes and need to curb your sugar intake, artificially sweetened beverages are convenient.

But we all know women who, equating diet sodas with a perfect, slim figure, live on diet sodas from morning to night. The problem is, a steady diet of diet soda can deprive you of important vitamins (like C, from fruit juice) and minerals (like calcium, from milk.) Although you can cut unnecessary calories by drinking diet sodas, they still contain the same phosphoric acid found in the real stuff and can jeopardize your bones if consumed frequently or in large quantities, says Harper. So diet sodas shouldn't be consumed with abandon.

What's more, relying on diet sodas to lose weight is like relying on any diet gimmick—it only works if you *also* learn to eat wisely and get regular exercise.

Here are some tips for using diet sodas sensibly.

Stop at one or two. As with regular soda, limit yourself to an average of no more than two glasses a day, Harper says.

Focus on food, not soda. "If you're counting calories, an occasional diet soda is an acceptable alternative to regular soft drinks," says Dr. Applegate. "Use the savings of calories to make room for more nutrient-dense foods, however—pick up a piece of fruit, for example, or munch on some baby carrots."

If you get a headache, stop. Some women complain that aspartame, the artificial sweetener in many diet sodas, triggers headaches, aggravates insomnia and worsens depression. According to the Food and Drug Administration, the sweetener is considered safe. But if you drink a lot of diet soda and have unexplained headaches, insomnia or depression, it makes sense to quit.

COFFEE AND TEA: TAKE A BREAK

Studies suggest that too much caffeine, like too much phosphorus, may undermine your bones. Caffeine is a diuretic, so if you drink a lot of it, you urinate more and excrete more calcium in the process.

Too much caffeine can also make you jumpy and temporarily raise your heart rate, says Dr. Peterson. It can worsen the pain and tenderness that accompany fibrocystic breast disease. It can increase stomach acid secretion—which can make things more painful for you if you have ulcers. And it can cause diarrhea if you have inflammatory bowel disease, since it has a mild laxative effect.

"If you're in good health, however, a cup or two of coffee or tea a day is fine," says Dr. Peterson.

Here's some advice on how to enjoy your morning java or

afternoon tea without compromising your health.

Add milk. You can have your strong bones and drink your coffee, too, if you drink it with milk. Researchers at the University of California at San Diego found that women who drank two cups of coffee a day had lower bone densities than those who drank fewer cups. But women who drank a glass of milk in addition to their coffee had bones as tough and strong as those of abstainers.

Say, "Latte, please." If you find coffee with skim milk about as appetizing as a mud puddle, try a creamy-tasting café latte. Add 6 to 8 ounces of steamed skim milk to 1½ ounces of espresso and sprinkle with some cinnamon. (Despite its reputation as a high-voltage brew, espresso isn't that much higher in caffeine than regular coffee, according to the Specialty Coffee Association of America. One ounce of espresso contains 18 to 30 milligrams of caffeine, compared with the 12 to 36 milligrams you get in an ounce of regular coffee.)

Mocha, s'il vous plaît. Turn the latte into a café mocha by adding some chocolate syrup or powder.

Mix decaf with regular. If you can't seem to make it through the day on fewer than three cups of coffee, dilute yours. Make each cup half regular coffee and half decaf, Dr. Peterson suggests.

Wean yourself from the bean. No question about it, say experts—caffeine is addictive. That means if you try to quit all at once, you'll feel it. "People who discontinue caffeine abruptly may go through withdrawal," says Harper. Headaches and irritability are common symptoms.

So take the evolutionary, not the revolutionary, approach. Slowly wean yourself off caffeine. If you're drinking four cups of regular coffee a day, taper down to three cups the next week and two the following week. Substitute decaf or herbal tea, Dr. Peterson suggests.

Ice it. When it's too darned hot for hot tea, try Dr. Edelberg's refreshing recipe for iced herb tea: Bring a quart of water to a boil, add a half-dozen herbal tea bags and steep until the tea darkens. Add a squeeze of lemon or a half-cup of apple juice and refrigerate.

Pregnant? Do without. Some studies suggest a link between high caffeine consumption and miscarriage, though others find no such connection. Leaning toward the safe side, the

THE HEALING POWER OF TEA

Just the thing to soothe you when you're sick, tea may also be just the thing to keep you from developing serious illnesses to begin with.

A growing body of scientific evidence suggests that tea may significantly lower your risks of both cancer and heart disease. Researchers in Shanghai found that women who regularly drank green tea (the kind available in Asian grocery stores) were less likely to develop cancer of the esophagus than those who didn't. A Japanese study concluded that men who made a habit of drinking green tea had higher-than-average levels of "good" HDL cholesterol and lower-than-average levels of "bad" LDL cholesterol in their bloodstreams. And researchers at Rutgers University in New Jersey found that mice developed 70 to 90 percent fewer skin tumors when fed either green or black tea.

Although initial studies focused on green tea—the tea of choice in Asian countries—researchers are beginning to turn their attention to the black tea that's more popular in the United States.

Results are encouraging, says M. T. Huang, Ph.D., associate professor of pharmacy at the Rutgers University College of Pharmacy in Piscataway.

"We've done animal studies that show green tea and black tea have a similar effect against esophageal cancer," says Dr. Huang.

What is it about tea? The beverage, made from the leaves of a type of evergreen, contains chemicals called polyphenols. Like vitamins A, C and E, polyphenols are antioxidants, substances that prevent the cell damage that leads to cancer and the dangerous formation of arterial plaques in the blood vessels leading to the heart and brain.

Green tea, produced by steaming, rolling and drying the evergreen leaves, contains different polyphenols than black tea, which is produced by partially drying, crushing and then fermenting the tea leaves, Dr. Huang says.

Researchers aren't sure precisely how much tea you'd have to drink to get an edge against serious illness. Generally, though, experts say two to four cups a day are protective.

American College of Obstetricians and Gynecologists suggests pregnant women avoid caffeine. Switch to decaf or noncaffeinated drinks.

CUT THE COCKTAILS

If you get no kick from champagne, experts suggest you avoid the stuff. If mere alcohol does thrill you, however, studies suggest you're best off with no more than a drink every other day—if you drink at all.

Generally speaking, a drink or two every day appears to lower your risk of heart disease—probably because the alcohol raises levels of ''good'' artery-cleansing cholesterol in your bloodstream, say experts.

But for women, it appears that the potential harm from anything more than an occasional drink may overshadow any potential benefits.

At the very least, alcohol can add a significant number of calories to your diet, raising your risk of unwanted weight gain and related health problems. You get 106 calories in a 5-ounce glass of wine and 150 in a 12-ounce beer. If you have more than one glass, the calories really add up. The effect on your waistline may be even more pronounced than you expect, since alcohol appears to interfere with fat metabolism and promote fat storage—even in people who consume moderate amounts of the stuff.

If you aren't calorie-conscious, alcohol poses other considerations. Research indicates that women's muscles (including their heart muscle) are more sensitive to the muscle-wasting effect of alcohol. A study conducted at Jefferson Medical College in Philadelphia found that women are more vulnerable than men to alcohol-related muscle and heart damage (called cardiomyopathy). When damaged, the heart doesn't contract as forcefully.

Women respond to alcohol differently than men, say the researchers. Part of the reason is that we're smaller. But we also seem to be more sensitive to the effects of alcohol—the harmful amount for women seems to be about 60 percent of what's harmful to men.

Trade-off number three: Research also suggests that drinking daily can raise your risk of breast cancer. A four-state study of more than 15,000 women found that those who downed just one drink a day were 30 percent more likely to get breast cancer than those who abstained. Women who had three or more drinks daily ran twice the risk.

Heavy drinking—three or more drinks daily—can also damage your liver and raise your risk of throat, mouth, laryngeal, stomach and colorectal cancer.

Drinking too much can also leach calcium from your bone structure. So heavy drinkers run a higher risk of osteoporosis, according to the National Osteoporosis Foundation.

If you don't drink, don't start. If you rarely drink, don't worry. And if you're going to drink, remember these guidelines.

Have three drinks a week—if you drink at all. Try not to exceed more than three glasses of wine, bottles of beer or mixed drinks (or any combination thereof) in a week. A joint study of 85,709 women by researchers at several Boston hospitals and universities found that those who downed just one to three drinks a week seemed to escape the life-threatening risks associated with heavier consumption. (In fact, they lived longer than women who didn't drink at all.)

That's one to three drinks a week, not a day—a noteworthy distinction. Just because a glass of red wine is potentially beneficial doesn't mean a carafe is even better.

Chase it with water. If you do have a drink, follow it with a glass or two of water to help replenish lost fluids. At parties and social gatherings, alternate sparkling waters with alcoholic drinks, Busch suggests.

Teetotal throughout pregnancy. If you drink during pregnancy, you can leave your baby a legacy of fetal alcohol syndrome—the number one cause of mental retardation. Abstain.

56

HOLIDAY FEASTS

Smart strategies for special occasions

"To me, holidays are synonymous with food," says Mary H., who responded to our *Food and You* survey. "*Not* overeat during the holidays? I can't even imagine it!"

Mary's got plenty of company. What's Christmas without cookies and eggnog? New Year's without champagne? Hanukkah without latkes? Easter without chocolate bunnies and coconut eggs?

You get the point. To everything there is a season, and to every holiday there is a dish—a cultural favorite, or something Mom has been baking every year since you were a child—that makes the special day extra-special.

What happens, then, to your low-sodium diet or high-carb/low-fat weight-loss program once December 25 or February 14 rolls around? Nothing good, most likely.

"It's not easy to be disciplined about food," says Nathaniel Branden, Ph.D., author of *The Six Pillars of Self-Esteem* and director of the Branden Institute for Self-Esteem in Beverly Hills. "We associate food with gratification and with pleasure." And when it's our birthday or Christmas or the anniversary of Elvis's discharge from the Army, the natural urge is to party—which generally translates into too much of the wrong kind of food.

492

"Halloween is the worst," says Jennifer H., one of the women to whom we spoke. "I don't feel safe until I get the leftover Mounds bars and Reese's Peanut Butter Cups out of the house. It's like having a bag full of plutonium in the kitchen."

FOOD, FOOD, EVERYWHERE

The workplace is not off-limits to dietary indulgences. Quite the opposite. Rosemary H. told us: "Around here, most employees traditionally bring in food on their birthday—usually doughnuts. Unless I'm really committed to a strict diet, I end up eating one. I tell myself, 'What's one doughnut? I'll work out later.' Then I feel guilty."

If you look at your calendar, see that it's mid-December and think you're suddenly eating three times as much as you usually do, it's probably not your imagination. During the winter holidays, food is everywhere, and it would take the spiritual strength of a Mother Teresa to resist.

Many of us, like Mary, enter the holiday season fully expecting to overdo things, foodwise. According to a joint poll of 771 men and women conducted by CNN and *Prevention* magazine, more than two-thirds—69 percent—said that they planned to eat whatever they wanted on Thanksgiving, Christmas and Hanukkah because the holidays come just once a year. What's more, 40 percent anticipated packing on the pounds during that period, and 60 percent figured that they very likely would lose this weight.

The risk of holiday weight gain—not to mention heartburn, sluggishness, constipation and other problems associated with too much of a good thing—is real. "By indulging in the parade of goodies that starts at Thanksgiving and continues unabated until New Year's, the average person will gain five to seven pounds," says Jo Ann Carson, R.D., program director of clinical dietetics at the Southwestern Allied Health Sciences School at the University of Texas Southwestern Medical Center in Dallas. To gain even five pounds, all you have to do is consume an additional 17,500 calories over the approximately 35-day stretch between Turkey Day and Noisemaker Day. That boils down to a mere 500 extra calories a day—a cinch for most of us.

THE TIE THAT BINDS

Food exerts a powerful force over us under ordinary circumstances, and that power is intensified on special occasions.

"Emotionally, food represents comfort, happiness, peace and love. And when people get together during the holidays, food is usually a centerpiece of the celebration," says Ronette L. Kolotkin, Ph.D., director of behavioral programs at the Duke University Diet and Fitness Center in Durham, North Carolina. That's particularly true in less-than-loving families, says Dr. Kolotkin. "In families where there may be a lot of stress and tension and concern about who's not getting along with whom and who's not speaking to whom, food is often the glue that holds things together, helping family members rise above the conflict and tension."

Dr. Kolotkin also points out that for many, food helps us cope with unrealistic holiday expectations, when emotions are, for many women, at their peak. "The holiday season is a time when you're supposed to be happy, but we may feel sad at this time of year, especially if loved ones are far away. Many singles dread New Year's Eve because it's considered a 'couples event.' Food is one way to comfort and nurture ourselves."

"There's more access to food around holidays; it tends to be a very social time," says Ronna Kabatznick, Ph.D., psychologist and consultant to *Weight Watchers Magazine* and founder and director of Dieters Feed the Hungry, a Berkeley group that tries to refocus dieters' attention from themselves to helping others. "Neighbors invite you for drinks, family members invite you to dinner, co-workers invite you to office parties—and there's candy on people's desks at work." Not only are we playing the role of frequent guest but the role of hostess, too. "It's difficult for women in particular because we're usually the ones buying and preparing most of the food, and so we think about it more," adds Dr. Kabatznick. "These ongoing food temptations make it much harder to stick to your regular eating habits."

"I MADE IT JUST FOR YOU!"

If the presence of the food itself were not temptation enough, there's the additional pressure from the people making and serving it.

"Several years ago, I went to my grandmother's house for New Year's Eve," recalls survey respondent Cheryl S., who lost 25 pounds and succeeded in keeping it off. "She made two main dishes—pasta with broccoli and a ham. I decided to eat just the pasta. My grandmother looked at my plate and asked, 'Don't you like the ham?' and I said, 'Yes. I just prefer to eat the pasta.' She said, 'But I made both!' Finally I gave in and ate the ham, too, just to placate her. But I didn't feel good about it."

That's a story we can all relate to. As Cheryl suggests, holiday get-togethers often bring out the kid in us—in the worst sense.

"Nobody really has the power to make you eat more—only you can open your mouth and put food in it—but people around us *can* trigger certain emotions," acknowledges Dr. Kabatznick. "If your mother or mother-in-law makes you feel inadequate, or if you feel you've always had to compete with an older sister, and you don't know how to deal with those feelings, you may channel some of that emotional discomfort into overeating when you're with them."

HOW-TO'S FOR HOLIDAY EATING

Luckily, there's lots you can do to keep the food and the feeders in their place—and *still* enjoy that Thanksgiving reunion or birthday bash. Here's a menu of strategies that work.

Be selective. When you think about it, many of the foods we enjoy at holiday time—roast turkey, sweet potatoes, apple cider—are perfectly healthful when prepared simply and eaten in reasonable quantities, says Judy E. Marshel, R.D., director of Health Resources in Great Neck, New York, and former senior nutritionist for Weight Watchers International. Focus on the peas, broccoli and lean white meat and go easy on the gravy, butter, au gratin dishes and pie.

Plan ahead. If you're like most people, you probably know what to expect at holiday meals—turkey at Thanksgiving, ham

UNDOING THE JANUARY DIET DISASTER

New Year's Day. Time to take the annual vows of dietary chastity: Go on a diet. Eat less fat and more fiber. Swear off sweets. Give up eating meat. Whatever.

Noble enough intentions. But come the end of January, chances are 50-50 that your resolve has dissolved, says John C. Norcross, Ph.D., professor of psychology at the University of Scranton in Pennsylvania, co-author of *Changing for Good* and author of three major studies on New Year's resolutions.

Why the high failure rate? "People set goals for themselves, but they don't consider the specific actions they'll need to take," say Nathaniel Branden, Ph.D., author of *The Six Pillars of Self-Esteem* and director of the Branden Institute for Self-Esteem in Beverly Hills. "To be worthwhile, a resolution to lose weight needs an action plan."

Write it down. "Make a list of what foods you're going to eat, what foods are on your forbidden list and what foods you can eat only in very small quantities," says Dr. Branden. "Then keep a log of what you did or didn't eat and what you did or didn't do in terms of exercise—after all, few diets work if not combined with exercise. People get very absentminded about dieting—they 'forget' what they did or find a reason to make an exception. Research shows that people who keep records have a much greater chance for success than those who do not."

"If you say you're going to lose 50 pounds and keep them off, you probably won't be as successful as if you say you'll lose 10 pounds," says Dr. Norcross. "My advice is: Make realistic resolutions—or don't make them at all."

Ignore setbacks. Slips are bound to occur, says Dr. Norcross, so plan for lapses. Don't give up your goal as lost. "We've found that the average 'resolver' will slip 14 times over a two-year period. Interestingly, those who achieve their goals have as many slips as the unsuccessful ones. The successful people just keep going and stay the course. Think of your New Year's weight-loss resolution not as a hundred-yard dash during January but rather as a marathon throughout the whole year."

at Christmas—so it makes it easier for you to plan ahead. Says Mary: "Every year at Christmastime my mom makes cheesecake. I crave it, but I always worry about what it's going to do to my diet. But last year I planned ahead: The days before and after Christmas, I ate a little less of everything else. So I was able to enjoy the cheesecake (and whatever else I wanted) and not dread it or feel bad afterward."

"Like everything else in life, it helps to have a plan," says Dr. Kolotkin. "Look ahead. Think about how long the holiday season lasts and make some decisions about how you'll get through it. Make choices, go for your favorites, but watch out for overindulgence and avoid thinking, 'Oh, it's the holidays; the sky's the limit.' "

Visualize. "Just as a football player visualizes the plays of an upcoming game, I visualize how the party or family dinner will go," Mary also told us. "If I'm going to visit the home of a relative or friend, for example, I'll picture myself entering the dining room and visualize what I will and won't eat. For me, rehearsing the meal is very helpful."

"When you do a 'mental' dress rehearsal, it's like going through the experience, so that when you actually experience the event, it's easier and you make better choices because you've already practiced them," says Marshel.

Sample, don't splurge. "I use four different ways to deal with problem food," says Carson. "One, substitute something that's lower in fat and/or calories; two, eat smaller portions; three, eat the problem foods less frequently; and four, change the way you prepare it.

"Take eggnog, for instance," says Carson. "You could have apple cider punch instead, which would be lower in fat and calories. Or two, you could have just a taste of the eggnog instead of a whole cup. Three, instead of having it every time it's served, limit yourself to eggnog on Christmas Eve only. Four, you could prepare it with egg substitute instead of eggs and with skim or 1 percent milk instead of whole milk and cream." This is a recipe for success Carson uses—and recommends—*any* time of year.

Buffeting the effects of buffets. Just because the table has three kinds of meat, four kinds of bread and six pies doesn't mean you've got to eat everything that's available. "I stand away from the buffet table; otherwise, it's too easy to keep

SURFING THE WAVE OF OFFICE PARTIES

Baby showers. Promotions. The annual office Christmas bash or summer clambake. Like interoffice memos and cartoons posted above the fax machine, parties—whether they're pot-luck or poshly catered—are a part of office life. They're also one more meal you didn't count on eating that day—and not necessarily the most nourishing fare at that.

How do you cope without seeming like a party-pooper? Mindy Hermann, R.D., a nutrition counselor in Mount Kisco, New York, offers these suggestions.

- Eat lightly the day of the party, but don't arrive famished, says Hermann. If you are too hungry, it will be harder to control yourself once you're there.
- Wear something snug to the party to serve as a "restraining device" for your stomach.
- Use a small plate, or fill up a regular plate with salad or veggies that take up a lot of space before serving yourself the higher-calorie fare.
- Look before you eat. "Mentally plan what you'll have—and you'll also see that there really aren't that many temptations," according to Hermann. If you know the lasagna isn't that good, skip it. Potato chips? Nothing special; why bother? Pretty soon you will have line-vetoed 75 percent of the food.
- At a pot-luck buffet, sample before you select. Help yourself to just one or two tablespoons of the foods that strike your fancy. Then go back and have reasonable-size portions of the couple of dishes you like best.
- If nibbles are at hand, opt for pretzels or raw veggies, which are lower in fat and calories than the chips or cashews.
- Placate your appetite with fluids. Plain water will do the trick, says Hermann, but the bubbles in seltzer water or diet soda will help you feel full and avoid overeating. As for alcohol, it may lower your resolve, so if you do have wine, beer or a cocktail, keep an eagle eye on what goes on your plate.

> If you contribute food to the affair, take the opportunity to prepare a dish you'll enjoy without loading up on fat and calories—lasagna made with low-fat cheese or a crustless quiche with low-fat milk, egg substitute and a tad less cheese. You don't have to tell your secret, but if you do, expect some thanks from diet-conscious co-workers.

nibbling,'' says Washington dietitian Edith Howard Hogan, R.D., a spokesperson for the American Dietetic Association. "So take small portions, fill your plate once, eat it, and that's it. Then walk away from the table.''

Leave the scene of the crime. "The problem with holiday meals,'' says Cheryl S. "is that we do most of our socializing around the table, long after the meal is over, which means we're sitting there, picking at food. So I usually move away from where I've been eating and go talk to someone else away from the food. Or else I'll go and hang out with my little nieces and nephews who are playing in their room.''

"It's really tough if some good food is sitting in front of you—it's a cue to eat,'' says Susan Olson, Ph.D., a clinical psychologist and consultant to the Southwest Bariatric Nutrition Center in Scottsdale, Arizona. "So remove yourself from the cue, and when you do, do something fun.''

People mistake failure as a lack of willpower to change behavior, when in fact it's a lack of reward. People can't replace something fun and enjoyable such as food with something unenjoyable like chores and expect to be successful in changing their eating behaviors and expecting the changes to last.

Keep your hands (not your mouth) full. "I always tended to be nervous when I first arrived at a party, and I'd grab an alcoholic drink or an hors d'oeuvre just to have something in my hand,'' confesses Mary. (She's not atypical.) "Now I always carry a clutch purse in one hand and reach for a club soda with the other. That way, it's too awkward to eat anything.''

Marshel applauds Mary's technique. "It's so easy to start out with the best intentions to eat properly, but you need to give yourself every advantage so you don't succumb to party-food temptations.''

POLITE WAYS TO FEND OFF FOISTED FOOD

Although Dr. Kabatznick concedes that you and you alone decide what you will eat and when, saying no to holiday hosts and hostesses can be tricky. "As during any other time of year, you have you be vigilant, know what your emotional vulnerabilities are, and understand that eating is often connected to those times when you're feeling less strong or powerful," she says. But, she adds, this is a terrific opportunity to practice standing up for yourself, "a good skill to have any time of the year."

The relationship between food and love is covered in more detail elsewhere in this book, but during the holidays, the following advice can help.

Learn to say no. Here are Dr. Kabatznick's suggested polite-yet-firm responses to the persuasive entreaty, "Have some more . . . I made it just for you!"

"No, thank you." Simple yet often surprisingly effective.

"I'm full." How could anyone truly know otherwise?

"I appreciate all your effort, and I've enjoyed every bite!" And you probably have!

"If you want to give me more, I can take another portion home in a doggie bag." What you do with it afterward is up to you.

"Keep saying no, and the person doing the coaxing will soon lose their power over you," says Dr. Kabatznick.

Dr. Kolotkin adds that, when all else fails, there's always the medical excuse, real or otherwise. "Many people with serious weight problems tell me the only way they've ever gotten people to stop pushing food is by saying they have an allergy or that they're concerned about their cholesterol or that their doctor advises against something," she says. If your weight has fluctuated over the years and your friend or family member doubts your diet convictions, a health explanation might get you off the hook more easily than a weight-loss rationale.

Enlist the support of the server. With someone you know well, Dr. Kabatznick says: "Tell them, 'This is not helpful. I need your support. I want you to know I'm in the process of changing my eating habits.' You can often turn an adversary into a supporter." Pointing out the behavior may be all that it takes, adds Dr. Kabatznick. The person may simply be coaxing you out of habit.

Talk to yourself. It works, says another one of our *Food and You* respondents. "At holiday family get-togethers, I'll go to another room and say under my breath, 'I'm in control of my life.' Certain people in my family can make me feel bad about myself, so I keep repeating those words. It's corny, but it really works. I try to make every choice, including food choices, my choices, no one else's."

"Positive self-talk is a very crucial way of reminding yourself that you're the adult in any given situation, that you don't have to give others the power to control you," says Dr. Olson. You can expect to make mistakes; it's part of the process and you can learn from them.

"At holiday time, there are all kinds of 'shoulds,' and you have to be on the lookout for them," adds Dr. Kolotkin. "Many adults feel like children in the presence of their family, but you don't have to feel locked into your typical behavior."

Take it—and leave it. Chances are there's so much going on at the dinner table that few people will really notice what you have or haven't eaten. So if what you do or do not put on your plate becomes an issue, just take what's served. "If worse comes to worst, you can take the food and not eat it or drink it," says Dr. Kabatznick. "I usually take a little bit of everything and leave some food uneaten," adds Cheryl S.

HOLIDAY FITNESS: AN OXYMORON?

In a corollary to the basic laws of physics, you could say that every dietary action has an appropriate mental or physical counteraction. Here are some nonfood strategies to round out your holiday eating plan.

Work out, give gifts, have fun. As we so often forget, the holidays are about more than food—they're meant to be opportunities to share time with loved ones, celebrate a notable event and leave you feeling good. Don't overlook the power of exercise to help you accomplish all three.

"Exercise is the best single thing you can do during the holidays," says Dr. Kabatznick. "If you're spending the holiday with children, consider going sledding or ice-skating—

it's a non-food-centered way of spending time. If you're with adults, go hiking or visit a museum. Consider working in a soup kitchen or food pantry where holiday nourishment has a different meaning for people. You're giving something of yourself instead of taking in excess food and calories. When you use your body in a positive, healthy way—and not just as a vehicle for food and drink—you feel better about yourself.

"Exercise is a tension-reliever, plus it gives you food 'credits' so you can overindulge a bit. Swim extra laps. Walk an extra mile or two a day. Enjoy your body in ways that don't have to do with food," she says.

Take time out. "During the holidays, it's important to be tuned in to your feelings and to give yourself what you need," says Dr. Kolotkin. "Many women, for example, get caught up in constantly doing for others, especially when get-togethers call for extra work. What you need is some time out—an hour or even just a few minutes here and there—to be alone and see how you're feeling. You might sense a pain across the back of your neck or other feelings of tension that arise if you're really annoyed. If that happens, go for a walk or lie down for a while. At family get-togethers in particular, lots of emotions come into play, and you need to take time to center yourself so you don't turn to food for solace."

Enjoy eating. "For the longest time, I felt I didn't deserve holiday food," says Mary. "And when I first reached my goal weight, I panicked thinking about the upcoming holidays and what I would eat. But then I thought: Food *should* be a good and loving part of the holidays, so I changed my attitude and stopped fearing food. Now I believe you're *supposed* to have the dessert and all the things that are traditional—it took me years to feel that way. But now I do."

"There's nothing wrong with giving yourself an occasional treat, as long as you're in control of it," says Dr. Branden. "Let's face it: Food is a big pleasure in life for a lot of people—and that's okay." The trick is to indulge without *over*-indulging.

57

TRAVEL LIGHT, EAT LIGHT

Eating wisely on the road

More singles, couples and families are taking multiple vacations in the course of a year. And more women than ever are traveling on business. Whether it's a weekend at the shore or a two-week honeymoon cruise, a sales conference in Rome, Italy, or Rome, Wisconsin, the best-laid food plans frequently go awry once the tickets are bought and the suitcases are packed. For business and leisure travelers alike, culinary temptations abound, meaning that t-r-a-v-e-l can easily spell t-r-o-u-b-l-e for any woman concerned about healthful eating. With a little forethought, however, eating healthy can be part of the fun and adventure of travel.

"With vacation travel, people get into the mindset of turning off the calorie-conscious button. You get into the 'special occasion' groove—'I'm on vacation, so I can eat with a no-holds-barred attitude,' " says Hope S. Warshaw, R.D., author of *The Restaurant Companion: A Guide to Healthier Eating Out.*

And who *doesn't* want to sample the culinary delights once she reaches her final destination? "When you go on vacation—whether to another country or another part of this country—you want to try a specialty of the region, like catfish and cracklin's in South Carolina," says Maria Simonson, Ph.D., Sc.D., professor emeritus and director of the Health, Weight and Stress Clinic at Johns Hopkins Medical Institutions in Baltimore. Dr. Simonson has been a consultant on nutrition and safety to various airlines for the past 20 years, and when it comes to enjoying the local fare, she's no exception. "When I was in Morocco, boy, did I go for the couscous with meats and fats!"

And why not? Doing—and dining—as the Romans do is all part of the adventure.

For women traveling on business, food is a security blanket of sorts. Points out 46-year-old Ellen M., who works in advertising and travels on business about once a month: "When you're traveling, especially when you're traveling alone, and there's so much pressure and tension—to get to appointments on time, to not get lost, to get the business—food becomes a reward."

Yet if you have special dietary or health needs, impulsive selections are not in your best interest. Planning ahead *is*. "I've had hypoglycemia for 15 years," says one woman. "If I'm concerned I won't be able to find sugar-free or fat-free snacks, I've been known to pack provisions like nuts, crackers, herbal teas and preservative-free snacks that don't require refrigeration." Judy E. Marshel, R.D., director of Health Resources in Great Neck, New York, and former senior nutritionist for Weight Watchers International, recommends packing cheese and crackers. Dr. Simonson suggests any foods you take be supervised by your doctor or nutritionist. So advance planning for travelers with special requirements is crucial. "Treating yourself is asking for trouble," she says.

FUELING UP FOR THE LONG HAUL

Auto travel has its own set of food foibles. Unless you plan ahead, your options are apt to be limited to fast-food places along thruways, food mart/service stations or rest area vending machines—not exactly known for their health-concious selections. Here's what nutritionists advise.

Take a cooler. "Take a cooler and pack it with healthy foods—fruit, low-fat cheese sticks, low-fat crackers, trail mix, mini-bagels and so forth," says Washington, D.C., nutritionist

Edith Howard-Hogan, R.D., a spokesperson for the American Dietetic Association. "Instead of stopping for soda, take along individual-sized bottles of sparkling water, juice or other low-calorie or calorie-free beverages."

Similarly, Marshel suggests adding low-fat or nonfat yogurt and cut-up raw vegetables—celery, carrots, cucumbers and peppers—and some flavored seltzer water to your cooler. A separate stash of low-sodium pretzels and/or flavored rice cakes also comes in handy during those lengthy drives.

Brown-bag it. If your trip will span lunchtime, pack some sandwiches the night before and stash them with your fruit and other goodies. Marshel recommends either a turkey sandwich without mayonnaise or a low-fat cheese sandwich with lettuce and tomato. That way, you're less likely to find yourself forced to choose among hamburgers, fried chicken nuggets and french fries at roadside eateries.

Plan some pit stops. "People often complain about constipation after long car trips," says Hogan. "But if you stop every two hours, get out, walk around briskly and drink some water, that can help prevent constipation."

EAT *BEFORE* YOU BOARD

These days, airports are to mass transit what bus stations were in the past—for many, air travel is the mode of choice for distances too far to drive. Still, except for the most frequent fliers, being on a plane puts most of us into a "let's have fun!" mode. When the smiling flight attendant offering honey-coated peanuts and drinks appears, our guard is down.

Then comes the actual meal. With competition among airlines at an all-time high, a growing number of airlines are responding to consumer demands for better, more healthful food. "Historically, airline food has been high in fat and calories," concedes Todd Clay, manager of corporate communications for Delta Air Lines in Atlanta. "But we've upgraded many of our special meals."

In addition to the standard fare, most airlines offer passengers a variety of special meals—diabetic, kosher, vegetarian, low-sodium, low-fat, low-cholesterol, Hindu and Muslim, according to Evelyn Tribole, R.D., author of *Eating on the Run*.

American Airlines, for example, has worked with the American Heart Association and the Dallas-based Cooper Clinic to come up with its heart-healthy American Traveler meals, which tend to be lower in fat and cholesterol than its typical fare.

Delta offers 19 different special meals; one out of four special meals ordered are vegetarian.

Some frequent travelers report the special meals look and taste better than the standard fare, says Hope Warshaw.

"Whether you're indeed a vegetarian or just want something other than the standard meal, you can usually get a fruit plate or a vegetarian platter," says Nancy Mills, a travel journalist in West Los Angeles who launched the newsletter *Travelin' Woman* in early 1994 to accommodate a growing market of female business and vacation travelers.

Order in advance. An aircraft is not a restaurant: If you want a low-cholesterol meal on a flight, order it when you book your ticket. Adds Warshaw, "People who travel regularly should set it up with their travel agent, so when the flight is arranged, the special meal is, too." That way, you won't forget to put in your request every time you book a trip.

On breakfast flights, you may have a choice between eggs—the standard option—and high-carb, low-fat options like cereal or bagels, calcium troves like nonfat yogurt and fiber-packed fresh fruit. On some airlines, such as American Airlines and Delta, lunchtime salads go beyond the ordinary to Cobb salad and Oriental salad. Dinnertime choices may include white-bean chili, chicken chili, vegetarian lasagna and a spicy Southwestern pasta salad, according to airlines spokespeople. Choices vary from week to week, of course.

BYOF (bring your own food). To avoid finding yourself being set up to eat certain foods just because they're all you have access to, Warshaw emphasizes advance planning, "because you never know if your flight will be delayed or canceled." Her portable, nonperishable suggestions: small boxes of raisins (or other dried fruit), mini-boxes of animal crackers, or fig bars.

The other option is to eat before you board. Prior to takeoff, Warshaw is likely to be found at one of the airport eateries. "In some airports, the food choices there are healthier than on the plane—frozen yogurt stands, sandwiches made to order, soft pretzels, plain, unbuttered popcorn and so forth. So if you haven't ordered a special meal on the plane, eat on the ground or take food with you.'' That's advice that frequent flier Sue lives by. ''I almost always take pretzels or fruit with me,'' she told us in our food survey. ''It's the one time out of ten when I forget to bring a snack of my own that I end up eating the peanuts.''

Order juice—and lots of it. ''When the flight attendant comes by for drink orders, I ask for one or two glasses of water,'' says Sue R., a survey respondent who works in communications. ''It helps keep me from getting dehydrated during the flight.'' In fact, adds Hogan, ''drinking one glass of water or juice per hour of flying time prevents or minimizes jet lag.'' In contrast, drinking alcoholic beverages while breathing dry aircraft air dries you out and contributes to jet lag, she says.

''Any time you can get extra fluid, fruit juice or water, for example, into your diet, you should,'' says Marshel. ''When you're flying, you can order orange or grapefruit juice. Tomato or mixed-vegetable juices are okay, too, but may contain fair amounts of sodium, so avoid them if your blood pressure is aggravated by excess sodium.''

Drinking fluids helps prevent dehydration. Juices provide fluid and help supply antioxidants like vitamins A and C that may help protect you against free radical damage triggered by breathing ozone at altitude, adds Marshel.

Conserve your calories. When it comes down to it, you don't have to eat on the plane at all, especially if a big meal is on the agenda that evening. Why waste calories? Just ask the flight attendant to keep bringing you water, club soda or tomato juice to sip until you get to your destination.

CRUISE SHIPS: NAVIGATING THE 18-HOUR BUFFET

Cruise ships are known for their never-ending food, so be careful. Says Hogan, ''Just because it's part of the package deal, you don't have to accept every offer of food. Eat at normal mealtimes—three meals a day and maybe one or two light snacks. Or, if you want to take advantage of all the food, have five mini-meals instead of five big ones.''

Hogan is well aware that rich desserts are popular cruise-ship fare. But while her shipmates are indulging in the choc-olate mousse, she'll top off her meal with a delicious cup of "skinny" cuppuccino or café latte, made with low-fat milk.

Hogan also makes a point of getting her fill of fiber while on board. "When I'm on a cafeteria-type food line on a cruise ship," she says, "I grab a couple of pieces of fresh fruit to take back to my cabin to eat later."

As for the ship's midnight buffet, Marshel suggests you save up some of your calories from the day. "Plan for it," she says. "You might have half a sandwich instead of a whole one for lunch, for example, so that late in the evening you can have some vegetables with dip, or even more than that, if you wish."

FUNDAMENTALS FOR THE FREQUENT (OR INFREQUENT) TRAVELER

Whether at home or away, your body needs certain basics; if they're neglected, you can be uncomfortable. Here are a few strategies to keep your dietary aims on course once you reach your destination.

Think fluids and fiber. "Because travelers deviate from their normal routine, constipation can be a problem while away from home," notes Marshel, who, during her 14 years as a senior nutritionist for Weight Watchers, traveled regularly to consult with nutritionists and doctors throughout Europe. "To avoid constipation, keep up your exercise routine; focus on eating whole-grain bread and cereals, drink plenty of water and juices and eat fresh fruits and vegetables. It's especially good to have fruit instead of rich desserts, which tend to be constipating."

In our *Food and You* survey, Connie L. said she tries to eat oatmeal or other whole-grain cereal for breakfast to help stay regular while traveling. "I can usually find oatmeal on most breakfast menus," Connie told us.

Balance intake with exercise. "I always say that planes, trains, ships and cars are all great fuel users, but you as a passenger don't burn much of your own fuel calories when traveling," notes Hogan. "So you must build exercise into your daily plan." It will not only help you burn calories but will energize you and help you sleep better and avoid constipation.

Do drink the (bottled) water. "When I was living in Paris for six and a half years, I got used to drinking bottled water, and now I insist on it whenever I travel," says Elaine G., another survey respondent. "Water is one of the most likely suspects for contamination in certain foreign countries, such as Mexico," says Marshel. "But you should have no problem finding bottled water—every mini-bar serves flat or carbonated water." (Don't forget, Marshel adds, that ice cubes are usually made from local tap water and for that reason should also be avoided.)

Book a place to cook. No, you don't want to spend your vacation planning and preparing all your meals. But you might want to book accommodations in a condo or one of the growing number of suite hotels that have mini-kitchens in the room. That way, you can be sure to start your day off right with a good breakfast. Hogan offers these best breakfast bets: juice or maybe some dried fruit ("I love dried apricots, and they have beta-carotene"), instant oatmeal or cream of wheat ("It's loaded with iron"), and skim milk for a calcium boost.

"My husband and I take annual ski trips to Colorado with another couple," says Sue. "We always rent a condo so we can share a kitchen with the other couple, and we make breakfast together, a very important meal when you're going to be skiing all day. We make a point of eating lots of carbohydrates, such as whole-grain bagels and Grape-Nuts cereal, and we drink plenty of liquids—lots of juice and water. We avoid caffeine because, at that altitude, it sometimes gives us headaches. We also pack fresh fruit and fiber bars to carry in our fanny packs."

"My husband and I vacation on Cape Ann, Massachusetts, about twice a year, and we always stay at the same motel that has a kitchenette in every room," Connie told us. "We like to have a light, healthy breakfast—some grapefruit or fresh oranges, coffee with steamed low-fat milk and maybe some whole-grain bread with low-fat cheese. Later on—and for us the highlight of the weekend—we go shopping in the outdoor market in the Italian section of Boston. We buy lots of different kinds of fresh fish and seafood, garlic and other fresh herbs and vegetables, and some canned tomatoes, and then throw together a big fish stew for dinner. It's one of the best meals we eat all year long—and it's super-healthy.''

INDEX

Note: **Boldface** references indicate primary discussion of topics.

dental problems during, 209

diabetes and, 110

exercise during, 276–77

fiber intake during, 276

food cravings during, 277–78

hemorrhoids from, 150

hypertension during, 157

metabolism during, 243

morning sickness during, 272

nutritional needs after, 278–79

nutritional needs before, 271–73

in vegetarians, 277

vitamin A and, 276

vitamins during, 276, 277

weight gain during, 274

Premenstrual syndrome (PMS), **261–69**

causes of, 261–63

chocolate cravings with, 253, 264–66

dietary help for, 263–69

herbal teas for, 267–68

nondietary help for, 269

serotonin and, 262, 265, 266

symptoms of, 263

  headaches, 267–68

  insomnia, 267–68

  water retention, **224–27**, 266, 268, 329

Prenatal vitamins, 276, 277

Pressure cookers, 452

Pritikin Program, weight loss and, 333

Processed foods

  nutrient loss in, 92

sodium in, 159–60, 225–26, 444

Produce, nutritional value of, 428–29

Protein

calcium loss from, 285–86

diets high in, 341–43

in high-carbohydrate diets, 333–34

for hypoglycemia, 164

for mental alertness, 117

metabolism and, 247

in prepregnancy diet, 273

in restaurant meals, 465

sources of, 293

sweet cravings and, 371

Psychotherapy, for eating disorders, 67, 68

Q

Quizzes

on eating disorders, 65–66

food/mood, 8

food personality, 414–21

sneak-eating, 28

R

Ragweed allergies, cross-reactions to food and, 131

Recreational eating, **21–24**

Rectal bleeding, from hemorrhoids, 150, 151

Relationship problems, avoiding, with food, 49

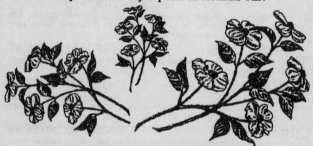